W0007788

FUNCTIONAL NEUROIMAGING IN CLINICAL POPULATIONS

FUNCTIONAL NEUROIMAGING IN CLINICAL POPULATIONS

edited by

FRANK G. HILLARY
JOHN DeLUCA

Foreword by Stephen M. Rao

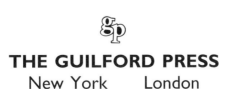

THE GUILFORD PRESS
New York   London

©2007 The Guilford Press
A Division of Guilford Publications, Inc.
72 Spring Street, New York, NY 10012
www.guilford.com

Printed in the United States of America

This book is printed on acid-free paper.

Last digit is print number: 9 8 7 6 5 4 3 2 1

Library of Congress Cataloging-in-Publication Data
Functional neuroimaging in clinical populations / edited by Frank G. Hillary, John
DeLuca ; foreword by Stephen M. Rao.
    p. ; cm.
   Includes bibliographical references and index.
   ISBN-10: 1-59385-479-X   ISBN-13: 978-1-59385-479-9 (cloth: alk. paper)
   1. Brain—Imaging.   2. Brain—Wounds and injuries—Diagnosis.   3. Brain—
Diseases—Diagnosis.   4. Mental illness—Diagnosis.   5. Aging—Physiological
aspects. I. Hillary, Frank G. II. DeLuca, John, 1956–
   [DNLM: 1. Brain—pathology.   2. Diagnostic Imaging—methods.   3. Aging—
physiology.   4. Brain Injuries—diagnosis.   5. Mental Disorders—diagnosis.   WL
141 F9797 2007]
   RC386.6.D52F86 2007
   616.8′04754—dc22   2007011923

To my family and to my graduate school mentor,
Dougas L. Chute

—F. G. H.

To my children, Jessica, Danielle, and Robbie,
who inspire me to achieve and be the best I can be
—J. D.

About the Editors

Frank G. Hillary, PhD, is Assistant Professor in the Department of Psychology at Pennsylvania State University and holds faculty positions in the Departments of Neurology and Psychiatry at Hershey Medical Center in Hershey, Pennsylvania, and in the Department of Radiology at the University of Medicine and Dentistry of New Jersey–New Jersey Medical School in Newark. He completed his postdoctoral training at the Kessler Medical Rehabilitation Research and Education Corporation in West Orange, New Jersey. During this fellowship, his training focused on the clinical application of functional magnetic resonance imaging (fMRI) to clinical samples, and he was honored with the Outstanding Postdoctoral Research Award. Dr. Hillary's research uses various MRI techniques, such as magnetic resonance spectroscopy, diffusion tensor imaging, and fMRI, to examine neural plasticity and recovery from brain injury and disease in humans. His current work examining the influence of brain trauma on the fMRI signal is funded by the National Institutes of Health.

John DeLuca, PhD, is Director of Neuroscience Research and Vice President for Research Training at the Kessler Medical Rehabilitation Research and Education Corporation; Professor in the Departments of Physical Medicine and Rehabilitation and Neurosciences at the University of Medicine and Dentistry of New Jersey–New Jersey Medical School; and a licensed psychologist in New Jersey and New York. Dr. DeLuca is currently studying disorders of memory and information processing in a variety of clinical populations, including multiple sclerosis, aneurysmal subarachnoid hemorrhage, chronic fatigue syndrome, and traumatic brain injury. He has published more than 300 articles, abstracts, and chapters, and serves on the editorial boards of several journals, including the *Archives of Physical Medicine and Rehabilitation*, *Rehabilitation Psychology*, and *Neuropsychology Review*. He also was editor for a special issue on multiple sclerosis for the journal *NeuroRehabilitation*, and one on chronic fatigue syndrome for *Applied Neuropsychology*. Dr. DeLuca is listed in *Who's Who in Science and Engineering, 1994–1995*, and received early career awards from both the American Psychological Association (Division 40, Clinical Neuropsychology) and the National Academy of Neuropsychology, as well as the Distinguished Researcher Award from the New Jersey Psychological Association in 2005.

Contributors

Anto Bagic, MD, Center for Advanced Brain Magnetic Source Imaging, Departments of Neurology and Neurological Surgery, University of Pittsburgh Medical Center, Pittsburgh, Pennsylvania

Peter A. Bandettini, PhD, Laboratory of Brain and Cognition, National Institute of Mental Health, Bethesda, Maryland

Vince D. Calhoun, PhD, The MIND Institute and Department of Computer and Electrical Engineering, University of New Mexico, Albuquerque, New Mexico; Department of Psychiatry, Yale University, New Haven, Connecticut

Nancy D. Chiaravalloti, PhD, Department of Physical Medicine and Rehabilitation, University of Medicine and Dentistry of New Jersey–New Jersey Medical School, Newark, New Jersey; Kessler Medical Rehabilitation Research and Education Corporation, West Orange, New Jersey

Steven C. Cramer, MD, Departments of Neurology and Anatomy and Neurobiology, University of California, Irvine, Orange, California

Bruce Crosson, PhD, Brain Rehabilitation Research Center, Malcom Randall VA Medical Center, and Department of Clinical and Health Psychology and McKnight Brain Institute, University of Florida, Gainesville, Florida

John DeLuca, PhD, Departments of Physical Medicine and Rehabilitation and Neurosciences, University of Medicine and Dentistry of New Jersey–New Jersey Medical School, Newark, New Jersey; Kessler Medical Rehabilitation Research and Education Corporation, West Orange, New Jersey

Mark D'Esposito, MD, Helen Wills Neuroscience Institute, University of California, Berkeley, Berkeley, California

Neal M. Fitzpatrick, BS, Department of Psychology, Pennsylvania State University, University Park, Pennsylvania

Adam Gazzaley, MD, PhD, Departments of Neurology and Physiology, University of California, San Francisco, San Francisco, California

Helen M. Genova, BS, Kessler Medical Rehabilitation Research and Education Corporation, West Orange, New Jersey; Integrative Neuroscience Program, Graduate School of Biomedical Sciences, Rutgers University–Newark, Newark, New Jersey

Cheryl L. Grady, PhD, Rotman Research Institute, Baycrest Centre for Geriatric Care, University of Toronto, Toronto, Ontario, Canada

Balázs Gulyás, MD, PhD, Psychiatry Section, Department of Clinical Neuroscience, Karolinska Institute, Stockholm, Sweden

Frank G. Hillary, PhD, Department of Psychology, Pennsylvania State University, University Park, Pennsylvania

Brenna C. McDonald, PsyD, Department of Radiology, Indiana University School of Medicine, Indianapolis, Indiana

Anthony R. McIntosh, PhD, Rotman Research Institute, Baycrest Centre for Geriatric Care, University of Toronto, Toronto, Ontario, Canada

Ralph-Axel Müller, PhD, Department of Psychology, San Diego State University, San Diego, California; Department of Cognitive Science, University of California, San Diego, La Jolla, California

Elizabeth R. Orr, MS, Department of Neurology, University of California, Irvine, Orange, California; Department of Kinesiology, California State University, Long Beach, California

Godfrey D. Pearlson, MD, Olin Neuropsychology Research Center, Institute of Living, Hartford, Connecticut; Department of Psychiatry, Yale University, New Haven, Connecticut; Department of Psychiatry, Johns Hopkins University, Baltimore, Maryland

J. Daniel Ragland, PhD, Department of Psychiatry and Behavioral Sciences, Imaging Research Center, University of California, Davis, Sacramento, California

Joseph H. Ricker, PhD, Department of Physical Medicine and Rehabilitation, University of Pittsburgh School of Medicine, Pittsburgh, Pennsylvania

Rachelle W. Rodriguez, FNP, Department of Neurology, University of California, Irvine, Orange, California

Bart Rypma, PhD, School of Behavioral and Brain Sciences, University of Texas Southwestern Medical Center, Richardson, Texas

Susumu Sato, MD, National Institute of Neurological Disorders and Stroke, National Institutes of Health, Bethesda, Maryland

Andrew J. Saykin, PsyD, Department of Radiology, Indiana University School of Medicine, Indianapolis, Indiana

Nils Sjöholm, PhD, Section for Nuclear Medicine, Department of Oncology, Karolinska Institute, Stockholm, Sweden

Gerald T. Voelbel, PhD, Department of Physical Medicine and Rehabilitation, University of Medicine and Dentistry of New Jersey–New Jersey Medical School, Newark, New Jersey; Kessler Medical Rehabilitation Research and Education Corporation, West Orange, New Jersey

Foreword

Prior to 1980 almost all of our understanding of the organization of human brain function came from the study of patients with focal brain lesions (e.g., brain tumors, strokes, penetrating head injuries). During the final two decades of the 20th century, we greatly expanded and complemented this knowledge by examining human brain function using noninvasive neuroimaging tools, such as positron emission tomography, functional magnetic resonance imaging, electroencephalography, and magnetoencephalography. During this growth phase of functional neuroimaging, virtually all studies were conducted in healthy individuals. Many of us, however, had the sense that the field would come full circle—namely, that functional neuroimaging tools would eventually become critical to our understanding of patients with brain disorders. With the advent of the 21st century, this prediction has been realized with a rapid growth in the number of functional neuroimaging publications focused on clinical populations.

This timely book edited by Frank G. Hillary and John DeLuca represents a distillation of our progress in this emerging field. The first section of the book provides the reader with chapters that summarize critical technical background information on each imaging tool. This is followed by chapters that discuss the strengths and limitations of applying these tools to the study of clinical populations and methods for understanding how brain disease can disrupt neural systems engaged during task activation. The remaining chapters discuss the application of functional neuroimaging tools to a wide range of clinical disorders.

Ultimately, whether functional neuroimaging tools will become routine procedures for the diagnosis and management of clinical disorders will be determined by the state of the scientific evidence. By carefully reading this book, you can determine how far the field has come and how much farther it must go to achieve this lofty goal.

STEPHEN M. RAO, PhD
Director, Schey Center for Cognitive Neuroimaging
The Cleveland Clinic

Preface

Historically, much of what has been learned about brain functioning in the neurosciences has occurred via experimentally induced lesions in animals and in naturally occurring damage in human clinical populations. Functional neuroimaging now offers innovative and largely complementary methods for further testing the established theories and novel hypotheses uncovered during the "lesion studies" of the past several decades and presents a unique opportunity for the clinical neuroscientist to examine brain activity during actual behavioral performance.

With the long-standing availability of positron emission tomography (PET) and emerging popularity of functional magnetic resonance imaging (fMRI) over the past decade, functional imaging has become an indispensable part of clinical and cognitive neuroscience. Additionally, while other techniques such as near infrared spectroscopy (nIRS) and magnetoencephalography (MEG) have not been used as much as PET and fMRI, these other techniques are also making critical contributions to the understanding of brain disorders.

These functional imaging techniques have fostered a veritable explosion of studies in the clinical neuroscience literature using imaging to examine various cognitive, sensory, and motor deficits associated with neurological insult. Thus we saw the need for this volume, which represents an initial attempt to compile this first generation of clinically oriented functional imaging studies and demonstrates the opportunities available in clinical neurosciences created by this technology.

This book is organized into three parts. Part I, Principles of Functional Neuroimaging, comprises three chapters that describe the basic principles underlying several of the most common functional imaging techniques. Balázs Gulyás and Nils Sjöholm (Chapter 1) discuss the principles and operations regarding PET. This comprehensive chapter outlines, very specifically, the basis of PET measurement, the physical principles, the methods, and the potential problems in using this technology. This chapter closes with examples of how PET has been used to make advancements in oncology, neuropsychiatry, and psychopharmacology. In Chapter 2 Peter A. Bandettini, one of the preeminent scholars regarding the principles of fMRI and its application, describes the bases of the fMRI signal and the physiological influences on its measurement, fMRI designs, and more recent clinical applications of fMRI. This chapter is critical because so much of the work in functional imaging today employs MRI-based techniques. Part I ends with Anto Bagic and Susumu Sato's (Chapter 3) discussion of the principles of electroencephalography (EEG) and MEG. These authors provide a comprehensive summary of the basic principles behind examining neural impulses and emphasize the critical advantages in using these methods for the direct examination of neural firing. Bagic and Sato also provide a historical perspective for EEG and its early clinical contributions to understanding epilepsy, and present more recent and very promising developments using MEG for clinical research.

Part II, Neuroimaging Methods, provides two chapters detailing special considerations for using functional imaging techniques in clinical samples and advanced statistical analyses that allow for examination of the changes in neural networks in response to brain injury and disease. These chapters are geared toward outlining basic methods as well as the challenges faced by applying functional neuroimaging techniques to clinical populations. Adam Gazzaley and Mark D'Esposito (Chapter 4) discuss functional imaging methods generally and, based on recent data from their laboratories, offer critical considerations for examiners using blood flow-based measurements (e.g., nIRS, fMRI) in populations where there are changes in baseline cerebral blood flow. The methodological issues covered in this chapter are important for anyone considering using BOLD (blood-oxygen-level-dependent) fMRI in clinical or "special" samples. Anthony R. McIntosh and Cheryl L. Grady (Chapter 5) examine advanced analyses using functional imaging data, with a focus on network analyses. These authors describe alternative methods for examining functional imaging data that allow clinical examiners to better understand how neural systems as a whole are affected by brain injury and disease. The advanced methods discussed here have already begun to contribute to the clinical neurosciences and are certain to play an increasingly important role in the next generation of clinical functional imaging studies.

Part III, Clinical Applications, comprises 10 chapters, each describing the use of functional imaging to examine clinical questions in a specific population or disorder. Ralph-Axel Müller (Chapter 6) details the functional imaging literature in neurodevelopmental disorders. Müller tackles this very large literature by examining a subset of these studies: the neurodevelopmental disorders considered to be largely genetic in origin. Using autism spectrum disorders as the primary focus, Müller integrates the available functional imaging literature and provides important insights into how functional imaging has advanced the understanding of basic neurodevelopmental processes. In Chapter 7 Brenna C. McDonald and Andrew J. Saykin provide an integrated overview of the current work using fMRI to examine presurgical planning and patient outcomes in individuals with seizure disorders. This chapter nicely demonstrates the advancements permitted by integrating functional imaging into the neurosurgical process in order to maximize diagnostic accuracy and evaluate the factors determining recovery of memory and language functioning, two areas most dramatically affected by temporal lobe epilepsy and resection of temporal lobe seizure foci. Bruce Crosson (Chapter 8) continues the discussion by shifting the focus to the use of functional imaging to examine the aphasias due to stroke. This chapter aims to clarify the complicated language recovery literature, including parsing out potentially competing imaging results. Crosson also provides an overview of current techniques and difficulties in examining language recovery, including methods for examining spoken language in the fMRI environment. Chapter 9, by Helen M. Genova, Neal M. Fitzpatrick, and Frank J. Hillary, offers an overview of the various imaging techniques used to examine the acute and chronic consequences of traumatic brain injury (TBI), including proton magnetic resonance spectroscopy and more traditional functional imaging techniques such as PET and fMRI. The authors integrate the cognitive findings to date that document altered neural activation following TBI while emphasizing those areas of cognitive function typically affected by TBI, including attention, memory, and executive functioning. Gerald T. Voelbel, Nancy D. Chiaravalloti, and John DeLuca (Chapter 10) review the literature on functional neuroimaging studies conducted in persons with multiple sclerosis (MS). They examine studies addressing motor functions, fatigue, and cognition, and present an interesting discussion on the challenges of interpreting functional imaging data in MS with regard to issues of neuroplasticity and cerebral reorganization. Chapter 11, by Vince D. Calhoun and Godfrey D. Pearlson, first focuses on the specific methods used for examining the effects of alcohol intoxication on the neural substrate, then provides examples and data illustrating how intoxicating substances may influence neural activity during tasks requiring visual perception, such as driving. J. Daniel Ragland (Chapter 12) provides an excellent theoretical overview of schizophrenia and outlines the functional imaging literature in the context of two theories regarding the pathophysiology of the disorder: hypofrontality theory and the left-hemisphere temporal lobe model. Through the integration of the available functional imaging literatures, Ragland offers a combined model suggesting a "frontotemporal" network subserving the functions commonly affected by schizophrenia. In Chapter 13 Bart Rypma integrates the literature on aging with specific emphasis on examining age-related performance decrements that have been observed in studies on normal aging. Rypma examines those changes linked to both peripheral and central processes with the aim of demonstrating that many of the age-related decrements in cognitive functioning that have been observed can be related to diminished processing speed and efficiency. Elizabeth R. Orr, Rachelle W. Rodriguez, and Steven C. Cramer (Chapter 14) integrate the current literature using functional imaging to examine stroke and stroke recovery, with a focus on recovery of motor function. The authors discuss the advancements in understanding and treating stroke using functional imaging, including understanding spontaneous recovery mechanisms as well as those changes attributable to therapeutic interventions. Methodological considerations for using functional imaging techniques in examining stroke are also discussed. Finally, in Chapter 15 Joseph H. Ricker provides a very nice overview of the implications of using functional imaging for neurorehabilitation. Consistent with the previous chapter, Ricker offers important insight into how "change" may be interpreted, given that spontaneous recovery following any neurological insult is expected.

This book represents several years of work pulling together a great number of authors from diverse backgrounds. We thank those who lent their expertise to this volume. We especially thank Rochelle Serwator of The Guilford Press for her guidance and support throughout this project. Without her constant optimism, this volume might not have become a reality. Finally, we also thank our students, who continually challenge us intellectually and have, in many ways, influenced our thinking about how the brain adapts to injury and disease and how best to help the patients who are afflicted with neurological disorders.

Contents

PART III. CLINICAL APPLICATIONS

PART I

PRINCIPLES OF FUNCTIONAL NEUROIMAGING

CHAPTER I

Principles of Positron Emission Tomography

Balázs Gulyás
Nils Sjöholm

Positron emission tomography (PET) is a powerful biomedical imaging technique widely used in neuroscience research, clinical applications, and neuropsychopharmacological drug development. In contrast to other imaging techniques that yield a detailed anatomical image of the body, the strength of PET lies in the facts that (1) it can provide detailed information of biochemical or physiological processes, (2) the information can be given in a precise anatomical context, and (3) the technique is capable of quantifying the measured parameters.

PET and Other Imaging Techniques

Imaging is a widely used approach in biomedical research to reveal structural, chemical, and functional information. As for the relationship between the energy source and the resulting image, the most common imaging techniques, used in biological and medical research and diagnostics, are based on three major principles: reflection, transmission, and emission.

The various techniques used in the exploration of the nervous system cover extensively both the spatial and temporal domains. The tomographic principle-based techniques, including computed tomography (CT), single-photon emission computed tomography (SPECT), PET, and magnetic resonance imaging (MRI), occupy a significant segment of the spatiotemporal domain available for investigative techniques in the neurosciences, including the millimeter–centimeter range in the spatial, and the second–hour range in the temporal domain. The spatial resolution of a PET scanner is limited by a number of factors, most importantly by the length of the path a positron travels before it meets an electron and by the intrinsic spatial resolution of the detectors. The temporal resolution of the scanner is primarily limited by the statistically sufficient number of counts, and by using short-half-life radiotracers—for example, $[^{15}O]$ water or $[^{15}O]$ butanol—it can be a few seconds.

As compared with other biological imaging techniques based on the tomography principle, the strength of PET is not in its spatial resolution: MRI and CT can provide us with anatomical images of high spatial resolution. PET, similarly to SPECT (and, to some extent, to magnetic resonance spectroscopy; MRS), is advantageous in monitoring biochemical changes in the living body (Greitz et al., 1985; Carson et al., 1997; von Schulthess 2000, 2003; Wahl & Buchanan, 2002; Cherry et al., 2003; Wernick & Aarsvold, 2004; Bailey et al., 2006; Valk et al., 2005). Although SPECT is more widely used in daily clinical practice for identifying regional metabolic, blood flow, or receptor systems-related changes, it is not capable of absolute quantification of the biochemical or physiological changes it detects. In contrast, with PET one can generate precise radioactivity distribution maps of the target and, consequently, can quantitatively measure a large battery of biochemical or physiological parameters (Table 1.1).

TABLE 1.1. A Comparison of Various Biomedical Imaging Techniques Based on the Tomographic Principle

	CT	MRI	SPECT	PET
Physical foundations	X-ray	Nuclear magnetic resonance	Photon emission	Positron emission and coincidence detection
Contrast or tracer material	Contrast materials (IV, oral, rectal, inhalation)	Gadolinium-based contrast agents	Photon-emitting radionuclide	Positron-emitting radionuclide
Most commonly used isotopes (PET, SPECT) or investigated atoms (MRI)	—	^{1}H, ^{23}Na ^{31}P	^{123}I, ^{131}I, ^{99m}Tc, ^{133}Xe	^{11}C, ^{13}N, ^{15}O, ^{18}F
Primary modality	Morphology	Morphology	Biochemistry	Biochemistry
Best spatial resolution	1 mm	< 1 mm	4–5 mm	2–4 mm
Biological dose equivalent of a usual investigation	2–8 mSv	—	6–10 mSv	2–10 mSv

Constituents of a PET Center

A fully fledged PET center reflects the complex and sophisticated nature of the technique: It should be able to (1) produce radionuclides, (2) synthesize them into radiotracers, (3) administer the tracers to humans or experimental animals under strict quality control conditions, (4) scan the administered radiotracer's distribution in the body of the patient or experimental animal, and (5) create physiological and biochemical parametric maps from the raw radioactivity distributions and analyze the resulting images often parallel with other (e.g., anatomical) scans (Gulyás & Müller-Gärtner, 1998).

A complete PET center therefore consists of (1) a cyclotron facility, (2) a radiochemistry laboratory, (3) a quality control unit, (4) a scanner, and (5) image-processing, analysis, and archiving tools.

Because of the relatively longer half-time of the ^{18}F isotope (110 min), the isotope itself or ^{18}F-labeled PET tracers (predominantly fluorodeoxyglucose; FDG) can be transported greater distances. This feature has made the "distribution concept" possible: ^{18}F or ^{18}F-labeled isotopes can be generated/synthesized in a cyclotron-radiochemistry center and distributed to PET users at greater distances.

Physical Foundations of PET

Essentially, the technique is based on the physical principles of (1) positron emission and (2) coincidence detection (Eriksson et al., 1990; Burger & Townsend, 2003). The radionuclides, most commonly used for PET, are emitting a beta particle or positron (β^+) shortly after their generation by a particle accelerator. For this reason, they are also called beta emitters. A number of the most useful beta emitters have a short half-time and can easily be built into biologically active molecules; with these characteristics they are often called bioisotopes (Table 1.2).

The large variety of radionuclides used in nuclear medicine and biological imaging research can be produced in a direct way in particle accelerators (a linear accelerator or a cyclotron) or, less frequently, in reactors. Indirectly, by secondary decays, they can also be produced by generators. The bioisotopes used for PET can most efficiently be produced by a cyclotron. In a cyclotron, protons or deuterons are forced by electromagnets to run along a circular path and accelerate to a high energy level. The high-energy particles are then extracted and directed to a target material, wherein the impact of the energy-rich particles results in the production of proton-rich radionuclides. These radionuclides can relatively easily be extracted from the target and transferred to dedicated chemical equipment, in which the nuclides can be synthesized into biologically active molecules. Less frequently, the generated nuclides (more precisely, their molecular forms) can themselves be extracted and

TABLE 1.2. Bioisotopes Used in PET

Isotope	^{11}C		^{13}N		^{15}O		^{18}F	
Half-time (min)	20.3		9.98		2.05		110	
Nuclear reaction	$^{14}N(p,\alpha)$	^{11}C	$^{12}C(d,n)$	^{13}N	$^{14}N(d,n)$	^{15}O	$^{18}O(p,n)$	^{18}F
Content of cyclotron target	N + O		H2O		N + O		$H_2^{18}O$	
Specific radioactivity (Ci/μmol)	9×10^3		19×10^3		90×10^3		1.7×10^3	
Maximal energy (MeV)	0.97		1.20		1.74		0.64	
Positron range (mean range; mm)	1.17		1.5		<2.5		<1.0	
Effective radius (maximum range; mm)	3.9		5.1		8.0		2.6	
Effective dose equivalent (for 100-MBq tracer)	0.4 mSv		0.25 mSv		0.1 mSv		2.5 mSv	
Available forms	$^{11}CO, ^{11}CO_2$		$^{13}N, ^{13}NH_3$		$^{15}O_2, C^{15}O$		$H^{18}F, ^{18}F_2$	
Critical organ in the body	liver		liver		lung		bladder	

administered—as radiotracers—to the patient or the experimental animal (e.g., O_2, CO, or CO_2).

The radionuclide-labeled (or radiolabeled) molecule contains a positron-emitting isotope, which, by emitting a positron from its nucleus, decays. The positron is the antiparticle of the electron: The two particles have the same mass but different charges; the electron has a negative, whereas the positron has a positive charge. The positron, emitted from the nucleus of the radio-nuclide of the radiolabeled molecule administered to a subject or animal, interacts with the surrounding tissue. When it meets an electron, the two particles "annihilate" each other: They generate two photons of 511-keV energy, in line with the $E = mc^2$ formula. The average distance traveled by the positron before annihilation is the positron range; it varies between 1 and 2.5 mm for the commonly used PET radionuclides.

The two photons leave the locus of the annihilation along one axis in two opposing directions. The generated 511 keV photons can be detected by a pair of detectors placed alongside the line of response on two sides of the annihilation event. Because the detectors have surface areas, two of them, facing each other, can define a volume, the "detector channel," inside which the annihilation event can be detected if the line of response remains within the detector channel (Figure 1.1).

The detectors consist of two components: a scintillation crystal and a photomultiplier tube. In the scintillation crystal the 511 keV gamma photons are converted into photons in the range of visible light. Several materials can scintillate or produce light as a result of this interaction with gamma photons; the most widely used of these in PET technology are NaI and BiGe. The light generated in the scintillation crystal enters the photomultiplier tube, which converts light signals of a few hundred photons into a measurable electric signal without significantly increasing noise. The electric signals, originating from two opposing detectors, enter a coincidence circuit, and if their entrance times are close to each other (usually less than 14 ns; "coincidence time window"), the coincidence logic accepts the two signals as the result of an annihilation event inside the respective detector channel (Figure 1.1).

The two detectors may detect two incoming signals from a single annihilation event that took place inside the volume of the detector channel. In this case we refer to a "true coincidence event." But the detectors can also detect incoming signals from two independent annihilation events so that one gamma photon from one event reaches one detector, and another gamma photon from another uncorrelated event reaches the other detector within the coincidence circuit's predefined time interval. Such coincidences are random coincidences. It is also possible that one of the two gamma photons, generated by an annihilation event, will not follow a straight path, owing to scatter: The photon changes its straight path after colliding with a particle (e.g., an electron). Such events are scatter events, which still represent a single annihilation, but not inside the detector channel volume of the two detectors that detect the resulting gamma photons. Ideally, in the generation of PET images we should consider true events.

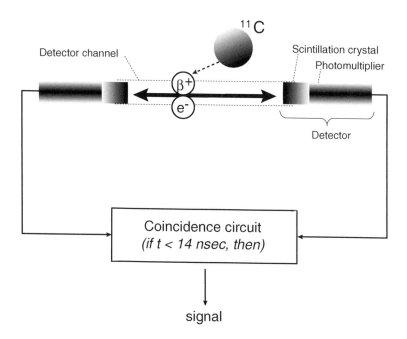

FIGURE 1.1. The physical basis of positron emission, positron-electron annihilation, and coincidence detection with the help of a functionally coupled detector system.

The PET Scanner

Because most detector blocks are only a few centimeters wide, in a PET scanner several detectors are built in rings (Figure 1.2A). The detector channels in a detector ring are not determined mechanically or geometrically. Usually, in a detector ring one detector can be coupled functionally (by way of the coincidence logic) with at least two-thirds of the detectors in the ring (Figure 1.2B).

In the early scanners the rings were separated from each other by lead septa, in order to guard the detectors in the individual rings from scatter arising from outside the plane of a given ring. In these scanners the detectors in a ring were coupled functionally to other detectors in the very same ring. In later-generation scanners the detectors are not necessarily coupled only with other detectors in the same ring: owing to the development of advanced software methods to improve scatter correction, coincidences between neighboring detector rings can also be accepted in order to increase sensitivity, that is, accepting photons traveling in planes oblique to a given receptor ring. In this way cross slices between neighboring rings can be defined. Even detectors in rings far away from each other can be coupled, and coincidences for large axial acceptance angles can be registered. The field of view (FOV) of the detector rings can be limited by using annular shields or septa. By using septa between the rings, the FOV of a detector ring can be stipulated to those annihilation events that occur inside the ring (2-D acquisition mode). In this case the signal-to-noise ratio is high, owing to the exclusion of a large part of random and scatter coincidences. By removing the septa, the field of view of the individual detector rings expands axially and the sensitivity of the system increases; however, the signal-to-noise ratio, especially in the axial end slices, decreases. In this case we refer to 3-D acquisition mode.

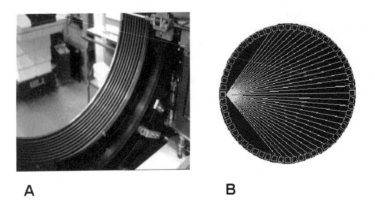

A   **B**

FIGURE 1.2. (A) Detector rings inside the scanner. (B) The possible arrangements of detector channels, related to one given detector, in a detector ring.

The diameter of the detector rings, defining the gantry of the scanner, can vary, depending on the primary use of the scanner; it can be rather small in dedicated animal scanners (rat-PET, monkey-PET), whereas it varies between 30 and 60 cm in dedicated brain scanners and whole-body scanners. Multiring systems provide a larger FOV and hence faster examination times. In the case of brain imaging it is usually possible to cover the entire brain without having to move the patient. In recent commercial scanners the axial FOV of the scanners is between 10 and 30 cm (the one used at Stockholm's Karolinska Institute has a FOV of 15 cm), but larger FOVs have become increasingly common in recent years. Although a large FOV is desirable, it is commonly the higher cost, due to the need of more detectors, that limits the number of rings used in a PET scanner.

Many commercial positron camera systems of today resemble each other in more than one way. In fact, most scanners are built according to the same architectural principles and vary only in design and materials used. However, it is the selection of individual components that determines the overall performance of a positron camera system. By far the most important factor regarding high resolution and image quality are the physical properties of the detectors and crystals used. Because image quality is also dependent on good timing and high energy resolution, state-of-the-art electronics are needed. Well-developed software algorithms for attenuation correction and scatter correction are also needed in order to produce high-quality images.

Detector Arrangement

It is rare to speak of a single detector. Most textbooks refer to a block of detectors, meaning a large, grown scintillating crystal that has been sawed to form a detector matrix. In the case of the Karolinska Institute PET scanner, a Siemens Ecat Exact HR 961, the rectangular crystal is sawed into an 8×7 matrix. In this case each detector block is made up of 56 detectors. Coupled to every block of detectors are four photomultiplying tubes (PMTs) (Figure 1.3A). As mentioned earlier, the aim of the PMTs is to amplify the light signal, generated by a photon interaction inside the scintillating crystal, and convert it into an electric pulse that can be registered and processed by postprocessing electronics and computers.

The resolution is partly defined by the size of each detector. Present systems have detectors that are about 3×3 mm, giving a spatial resolution of approximately 4.5 mm FWHM (full width at half maximum) for whole-body scanners, and approximately 2.4 mm FWHM for dedicated brain scanners. A limiting factor for high-resolution systems is the average positron range in tissue, meaning the average distance a positron travels before it meets an electron and annihilates. For 18F in human tissue, this is about 2 mm. Another resolution-limiting factor is that the gamma rays created by the annihilation process do not part at exactly 180 degrees, but rather at 180 ± 0.25 degrees. Because a whole-body scanner has a larger diameter than a dedicated brain scanner, the angular deviation of 0.25 degrees has a larger effect.

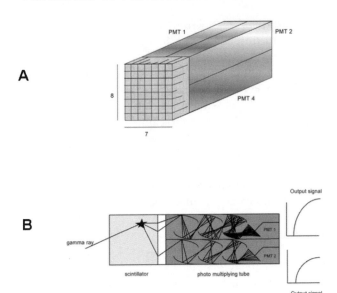

FIGURE 1.3. (A) Schematics of a detector block consisting of 56 individual detector crystals coupled to four photomultiplying tubes (PMTs). (B) Events inside a detector block. As a gamma ray interacts with the scintillator, a light flash is produced. The amount of light that passes through to each of the four PMTs is proportional to the location of interaction. The PMTs then convert the light into an electric pulse.

Inside a Detector Block

Photons interact with matter in three ways: (1) pair production, (2) Compton scatter, and (3) photoelectric effect. Pair production occurs when a high-energy photon, generally interacting with an atomic nucleus, produces an electron and a positron. However, for this process to occur, photons with energies greater than 1.022-MeV are needed. Hence, pair production is not relevant to PET because the only photons of interest are those at 511 keV. Compton scatter occurs when a photon, regardless of its energy, collides with other particles and thereby changes direction and loses speed. As a direct consequence, some of its original energy is lost. Scattered events leave unwanted effects on PET imaging.

Photoelectric effect is the complete absorption of a photon in the scintillating crystal on which the photon deposits all its remaining energy. In the case of PET, it is the photoelectric effect inside a scintillating crystal that produces a light flash. The light created is then led through the sawed detector matrix into the PMTs, where an electric pulse is generated (Figure 1.3B). Because the light flash spreads inside the crystal and gives a signal to more than one PMT, it is essential to develop an algorithm that can decide in which crystal the interaction has occurred. This algorithm is based on how much light output each of the four PMTs received. The outputs from the PMTs are also used in order to reject photons that have scattered before reaching the detector. This is possible because the amplitude of the created signal is proportional to the scintillator's light output, and therefore also to the energy deposited by the photon interaction. An energy window that lets only photons that have deposited energies within its limits can then be created. With good timing it is possible to determine at what time the pulse was generated, which in turn enables one triggering event to be coupled with another in order to form a line of response.

Because decay times and light output may differ between individual crystals and PMTs have different gains, these parameters must be assessed and correction maps generated to ensure a uniform response from the detectors. This is done during the detector setup and calibration procedure that is part of every facility's quality assurance program (NEMA NU2, 2001).

Crystals

The limiting factors of spatial resolution in today's scanners lie within the physical properties of the detector crystals being used. Although fast electronics are needed for good timing, it is the properties of the crystals being used that constitute the bottleneck of present scanners.

The main properties that determine whether a detector crystal is suitable for PET are (1) high light output, (2) fast decay time, and (3) high stopping power.

The amplitude of the electric pulse created by the PMTs is proportional to the amount of light input the PMTs receive. Because PMTs and electronics create background noise, it is important to use crystals with a high light output so that the registered signal is not blurred and drowned in the noise.

The decay time of the light flash generated by a photon interaction in the crystal sets a limit as to how many events can be registered within a given time frame. Fast crystals not only enable the system to register many events within short time frames, but also give better timing resolution. Ideally, the generated pulse would be a very high and narrow peak. Such a peak can be created only if the crystals are very fast and have a high light output. Fast crystals are therefore needed in next-generation PET scanners capable of calculating the time of flight (TOF). In this case the aim is not only to register a line of responses, but to calculate where along the line of response the positron emission most likely occurred.

Ideally, every photon interacting with a crystal should be stopped in the same crystal and not be scattered to a neighboring crystal. In order to achieve this, it is essential that the crystals used have high stopping power. High stopping power is achieved by using crystals with high density, and hence high atomic numbers. However, a drawback to the theory is that high-density crystals often have long decay times.

In today's scanners BGO (bismuth germanate) crystals are commonly used. The light output of these crystals cannot compare to the light output of

TABLE 1.3. Comparison of Properties of Scintillator Crystals for PET

Scintillator	τ (ns)	μ (cm^{-1})	Relative light output (%)
NaI (Tl)	230	0.35	100
BGO	300	0.95	15
GSO	60	0.70	25
LSO	40	0.86	75
LuAp	18	0.95	30
LaCl$_3$	26	0.36	120
LaBr$_3$	35	0.47	160

Note. Energy resolution taken at 662-keV (Surti et al., 2003). τ is the decay time and μ is the attenuation coefficient. The decay time determines the duration of the light flash, and the attenuation coefficient is a measure of stopping power.

NaI (sodium iodide) crystals but do provide an acceptable compromise of high light output and high stopping power (bismuth's atomic number is 83). However, they are too slow for TOF measurements.

Continuous research is widely exploring the potentials of new crystals. Luteium oxyortho-silicate (LSO) and lanthanum bromide (LaBr$_3$) are two crystals proven to have great potential for PET (Surti et al., 2003). Some companies already utilize LSO crystals, and LaBr$_3$ seems to be a suitable crystal for next-generation TOF scanners. Table 1.3 shows a comparison of various "classical" or novel scintillation crystals suitable for PET. NaI doped with thallium (Tl) is considered to be the standard for light output measurements, and its light output is therefore set to 100%.

Data Processing and Image Generation

Computer Background of a PET Facility

A PET facility puts a substantial demand on its computer equipment. In one sense, it is the computer system that is the organizer of the facility. Although the scanner is the base for all imaging, its only purpose is to create files with information on the radioactive distribution of the investigated object. It is then the computer's function to translate this information into images.

Many time-consuming computer operations, such as image reconstruction and scatter corrections, are performed by the software. This creates a demand for fast processors and extensive disk space. However, the rapid evolution of computer components continuously improves performance and reduces the amount of time needed to generate images.

Image Generation

The first step of image generation is to acquire information on the activity distribution of the investigated object. This information, called raw data, is stored in sinogram files. For accurate quantitative studies, two sinograms are needed. One sinogram carries information on activity distribution (emission sinogram), and the other sinogram carries information on the attenuation of the object (transmission sinogram). Whereas the emission sinogram is a result of injected activity in the object, the transmission sinogram is commonly generated by transmission rods circulating the object. Usually, these files are stored in a separate computer unit called the acquisition computer system (ACS).

The raw data is then copied from the ACS to the reconstruction unit, together with a normalization file and a blank file. The normalization file contains information on the uniformity of the scanner. Ideally, all detectors should register equal amounts of activity when measuring a circulating rod source, as the activity is then, over time, evenly distributed in every angle. Because the efficiencies of the detectors vary over time, the number of interactions they detect relative to each other must be either increased or decreased. Information on how much the efficiencies need to be tuned is then stored in the normalization file. The blank file contains information generated by a transmission scan without placing anything inside the gantry, hence the name "blank file." The blank is needed, together with the transmission file, in order to perform the 2-D attenuation measurement. The generation of normalization and blank files are part of every facility's quality assurance program.

The sinogram files contain all necessary information on the activity distribution needed for image reconstruction. This means that matrix size, zoom factor, filter, and filter parameters are all set just prior to the reconstruction and that the reconstruction can be done over again with different sets of reconstruction parameters. After the images have been created, they are archived together with all files needed for a later reconstruction. Archiving to a medium such as CD-ROM, DDS tapes, DAT tapes, or LTO tapes, which can store up to 200 GB of data, is common. For quality assurance, all data should be archived on two separate information carrier media, which are then stored at two different locations.

Most modern PET scanners are capable of performing data acquisition and reconstruction in both the 2-D and 3-D modes (see above). The two major differences between 2-D and 3-D PET imaging concern data redundancy and spatial variance.

Image Reconstruction

In PET, as in other tomography-based imaging techniques, the reconstruction of the sampled image data is based on the tomography principle (Defrise & Kinahan, 1998). The essence of this principle is similar to the well-known arithmetical puzzle: how to identify the figures of a grid when only their sums are familiar to us. A number of mathematical algorithms have been developed for the reconstruction process, of which the filtered backprojection (FBP) is the most commonly used in PET. Backprojection is a mathematical process whereby a number of one-dimensional projection data are reprojected in order to form a 2-D image. This situation is best described using a point source centered in the gantry, such as shown in Figure 1.4. The question is how a real-life radioactivity distribution can be reconstructed following data sampling by a detector ring system (Figure 1.4A, B).

In the specific case of a point source centered in the gantry, it is true to say that (1) each projected profile can be represented by a sharp and narrow peak, also known as a delta function, as well as (2) all profiles will be identical, regardless of their angles to the object being investigated (Figure 1.4C). If these profiles are then backprojected, a new 2-D image will arise. This image

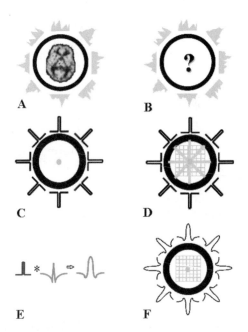

FIGURE 1.4. Schematic diagram showing the procedure of filtered backprojection. The original biological target has a radioactivity distribution pattern inside the scanner's gantry (A). The main question of data sampling and reconstruction centers on the reliability of the generated image (B). In the special case of a point source centered in the gantry, all projections, regardless of angle, will be the same (C). If these projections were to be backprojected, the reconstructed image would be smeared (D). Instead, a convolution between the profile and the reconstruction filter is applied (E), creating a filtered profile. The filtered profile can then be used to successfully reconstruct the original image (F).

will resemble the true object, but will be smeared and not very sharp; see (Figure 1.4D). This smearing artifact is due to the fact that the intensity of the point source decreases proportionally to 1/r (r = radius) from the center of the point source. By filtering each profile before backprojection, the smearing can be removed, hence the algorithm name "filtered backprojection." The filtering process is a convolution of the profile with the reconstruction filter (Figure 1.4E). After the convolution, a new wave profile is formed, and it is this profile that is used for the backprojection (Figure 1.4F). In order to get the true image after backprojection, it is essential that the number of projections is sufficient and that the linear sampling of the measured projections is dense enough.

Despite the best possible reconstruction algorithms, there are various inaccuracies, resulting from a number of factors. These include (1) the nature of the beta decay and the electron–positron annihilation, (2) the physical features of the detector system, (3) the nature of the reconstruction algorithms and procedures, and (4) the inherent biological features of the investigated object. Even an "ideal" point source of radioactivity would appear in the resulting image as a "smeared out" blob, the physical nature of which follows a Gaussian distribution (Figure 1.5). For these (and a few other) reasons, the spatial resolution of a PET scanner cannot surpass a certain lower limit.

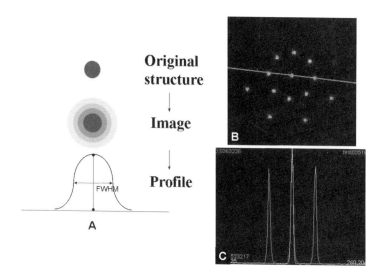

FIGURE 1.5. (A) Even an ideal point source of radioactivity appears on an optimally tuned PET system's image as a Gaussian distribution of radioactivity. The distribution's principal mathematical feature, the "full-width-at-half-maximum" (of the peak value) (FWHM) characterizes a scanner's spatial resolution. (B) Transaxial PET image of a radioactive phantom with thin line sources. (C) Radioactivity distribution of the thin line sources in the PET image, corresponding to the line in panel (B).

Inaccuracies in the Reconstructed Images Due to Attenuation and Scatter

When reconstructing images, it is also necessary to make attenuation and scatter corrections. Attenuation is caused when the annihilating photons interact with the surrounding tissue rather than the crystal detectors. For a whole-body exam, as many as 95% of all photons are attenuated within the body, leaving only 5% reaching the detectors. A cylinder with uniform activity concentration will appear denser in the outer regions, closer to the detectors, as compared with its center, if no attenuation correction is made. The activity profile of such a cylinder will therefore resemble the cross section of a bathtub (Figure 1.6). To obtain reliable images of the investigated object's radioactivity distribution, the emission scans should be "attenuation corrected." In order to achieve this, emission scans are complemented with transmission (or attenuation) scans, by using a rotating single photon source, such as ^{68}Ge, around the target object.

Photons that are scattered may well reach the detectors and deposit all their remaining energy therein, but they also contribute to giving false information to the system, inasmuch as they now represent a different line of response than the one they originated from. Photon scatter therefore increases smearing and blurring of the reconstructed image. In whole-body scanners as many as 50% of all detected photons may originate from scattered events. Because there is less matter in the brain, as compared with the thorax, the scatter-to-true ratio is about 25% in dedicated brain scanners. Taking attenuation and scatter into consideration, one finds that only approximately 2.5% of all photons contribute to a whole-body image and 3.75% to a brain image.

Postprocessing of the Images

In a number of cases data acquisition can be done continuously, that is, within one "time window." In this case the image is generated on the basis of the autoradiography principle. However, for finer analysis of the available information, data acquisition takes place in a sequence of shorter time windows, resulting in dynamic images. Typically, time frame sequences are not spaced evenly in a dynamic acquisition program, but they follow the temporal requirements of the tracer uptake follow-up: In the early phases, more frequent and shorter, and in later phases, less frequent and longer time frames are required.

The reconstructed images represent raw radioactivity maps, which can, of course, already be used for identifying certain basic information in the image. For a number of purposes, the raw data image can be used as it is; for example, diagnostic FDG-PET images need no special postprocessing and can be the basis of a "visual" diagnosis.

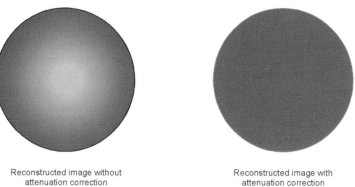

A

Uniform cylindrical phantom

B

Uniform cylindrical phantom

activity concentration

activity concentration

Activity concentration profile without attenuation correction

Activity concentration profile with attenuation correction

Reconstructed image without
attenuation correction

Reconstructed image with
attenuation correction

FIGURE 1.6. Illustration of the importance of attenuation correction. (A) The resulting concentration profile and reconstructed image of a uniform cylindrical phantom when no attenuation correction is applied. (B) The correct concentration profile and reconstructed image when proper attenuation corrections have been made.

For scientific purposes, however, the raw data images form only the first layer of information. Using additional measurements (e.g., arterial blood radioactivity concentration measurements), parametric images of physiological or biochemical processes can be determined, such as blood flow, oxygen consumption, or glucose metabolism.

In addition, the kinetic behavior of receptor radioligands or labeled drugs can be assessed. Using both "external cues" (blood and plasma metabolic and radioactivity measurements) and "internal cues" in the image (e.g., reference tissue measurements), quantitative parameters of the ligand's behavior in the brain or body can be calculated. These calculations of biochemical parameters require various mathematical models and are usually computation-intensive.

But image postprocessing can also improve image quality and parametric accuracy in many other ways, too. An important aspect of a parametric image is the signal-to-noise ratio, which can be improved in a number of ways. The reconstructed PET images are not noisy. The origin of the noise is multiple: partly biological (i.e., noise in the scanned biological target), partly physical (noise due to the nature of the annihilation process and noise arising from the scanner), and partly due to the reconstruction process. The measured signals therefore comprise both a "true biological signal" and noise of multiple origin. However, the intrinsic nature of the noise and that of the true signal are different from each other: The spatial origin and temporal integrity of the true signal are consistent in the dynamic images, whereas those of the noise are not. This provides us with the opportunity of using noise-reducing techniques aimed at improving the signal-to-noise ratio in the image.

One possible approach is based on the wavelet technique, which is widely used today in biomedical applications. With the help of wavelet analysis, the parametric accuracy of, for example, receptor binding images can significantly be improved. Another important question is the correction of the partial volume effect. The partial volume effect is an inevitable consequence of imaging of bodies with multiple compartments, each exhibiting a different absorption of the radioactively labeled tracer or ligand. Using dedicated software, the partial volume effect can be corrected to a great extent.

The spatial resolution of PET is inferior to that of anatomical or morphological imaging techniques used in diagnostic medicine (CT, MRI). In order to combine the advantages of morphological and functional imaging techniques, thereby improving the localization precision in the functional images, PET is often combined with CT or MRI scans. The registration of the two types of images requires software tools applicable for image registration.

Currently, a new version of PET, the PET/CT, combines the strengths of two well-established imaging modalities, CT for anatomy and PET for function, into a single imaging device. PET/CT scanners provide accurately aligned anatomical and functional images of a patient, allowing functional abnormalities to be localized and distinguished from normal uptake of the PET tracer, which increases a physician's confidence in arriving at a correct diagnosis.

Good Imaging Practice

To ensure good image quality, it has become common practice, among leading PET centers, to operate all equipment, including the PET scanner and any computer hardware connected to it, according to given protocols. The protocols, formerly known as SOPs (standard operating procedures), serve as a main guarantee that operational procedures are performed in exactly the same way, even though preformed by different persons. SOPs are not only used to regulate and document any activities related to the scanner, such as time intervals between service, but also constitute the spinal cord of all regulations and order of decision making relevant to the PET center. All routines for addressing an emergency, either technical or clinical, should be clearly stated in the SOPs. However, a PET center may choose to distinguish between SOPs that serve a technical purpose, such as good imaging practice (GIP) and good clinical practice (GCP). Apart from GIP and GCP, several more procedures can be described by good manufacturing practice (GMP) and good laboratory practice (GLP). These procedures are sometimes gathered in a more common description, GXP.

There are several regulatory institutions that handle regulations and recommendations regarding the information that each form of GXP should contain.

Foundations of PET Radiochemistry

The main objective of radiochemistry is to incorporate the isotopes, produced by a cyclotron, into molecules that can be used to label biochemical or physiological processes by inertly participating in physiological operations (e.g., [^{15}O] butanol or [^{15}O] water as blood flow tracers), by entering the organism's biochemical processes (e.g., FDG) or by binding to various binding sites in the body (e.g., central neuroreceptor ligands) (Stöcklin & Pike, 1993). The labeled molecules are, in general, radiotracers or radiopharmaceuticals, and those radiotracers that bind to specific binding sites in the body are called radioligands.

In comparison with other subdisciplines of chemistry, radiochemistry has its own special conditions. Owing to the rapid decay of the isotope, a radiochemical synthesis must be fast and effective. The synthesis time cannot exceed two to three half-lives of the isotope. Usually 20–50% end-of-batch efficacy is required; that is, the end product must contain 20–50% of the original radioactivity. Because of the increased radiation exposure, radiochemists must work under stricter safety conditions. The products should be purified and tested for purity before application.

All major positron emitters can be used for radiochemical synthesis, but the most commonly used radionuclides are ^{18}F and ^{11}C. The use of ^{13}N and

^{15}O is more limited, mainly due to the shorter half-lives of these radionuclides. ^{81}Rb, another possible PET radionuclide, is also of limited use, as it is a generator product and is exclusively used for heart studies.

Owing to the short half-life time of the radionuclides, the PET data acquisition time is also limited. This, in turn, puts limitations on the various radiotracers' usefulness in tracking the kinetics of the injected/administered tracer. Data acquisition statistics deteriorate after three to four half-lives of the isotope. In line with this, the acquisition time with ^{15}O tracers can last for up to 2–4 min, with ^{11}C tracers up to 60–90 min, and with ^{18}F tracers it can, in theory, last for up to 5–6 h. However, in diagnostic neuroimaging routine investigations the acquisition times are much shorter (^{15}O, 1–2 min; ^{11}C, 10–20 min; ^{18}F, 10–30 min).

Among the PET radionuclides, the frequently utilized ^{18}F has earlier been used in a single form: FDG. More recently, a burgeoning variety of radioligands are available with the radionuclide (Table 1.4). The longer half-life of ^{18}F (110 min), among other PET radionuclides, provides the radiochemist with relatively long synthesis times, and it also guarantees the tracking of tracer kinetics with the PET scanner for up to 5–6 h. Because of the longer half-life of this radionuclide, ^{18}F radiopharmaceuticals can be transported longer distances—for instance, to PET scanners not adjacent to a cyclotron and a radiochemistry laboratory. This possibility is widely used in the FDG distribution concept: One PET/radiochemistry center can provide FDG for a number of PET scanners at longer distances (see above).

Although a large number of ^{18}F-labeled radiotracers have been synthesized and tested for PET, relatively few of them have become widely used PET radiopharmaceuticals. The most frequently used radiopharmaceutical of all radiotracers, 2-[^{18}F] FDG is the workhorse of clinical PET studies. FDG is a most faithful indicator of tissue glucose consumption (i.e., energy metabo-

TABLE 1.4. A Selection of PET Radiotracers, Labeled with the Four Most Common Radionuclides

Oxygen	Nitrogen	Carbon	Fluorine
Butanol	Ammonia	Acetate	Altenserine
Carbon monoxide		Carfentanil	Flumazenil
Carbon dioxide		Cocaine	Fluorine ion
Oxygen		Deprenyl	Fluorodeoxyglucose (FDG)
Water		FLB457	Fluorodopa (F-dopa)
		Flumazenil	Fluoroethylspiperone
		Leucine	Fluorouracil
		Methionine	Haloperidol
		N-Methylspiperone	
		Raclopride	
		WAY-100635	
		Thyrosine	

lism). For this reason, FDG can be used as an ideal diagnostic indicator of normal and pathological glucose metabolism, including regional decreases and increases in various anatomical structures. Similar to glucose, FDG passes the blood–brain barrier, enters the brain, and undergoes the first metabolic step, resulting in FDG-6-phosphate. But unlike glucose-6-phosphate, which can enter further metabolic steps, FDG-6-phosphate cannot enter further metabolic processes and falls into a "metabolic trap." The labeled metabolite can thus faithfully represent the transport and uptake of glucose in the body (Figure 1.7). In addition to FDG, the number of ^{18}F-labeled PET ligands has steadily been increasing in recent years (Couturier et al., 2004; Varagnolo et al., 2000).

For a long time, ^{11}C has been used in the widest variety of PET radiochemistry applications (Halldin et al., 2001a, 2001b, 2004). The range and number of the applications of C-11-labeled receptor ligands and drugs have steadily increased during the past years, as witnessed by the increasing number of publications in this field. An important prerequisite for radioligand development is that the molecule maintain its properties after labeling. This is one of the reasons for the common use of the short-lived positron-emitting radionuclide carbon-11. The substitution of naturally occurring carbon-12 with carbon-11 does not change the biochemistry or the pharmacology of the ligand molecule.

The most widely used approach for labeling ligands using carbon-11 is [^{11}C]methylation. A typical total synthesis time for a ^{11}C-labeled radioligand including high-performance liquid chromatography (HPLC) purification is 30 min. The reaction may require the presence of base for the generation of the nucleophile. Moreover, [^{11}C]acylations with [^{11}C]acylchlorides and [^{11}C]cyanation with [^{11}C]cyanide are two common types of reactions.

[13]N is mainly used in one form—ammonia—for PET studies on the heart. The use of [15]O tracers is limited mainly to research purposes (measuring

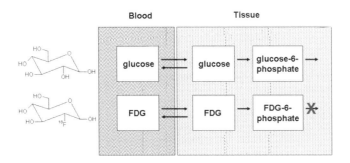

FIGURE 1.7. The metabolic routes of glucose (upper row) and its ^{18}F-labeled PET tracer analogue, FDG (fluorodeoxyglucose: 2-deoxy-2[^{18}F]fluoro-D-glucose) (lower row).

global and regional cerebral blood flow), owing to the short half-time of the radionuclide (approximately 2 min). Finally, apart from the "classical" bioisotopes, ^{82}Rb can also be used as a heart tracer in diagnostic PET studies, but its use is limited as the radionuclide is not a cyclotron, but a generator, product.

Administration and Quality Control of the Administered Drug

The end product of a radiochemical synthesis should be chemically and radiochemically clean, sterile, and free from pyrogens. The radiopharmaceutical control of the administered drug should be performed and testified to by independent experts not participating in the preparatory processes and the synthesis of the radiotracers.

The most common means of administering a radiotracer is by way of an intravenous bolus injection, but labeled drugs or radiotracers can also be administered by inhalation. In theory, peroral administration is also possible, but in practice it has been used rather rarely. The amount of administered radioactivity is limited by radiation safety regulations, and it also depends on the isotope and the sensitivity of the scanner. The injected radioactivity doses are in the range of 5–10 mCi for ^{18}F and ^{11}C tracers. An important precaution is related to radioligands with specific activity (SA). For instance, the typical specific activities of ^{11}C-labeled radioligands are on the order of 10 Ci/μmol (370 GBq/μmol). In this range of specific activity, only one of a thousand tracermolecules contains ^{11}C, whereas the rest contain ^{12}C. Owing to the decay of the radionuclide, the ratio of the labeled versus unlabeled molecules changes rapidly in the product, and this fact has important consequences in

---

TABLE 1.5. Physiological–Biochemical Parameters Measurable with PET

- Blood flow
- Blood volume
- Protein synthesis
- Molecular diffusion
- Tissue pH
- Metabolism of oxygen, glucose, amino acids, fatty acids, fluor, etc.
- Receptor and transporter systems: uptake, binding, occupancy, distribution volume, etc. (dopamine, serotonin, noradrenaline, glutamate, GABA–benzodiazepine, etc.)
- Pharmacodynamics and pharmacokinetics of labeled drugs

research studies. Because the administered radiolabeled drug (tracer, ligand) is given in tracer doses (nanogram–pikogram amounts), no pharmacological effects can be expected.

Using additional physiological information and mathematical models from the radioactivity distribution maps, obtained by the PET scanner, a large number of biochemical parameters can be calculated, including several parameters related to the distribution and density of receptor systems and the ligands' or radiolabeled drugs' interaction with the receptors can also be measured (Table 1.5).

Measuring and Modeling Radiotracer Effects in the Brain

The great advantage of the PET technique is that it is capable of obtaining "absolute" (i.e., quantified) measurements of regional radioactivity concentrations, which, in turn, with the help of appropriate kinetic models, can be transformed into quantitative parametric maps of related receptor parameters.

The quantitative measurements with PET require the determination of tissue and blood/plasma radioactivity concentrations and the a priori knowledge of a number of experimental parameters, including basic features related to the tracer, the biochemical and physiological characteristics and metabolic stability of the ligand, and those of the scanner. In a next step, a multi-compartmental model describing the distribution and metabolism of the ligand in the brain and, eventually, in other body compartments, is developed, tested, and validated. With the help of appropriate tracer kinetic models the requested biological variables (e.g., receptor occupancy data) can be described in quantitative terms in precise anatomical context in the brain or body organ covered by the PET scan.

Clinical Applications of PET

During the past two decades, PET has established its unique place among nuclear medicine techniques in clinical diagnostic practice. The overwhelming majority of diagnostic PET investigations are based on the use of metabolic markers—foremost, FDG (Plate 1.1), and only a small number of diagnostic PET examinations utilize other measuring modalities of PET, including regional blood flow or receptor binding measurements. Metabolic measurements with PET focus on regional increases or decreases of metabolism as a result of pathological increases in metabolism (most commonly observed in tumors) or pathological decreases in metabolism (observed, for instance, in degenerative diseases or lesions in local circulation) (Ruhlmann et al., 1999).

The rationales behind the great advantage of clinical diagnostic PET investigations are multiple:

- In several disease groups, PET has a unique sensitivity and specificity, as compared with other diagnostic imaging techniques, as it can, for instance, reveal metastatic diseases that other imaging techniques simply cannot detect.
- Follow-up PET investigations can show the progress of disease as well as treatment effects.
- PET (especially the novel PET-CT) can replace a number of other diagnostic investigations and has therefore the potential to significantly reduce multiple medical costs and minimize patient discomfort.

As a clinical diagnostic technique, PET is most frequently used in oncology, followed by neurology and cardiology. The common uses of PET in clinical practice are shown in Table 1.6, whereas the most frequent diagnostic applications are shown in Table 1.7. As already mentioned, the sensitivity and selectivity of PET is, in most cases, superior to those of morphological imaging techniques, and the combination of PET with CT or MR can further improve diagnostic efficacy.

The most common diagnostic approach is related to the detection of metabolic increases, as in the case of tumors. Tumor growth in most cases is accompanied by regional metabolic increases, which can easily be detected with FDG, but also with other metabolic tracers, such as [^{11}C] methionine. In exceptional cases, for instance, in low-grade astrocytomas, the tumor can be less active metabolically than its environment. PET as a diagnostic technique can also be used in central nervous system (CNS) diseases resulting in metabolic decreases, such as Alzheimer's disease, epilepsy, Creutzfeldt–Jakob disease, or stroke (Plate 1.2).

TABLE 1.6. Clinical Uses of PET in Oncology

- Identifying and localizing primary tumor
- Differentiating benign versus malignant processes
- Establishing local extent of tumor
- Establishing grade of malignancy, staging
- Posttreatment restaging
- Detecting regional spread
- Identifying distant metastases
- Guiding locus of biopsy
- Treatment planning
- Treatment monitoring
- Detecting residual tumor after surgical intervention
- Detecting and localizing suspected recurrence
- Differentiation of residual soft tissue (scar) versus tumor

---

TABLE 1.7. The Most Frequent Diagnostic Applications of PET

Oncology	Neurology	Cardiology/cardiosurgery
Brain cancer	Epilepsy	Cardiac viability
Breast cancer	Dementia	
Colorectal cancer		
Esophageal cancer		
Head and neck cancer		
Lung cancer		
Thyroid cancer		
Cervical cancer		
Solitary pulmonary nodule		
Lymphoma		
Melanoma		

PET in Basic Neuroscience Research

Basically two aspects of PET have made it a distinguished research tool in the neurosciences. Using PET with metabolic and/or blood flow tracers, one can localize various sensory, motor, or cognitive functions in the brain, and when using PET with receptor radioligands, the receptor architecture of the brain can be mapped.

The localization of brain functions with PET is based on the assumption that increased neuronal activity requires metabolic increases and, consequently, increased regional cerebral blood flow, which in turn can be detected with the help of blood flow tracers (Roland, 1993; Friston et al., 1997). The most commonly used blood-flow tracers are ^{15}O-labeled water and butanol. The localization of various brain functions requires carefully planned experimental designs, with the help of which one can identify brain regions responsible for certain neuronal operations. Using appropriate statistical analysis techniques, the cortical neuronal populations underlying sensory, motor, or cognitive processes in the human brain can be localized.

The mapping of neuroreceptor systems requires radioligands, most frequently labeled with ^{11}C, selective for one receptor or transmitter system, such as shown in Plate 1.3. The analysis of the human brain's receptor fingerprint in rest and under various drug or psychophysical challenge conditions can provide an insight into the neuronal–biochemical operations underlying cognitive processes or the biological nature of personality.

PET in Neuropsychiatric Drug Research

The development of a new drug is a time- and cost-intensive process, which may last for well over a decade and cost more than a half billion dollars. PET has a unique potential to speed up and facilitate drug development, with special relevance to the field of neuropsychopharmacology. With this technique, several vital parameters of the drug-candidate molecule can be measured in the preclinical phase, and the drug's physiological and therapeutic effects can be monitored in the clinical phase of the development process (Comar, 1995; Farde, 1996; Schwaiger et al., 2004; Lee & Farde, 2006).

For radiolabeled drug administration to humans in microdoses, approval can be obtained with less extensive safety and toxicology documentation than that which is required for the much higher doses that induce clinical effects. In this emerging field there are as yet no international guidelines for the preclinical documentation required. A common practice used by several national drug agencies is to approve PET studies with new radiolabeled drugs if the acute toxicity has been examined in a rodent and if a genotoxicity test is negative. For this reason it is now possible to use PET for examination of a large number of new molecules directly in human subjects.

In the preclinical phase of the development of a novel drug the most important questions that can be answered by PET are related to the distribution of the drug in the body following peroral or intravenous administration, its penetration through the blood–brain barrier and uptake in the brain, its regional distribution in the brain and binding to specific binding sites, and the kinetic behavior of the drug. A more detailed list of the potential uses of PET in drug development is shown in Table 1.8.

TABLE 1.8. Possible Applications of PET during Neuropsychopharmacological Drug Development

Pharmacokinetics (movement of drugs)

1. To confirm brain distribution (i.e., passage across the blood–brain barrier)
2. To confirm that the drug binds to central neuroreceptors (validation of principle)
3. To identify relationships between dose, plasma concentration, and central receptor occupancy
4. To provide additional information on absorption, bioavailability, distribution, and elimination

Pharmacodynamics (therapeutic and side effects)

1. Correlation between receptor binding and therapeutic and side effects
2. Correlation between regional binding and regional effects on physiological parameters (metabolism, blood flow, etc.)
3. Functional measurements between and after treatments with the drug

Drug testing

1. Validation of animal models for human conditions
2. Measuring species differences (tissue metabolism, receptor binding)
3. Comparison of the effects of various drug molecules

Therapy planning

1. Individual therapy planning
2. Optimizing therapeutic effects
3. Minimizing side effects

When testing a candidate drug's pharmacological effects, there are two possible and widely used experimental designs (Figure 1.8).

1. The most frequent approach is to study how an unlabeled drug inhibits specific binding of a well-characterized selective PET radioligand. In this case the unlabeled drug is entering into competition with a labeled ligand for occupying a receptor system. The amount of the unlabeled drug greatly exceeds the amount of the labeled drug. The unlabeled drug is given in a pharmacological dose (mg range), whereas the labeled ligand is given in a tracer dose (μg range or less), the two doses being different at least three to four orders of magnitude. The reason for this is that we would like to block a given receptor system as completely as possible by the unlabeled drug. This can be achieved either by giving the unlabeled drug before the administration of the labeled drug (pretreatment) or somewhat after it (displacement).

2. The alternative direct approach is to radiolabel a new potential drug and to trace its uptake, anatomical distribution, and binding in the brain. The PET technique is sensitive for determinations of concentrations as low as the

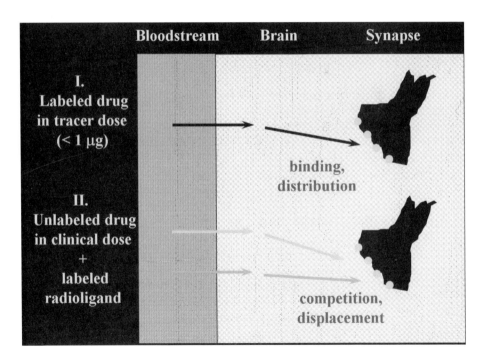

FIGURE 1.8. Two approaches used in drug development with PET. (I) A straightforward approach is to radiolabel a new potential drug and to trace its anatomical distribution and binding in the brain. (II) Indirect approach: A well-known labeled radioligand (used in tracer dose) is entering into competition with a drug (used in therapeutic dose) for the same receptor system.

subpicomolar range. Effective radiochemical labeling yields a drug that is labeled to a high specific radioactivity (SA), that is, with a high ratio of radiolabeled-to-unlabeled drug molecules. A consequence is that intravenous (IV) injection of less than a microgram of the radiolabeled drug is sufficient for a PET study in humans. The concept "tracer dose" is often used to emphasize the low mass that does not induce drug effects.

In addition to these "direct" uses of PET in neuropsychopharmacological drug development, the technique can also be used to assess the effects of a neuropsychopharmacological drug on metabolic or blood flow parameters, thereby assessing its therapeutic efficacy in relation to vital biochemical–physiological parameters. Furthermore, with PET the sites of pharmacological actions and physiological actions can be identified, providing cues for interpreting drug effects. The technique in combination with other measurements can also yield information about metabolic routes of drug metabolism.

In the clinical phase of drug development, the drug's effects on physiological parameters, as well as long-lasting therapeutic effects, can be assessed with the help of PET.

Using different metabolic and blood flow tracers (e.g., FDG and water or butanol, respectively), the biochemical or physiological effects of drugs, administered in pharmacological doses, can be assessed. The usual protocol in this case is a comparative PET protocol: The respective metabolic or blood flow parameter (cerebral metabolic rate of glucose; CMR_{glu} or cerebral blood flow; CBF) is quantitatively measured before and after drug administration. The administration is usually intravenous (bolus, prolonged infusion, or a longer treatment regime), but the drug can also be given perorally. This approach has been exemplified in exploring the effects of vinpocetine, a vinca alkaloid, which is known to effectively increase cerebral blood flow and cerebral glucose metabolism and exercise a neuroprotective effect. In a series of PET studies, we measured blood flow and metabolism before and after treatment with the drug and the differences (pretreatment–posttreatment) display the regional effects of the drug treatment (Plate 1.4A and B).

PET can also follow up the long-lasting therapeutic effects of drugs, including cytostatic drugs, antiinflammatory agents, and psycopharmacons. For instance, haloperidol, an antipsychotic drug, binds to the dopamine D2/D3 receptors in the brain. Treatment over a long period with haloperidol in patients with schizophrenia results, in most cases, in clinical improvement. Parallel with the patient's improvement, the patient's dopamine receptors in the striatum are occupied and "blocked" by the therapeutic drug and are, consequently, no longer available for a PET radioligand with high affinity to the dopamine receptors (Plate 1.4C and D).

Last but not least, PET can help us visualize the "fate" of labeled drug molecules in the human body. The injected radiolabeled drug molecule's fate can be multifold: (1) If it has high affinity to some binding sites or receptors in the body, a part of it binds to the specific binding sites or receptors, (2) whereas a certain amount of the molecules bind to plasma proteins and circulates in the blood for a while. (3) Some of the molecules can be deposited in some tissue compartments (e.g., lipophylic molecules in the fatty tissue). (4) The drug molecules can undergo metabolism (usually in the liver) and are finally chemically "decomposed," metabolized. (5) Both the mother molecule and the metabolites can be eliminated by way of kidney excretion (and stored in, and eliminated by, the urine), biliary excretion (and eliminated by stool), or other mechanisms (e.g., expiration). (6) With time, some of the drug molecules can be "redistributed" in the body—for example, cleaned from the brain and deposited in the bone marrow.

The Future of PET

Because of its unique features, PET is not a technique of the past nor of dedicated clinical diagnostic use alone. PET is a technique of the future with an extraordinary potential in all of its recent fields of application. Although the physical limits of the method are well known, the development of a tracer repertoire is essentially limitless and depends on the talent and imagination of the radiochemists. This potential paves the way for the exploration of the various receptor systems, as well as a large number of physiological and biochemical processes not yet explored with the technique. These possible developments can result in novel diagnostic protocols, new approaches to research into the functioning of the brain and body, and a revolution in drug development.

REFERENCES

Bailey, D. L., Townsend, D. W., Maisey, M. N., et al. (Eds.). (2006). *Positron emission tomography: Clinical practice*. New York: Springer.

Bailey, D. L., Valk, P. E., Townsend, D. W., et al. (Eds.). (2005). *Positron emission tomography: Basic sciences*. New York: Springer.

Burger, C., & Townsend, D. W. (2003). Basics of PET scanning. In G. von Schulthess (Ed.), *Clinical PET, PET/CT and SPECT/CT: Combined anatomic–molecular imaging* (pp. 14–39). Philadelphia: Lippincott Williams & Wilkins.

Carson, R. E., Daube-Witherspoon, M. E., & Herscovitch, P. (Eds.). (1997). *Quantitative functional brain imaging with positron emission tomography*. San Diego: Academic Press.

Cherry, S. R., Sorenson, J. A., & Phelps, M. E. (Eds.). (2003). *Physics in nuclear medicine*. Philadelphia: Saunders.

Comar, D. (Ed.). (1995). *PET for drug development and evaluation*. Boston: Kluwer.

Couturier, O., Luxen, A., Chatal, J. F., et al. (2004). Fluorinated tracers for imaging cancer with positron emission tomography. *European Journal of Nuclear Medicine and Molecular Imaging, 31*, 1182–1206.

Defrise, M., & Kinahan, P. (1998). Data acquisition and image reconstruction for 3D PET. In B. Bendriem & D. W. Townsend (Eds.), *The theory and practice of 3D PET* (pp. 11–53). Dordrecht, The Netherlands: Kluwer Academic.

Eriksson, L., Dahlbom, M., & Widén, L. (1990). Positron emission tomography—a new technique for studies of the central nervous system. *Journal of Microscopy, 157,* 305–333.

Farde, L. (1996). The advantage of using positron emission tomography in drug research. *Trends in Neurosciences, 19,* 211–214.

Friston, K. J., Frith, C. D., Dolan, R. J., et al. (Eds.). (1997). *Human brain function.* San Diego: Academic Press.

Greitz, T., Ingvar, D. H., & Widén, L. (Eds.). (1985). *The metabolism of the human brain studied with positron emission tomography.* New York: Raven Press.

Gulyás, B., & Müller-Gärtner, H. W. (Eds.). (1998). Positron emission tomography: A critical assessment of recent trends. Dordrecht, The Netherlands: Kluwer Academic.

Halldin, C., Gulyás, B., & Farde, L. (2004). PET for drug development. *Ernst Schering Research Foundation Workshop, 48,* 95–109.

Halldin, C., Gulyás, B., & Farde, L. (2001a). PET studies with carbon-11 radioligands in neuropsychological drug development. *Current Radiopharmaceutical Design, 7,* 1907–1929.

Halldin, C., Gulyás, B., Langer, O., et al. (2001b). Brain radioligands: State of the art and new trends. *Quarterly Journal of Nuclear Medicine, 2,* 139–152.

Lee, C.-M., & Farde, L. (2006). Using positron emission tomography (PET) to facilitate CNS drug development. *Trends in Pharmalogical Sciences, 27,* 310–316.

NEMA NU2. (2001). *Performance measurements of positron emission tomographs.* Rosslyn, VA: NEMA.

Roland, P. E. (1993). *Brain activation.* New York: Wiley-Liss.

Ruhlmann, J., Oehr, P., & Biersack, H.-J. (Eds.). (1999). *PET in oncology.* New York: Springer.

Saha, G. B. (Ed.). (2004). *Basics of PET imaging: Physics, chemistry, and regulations.* New York: Springer.

Schwaiger, M., Dinkelborg, L., & Schweinfurth, H. (Eds.). (2004). *From morphological imaging to molecular targeting.* New York: Springer.

Stöcklin, G., & Pike, V. W. (Eds.). (1993). *Radiopharmaceuticals for positron emission tomography: Methodological aspects.* Dordrecht, The Netherlands: Kluwer.

Surti, S., Karp, J. S., Muehllehner, G., et al. (2002). Investigation of lanthanum scintillators for 3-D PET. *Nuclear Science Symposium Records, 2,* 1177–1181.

Theodore, W. H. (Ed.). (1988). *Clinical neuroimaging.* New York: Liss.

Varagnolo, L., Stokkel, M. P., Mazzi, U., et al. (2000). 18F-labeled radiopharmaceuticals for PET in oncology, excluding FDG. *Nuclear Medicine and Biology, 27,* 103–112.

von Schulthess, G. K. (Ed.). (2003). *Clinical molecular anatomic imaging.* Philadelphia: Lippincott Williams & Wilkins.

von Schulthess, G. K. (Ed.). (2000). Clinical positron emission tomography (PET): Correlation with morphological cross-sectional imaging. Philadelphia: Lippincott Williams & Wilkins.

Wahl, R. L., & Buchanan, J. W. (2002). *Principles and practice of positron emission tomography.* Philadelphia: Lippincott Williams & Wilkins.

Wernick, M. N., & Aarsvold, I. N. (Eds.). (2004). *Emission tomography—The fundamentals of PET and SPECT.* Amsterdam: Academic Press.

CHAPTER 2

Principles of Functional Magnetic Resonance Imaging

Peter A. Bandettini

The thought of using magnetic resonance imaging (MRI) to map human brain activation noninvasively, rapidly, with full brain coverage, and with relatively high spatial and temporal resolution was, before 1991, pure fantasy. Functional MRI (fMRI) was introduced with a groundbreaking paper by Belliveau et al. (1992). That technique, involving sequential bolus injections of the susceptibility contrast agent Gadolinium-DTPA to characterize blood volume during rest and activation, was rendered obsolete by a completely noninvasive MRI-based technique utilizing endogenous functional contrast associated with localized changes in blood oxygenation during activation.

Between the early spring and late fall of 1991, the first successful experiments were carried out at the Massachusetts General Hospital (May 1991), University of Minnesota (June 1991), and Medical College of Wisconsin (September 1991) using endogenous MRI contrast to assess brain activation. These experiments were published within 2 weeks of each other in the early summer of 1992 (Kwong et al., 1992; Ogawa et al., 1992; Bandettini et al., 1992).

The mechanism of endogenous contrast on which these early results were based was pioneered by Ogawa et al. (1990a, 1990b), who coined the term "blood oxygen level dependent" (BOLD), as well as by Turner et al. (1991). In a prescient quote in 1990—2 years before the first successful fMRI experiments were published and about a year before the first successful experiments were performed—Ogawa et al. (1990a) predicted the beginning of a new brain activation method: "BOLD contrast adds to . . . functional MRI methodologies that are likely to be complementary to PET imaging in the study of regional brain activity" (p. 9872).

Another noninvasive technique for assessing brain activation with MRI that emerged almost simultaneously with BOLD contrast is known as arterial spin labeling (ASL) (Williams et al., 1992). The contrast in ASL arises from blood flow and perfusion, independent of blood oxygenation. Other techniques, allowing noninvasive assessment of activation-induced changes in blood volume (Lu et al., 2003) and oxidative metabolic rate (Davis et al., 1998b, Hoge et al., 1999), temperature (Yablonskiy et al., 2000a, 2000b), and diffusion coefficient (Le Bihan et al., 2006) have since been demonstrated. BOLD fMRI is currently the brain activation mapping method of choice because it is easiest to implement and the functional contrast to noise is higher than with the other methods. For most studies, the need for sensitivity (the main advantage of BOLD contrast) outweighs the need for further specificity, stability over long periods of time, quantitation, or baseline state information—all which are advantages that ASL has over BOLD.

Functional MRI (fMRI) can be thought of as having four basic components, which have been synergistically evolving over the years: hardware, methodology, signal interpretability, and applications. It is useful to also consider the professions that lend themselves to each of the components. Figure 2.1 shows each component and the corresponding professions. It is optimal

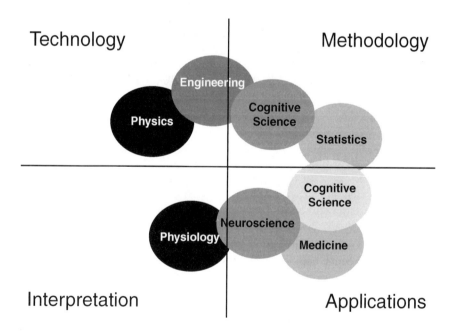

FIGURE 2.1. Schematic depiction of four primary components of fMRI advancement as well as the relative place that each areas of expertise holds. Communication is essential between areas of expertise. Also important is that the center of expertise mass in a cutting-edge fMRI group is positioned as close as possible to the center, interfacing with each component.

from a research standpoint to have a team's center of mass as close to the center as possible.

Hardware includes all that is used physically to perform MRI—the primary magnet, shim coils, gradient coils, radio frequency coil configuration—as well as the subject interface devices such as button boxes, projectors, eye-tracking devices, and headphones. Methodology includes pulse sequences, postprocessing methods, multimodal integration methods, and task or stimulus paradigm designs. Signal interpretability includes advancements in the understanding of the relationship between underlying neuronal activity and BOLD. Applications include not only those directed at understanding brain organization but also those that are aimed at complementing clinical diagnoses and helping to further characterize neurological and psychiatric disorders. Generally, advances in any one of these components have enabled further advances in the others, and the needs of one have in many instances driven the development of the others.

This chapter gives a brief overview of MRI, and the rest of the chapter focuses on fMRI. First a description of the history and development of fMRI is provided for perspective. Then the basic principles behind fMRI are outlined. Next, a few of the more significant and interesting recent innovations of fMRI are described. A discussion on the limitations of fMRI follows. The next section focuses exclusively on the emerging types of clinical applications of fMRI. The last section is a simple list of available resources to further one's knowledge and skill in fMRI.

Magnetic Resonance Imaging

The more familiar a researcher is with MRI, the more he or she will be able to effectively work within the context of continuous technical advances—and demands—in MRI and fMRI. New pulse sequences designed to minimize artifacts, increase resolution or stability, or extract a new kind of functional contrast arise on a regular basis, as do new processing methods tailored to these pulse sequences and the information they provide.

This section is not intended to be a detailed, comprehensive, or even balanced overview of MRI. The goal is to familiarize the nonphysicist with a few of the basic concepts behind MRI and to provide references to direct the reader to further, more detailed information if desired.

Resonance, Precession, and Relaxation

The creation of a magnetic resonance image requires that the object is within a strong magnetic field. Magnets for human use range in field strength from less than 0.5 to 9.4 tesla (less than 10,000 to 190,000 times the magnetic field of earth). The strength of most fMRI scanners is 3 tesla. The presence of a magnetic field causes the nuclear spins of certain atoms within the body to be oriented either parallel or antiparallel to the main magnetic field (B_0). Classically described, the nuclei *precess* about B_0 with a frequency, called the Larmor frequency (ν_0), which is directly proportional to B_0:

$$\nu_0 = \gamma B_0$$

The value, ?, is the gyromagnetic ratio, a fundamental physical constant for each nuclear species. Because the proton nucleus (^1H) has a high sensitivity for its magnetic resonance (MR) signal (a result of its high gyromagnetic ratio, 42.58 MHz/tesla) and a high natural abundance, it is the nucleus of choice for MRI. Magnetic *resonance* occurs when a radio frequency (rf) pulse, applied at the Larmor frequency, excites the nuclear spins, raising them from lower to higher energy states. Classically, this can be represented by a rotation of the net magnetization, M_0, away from its rest or equilibrium state. The amount of this rotation is given in terms of the flip angle, which depends on the strength and duration of the rf pulse. A 90° flip angle is associated with the magnetization being rotated completely into a plane perpendicular to B_0, thereby creating transverse magnetization (M_T).

Once the magnetization is rotated, the rf field is switched off and the magnetization once again freely precesses about the direction of B_0. According to Faraday's law of induction, this time-dependent precession will be able to induce a current in a receiver coil, the rf coil. The resultant exponentially decaying voltage, referred to as the free induction decay (FID), constitutes the MR signal. Because precession occurs at the Larmor frequency, the resulting MR signal also oscillates at a frequency equal to the Larmor frequency.

During the period of free precession the magnetization returns to its original equilibrium state by a process called relaxation, which is characterized by two time constants, T1 and T2. T1 and T2 depend on physical and chemical characteristics unique to tissue types and hence are the primary sources of tissue contrast in anatomical images.

Spin–Lattice Relaxation (T1)

Radio frequency stimulation causes nuclei to absorb energy, lifting them to an excited state. The nuclei in their excited state can return to the ground state by dissipating their excess energy to the lattice. This return to equilibrium is termed spin–lattice relaxation and is characterized by the time constant, T1, the spin–lattice relaxation time. The term "lattice" describes the magnetic environment of the nuclei. In order for the lattice field to be effective in transferring energy from the excited spins to the lattice, the lattice must fluctuate and the fluctuations must occur at a rate that matches the precessional frequency of the excited spins—the Larmor frequency. As energy is released to the lattice, the longitudinal magnetization (magnetization along the z-axis, M_z) returns to its equilibrium value. This return to equilibrium is characterized by the time constant T1. In brain tissue, T1 is about an order of magnitude longer than T2 or T2*.

Spin–Spin Relaxation (T2, T2*)

Immediately after an rf pulse, the magnetic moments (or spins) are precessing in phase. Because of natural processes that cause nuclei to exchange energy with each other, the moments begin to spread out in the transverse plane and lose their phase coherence. As a result, the net transverse magnetization (M_T) decays to zero exponentially with time, hence spin–spin relaxation. This decay is characterized by the time constant T2. However, processes other than inherent spin–spin interactions also cause the spins to dephase faster than the rate determined by tissue T2. The main magnetic field is not perfectly homogeneous. So nuclei in different portions of the sample experience different values of B_0 and precess at slightly different frequencies. This is described in more detail later, as it is the basic mechanism of BOLD contrast. When both natural processes and magnetic imperfections contribute to M_T decay, the decay is characterized by the time constant T2*, which is less than T2. T1, T2, and T2* are roughly dependent on field strength (Bottomley et al., 1984; Jezzard et al., 1996). T1 typically lengthens, whereas T2 and T2* shorten as field strength increases. T2* is also highly influenced by magnetic field homogeneity. The less homogenous the field is, from the microscopic level to the level of an entire brain, the shorter T2* becomes.

Image Formation

The goal of MRI is to measure the distribution of magnetization within the body, which depends on both the variation in the concentration of water (proton density) and the magnetic environment between different tissues (T1, T2, T2*). In a completely uniform field, all of the protons resonate at the same frequency. The rf coil used to detect the signal is sensitive only to the frequency, amplitude, and phase of the precessing magnetization, not to the spatial location. It cannot distinguish two spins at different locations that are precessing at the same frequency. To make an image, it is necessary to make the spin's precessional frequency depend on the *location* of the spin. This is accomplished by superimposing linear magnetic field gradients on the main magnetic field. The term "gradient" designates that the magnetic field is altered along a selected direction. Referring to the Larmor equation, it can be seen that if the field is varied linearly along a certain direction, then the resonance frequency also varies with location along this same direction, thus providing the information necessary for spatial localization. Obtaining a two-dimensional image requires basically three steps: slice selection (spatially selecting a frequency range of spins to excite by superimposing a gradient perpendicular to slice direction and applying an excitation rf pulse at the desired frequency range as determined by the gradient), frequency encoding (spatially encoding the location of spins along the *x*—or typically left to right—direction, and phase encoding (spatially encoding the location of the spins along the *y*—or typically top to bottom—direction.

The details of image formation are beyond the scope of this chapter. For excellent and much more detailed descriptions, see Schmitt et al., 1998; Mitchell and Cohen, 2003; Stark and Bradley, 1999; Haacke et al., 1999.

MRI Contrast

Though T1, T2, and proton density are intrinsic tissue parameters, one can alter tissue contrast in the image by the choice of the pulse sequence parameters. For example, with a spin–echo imaging sequence (Haacke et al., 1999), the type of image weighting is determined by the repetition time (TR) and the echo time (TE). The initial 90° rf pulse completely tips the existing longitudinal magnetization into the transverse plane, leaving zero longitudinal magnetization. If the spins were again excited at this time, no signal would be produced. Therefore, a time interval (TR) is allowed to elapse between excitations so that the spins can undergo T1 relaxation and recover at least part of their longitudinal magnetization. The maximum T1 contrast (the difference in signal as it relates to the different rates of signal recovery) between tissues occurs when TR is greater than 0 and less than some time when both tissues have completely recovered their longitudinal magnetization. A long TR ($\gg$ 5T1) allows enough time to elapse so that almost complete T1 relaxation occurs and therefore tissue contrast is no longer influenced by T1. The maximum magnetization to which the signal returns is determined by proton density. Likewise, the amount of T2 contrast is dictated by the choice of TE. The longer the time interval TE, the greater the degree of T2 relaxation. Therefore, spin–echo images that are acquired with intermediate TR (TR ~ T1) and short TE (TE < T2) are T1-weighted. With shorter TR values, tissues such as fat, which have short T1 values, appear bright, whereas tissues that have longer T1 values, such as tumors and edema, take more time to relax toward equilibrium and therefore appear dark. A short TE value diminishes the importance of tissue T2 differences. Similarly, images acquired with long TR (to diminish T1 differences) and intermediate TE (TE ~ T2) are T2-weighted. Therefore, tissues with long T2, such as tumors, edema, and cysts, appear bright, whereas tissues that have short T2, such as muscle and liver, appear dark. Images acquired with long TR (TR $\gg$ 5T1) and short TE (TE < T2) are called proton-density weighted images. Tissues with increased proton density appear moderately bright. It should be noted that both T1- and T2-weighted images are always partly weighted toward proton density as well.

Echo-Planar Imaging

A pulse sequence in MRI is essentially a specific set gradient, rf, and acquisition timings to enable a specific imaging speed, resolution, and/or contrast. Echo-planar imaging (EPI) (Schmitt et al., 1998; Stehling et al., 1991) is a unique type of pulse sequence, not commonly used clinically for anatomical imaging (due mostly to insufficient resolution), which places extreme demands on the imaging system, particularly the gradients. In fact, although EPI was conceived in the 1970s by Mansfield (Mansfield & Maudsley, 1977; Mansfield et al., 1976; Garroway et al., 1974), it was not incorporated in clinical scanners until the mid to late 1990s. With more conventional MRI methods, only one projection (or line in raw data space) is acquired with each TR interval, so that the image acquisition time is relatively lengthy, as the number of excitations equals the number of lines of data—corresponding to the resolution in the y direction. With the typically used "single-shot" EPI, all lines of data for each image are acquired after a single rf pulse (hence, one "plane" is acquired with one rf excitation and subsequent echo—thus, "echo-planar" imaging). Spatial encoding, performed in about 20–40 ms for each image during the FID, puts high demands on the gradients. To enable rapid gradient switching, high-powered gradient amplifiers are used. Before such technology was available, one solution to this challenge was to use small, low-inductance "local" gradient coils (Bandettini et al., 1992; Wong et al., 1992).

There are several advantages of EPI for fMRI. Because the acquisition is achieved in typically less than 40 ms for each image, most physiological motion is essentially "frozen" during the acquisition, which significantly reduces the effect of physiological fluctuations within the image, thus significantly improving the reproducibility of images relative to those acquired over several heartbeats or respiratory cycles. With EPI, time series fluctuations, although still present, are much less severe (and more spatially localized) than time series images collected with conventional techniques. Another advantage of EPI is, of course, its speed. An entire volume of data covering the brain can be obtained in about 1.5 s, allowing whole-brain rapid time series collection. A single shot also allows for a longer TR, providing more time for T1 relaxation to take place, and therefore more signal.

EPI has several disadvantages, which pulse sequence developers are still working to alleviate. First, because of the relatively long readout window per excitation rf pulse (40 ms rather than about 5 ms for conventional techniques), image distortions are worsened. Although these distortions are correctible (Jezzard & Balaban, 1995), correction methods have not been perfected. Second, EPI has relatively low resolution—but superior to magneto-encephalography (MEG), positron emission tomography (PET), and electro-encephalography (EEG), so this is relative to structural MRI (limited by the small amount of time for image acquisition before $T2^*$ or T2 causes the signal to disappear)—about 60–120 ms, respectively. Typical in-plane resolution is on the order of 3 mm². With techniques such as parallel imaging (discussed below), resolution can be improved to about 1.5 mm². At this resolution, image signal-to-noise is typically too low for performing fMRI at field strengths below 7 tesla. Signal-to-noise ratio (SNR) is a linear function of field strength and an inverse linear function of voxel volume. Another drawback of EPI is the high acoustic noise accompanying the gradient switching, interfering with many types of auditory activation paradigms. Alternative paradigm and imaging techniques have been proposed to circumvent this problem

(Seifritz et al., 2006; Amaro et al., 2002). In spite of these problems, EPI remains the pulse sequence of choice because of its high speed, high efficiency, and relatively high temporal stability.

Functional MRI

Development

During 1991, human brain activation studies were being performed by a handful of groups using techniques involving ionizing radiation or EEG. Although these techniques are still quite useful today, giving information complementary to that of fMRI, the degree of flexibility offered by fMRI as it came into common use in the early 1990s was a breakthrough in brain mapping experimentation. After 1992 an investigator could perform a brain activation study relatively easily: Simply put a person in the scanner, have him or her perform a task during time series image collection, and look for where the MRI changes. This was both a blessing and a curse for the burgeoning brain-mapping community.

This access to these powerful tools contributed to several phenomena:

1. Many poorly planned, executed, and analyzed experiments associated with overinterpretation of artifactual signal changes were published and are still published today, but to a lesser degree as the collective expertise of the imaging community is improving rapidly. It is worth mentioning that the impact of the major fMRI courses offered four to six times a year for as many as 50 people at a time at the Massachusetts General Hospital, twice a year at the Medical College of Wisconsin, and periodically elsewhere over the past decade have likely expedited the increase in sophistication of fMRI experimentation and perhaps significantly increased the overall impact of fMRI research over the years.

2. A frantic rush to pick the scientific "low-hanging fruit" in functional imaging began in earnest and continues in many contexts today. The collective sentiment of the imaging community appears to be that we are only scratching the surface of its potential. This is particularly true for clinical applications.

3. Some truly unique insights into how the human brain is organized, how it changes over time (from seconds to years), and how it varies across populations have been steadily advanced.

4. Most important, a much larger collective effort toward using brain mapping technology to understand the human brain and to apply fMRI to diagnosing and treating clinical populations was started.

The benefits of the last phenomenon are just beginning to be realized. In 1995 the first meeting devoted to human brain mapping took place in Paris, France, owing partly to the emergence of fMRI. The cornerstone technique of the Organization for Human Brain Mapping and the Cognitive Neuroscience Society is fMRI.

In 1992, after the first papers were published, only a handful of laboratories could perform fMRI because it required not only an MRI scanner but also the capability of performing EPI. Some early studies used non-EPI techniques with some additional artifact correction strategies, but EPI, and more generally, "single-shot" one-rf pulse-per-image techniques are the most common and successful. Until about 1996, the hardware for performing EPI was not available on clinical systems. Centers that performed EPI were those that had home-built low-inductance gradient coils or those that were fortunate enough to work in collaboration with small companies that created systems that allowed rapid gradient switching (Kwong et al., 1992). While EPI is now available for clinical systems, other "cutting-edge" technology, such as multi-echo EPI and ASL pulse sequences, are not. The most innovative technology for performing fMRI is at least several years ahead of what is available for clinical scanners. Vendors usually implement only that which has a clinical application, so sequences that are not yet ready for clinical application are not installed—a Catch-22 situation for all but physicists who can pulse program a scanner and who also do clinical research. Perhaps the situation may shift a bit as the overall clinical utility of fMRI becomes more apparent.

Figure 2.2 shows the results of a science citation index reference search on fMRI-related studies published since 1992. The growth appears to be exponential until 2000. It then appears to taper to a linear function. Studies published before 1996 were typically performed on systems developed in-house. After 1996 the number of groups performing fMRI expanded rapidly.

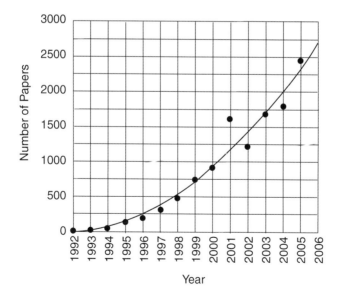

FIGURE 2.2. The relationship between the number of papers using fMRI per year (as searched for using Scopus and the search terms "fMRI" or "functional MRI"). The growth shows no sign of slowing.

After about 1996, with rapid proliferation of EPI-capable MRI scanners incorporating whole-body gradients, the standard platform for fMRI reached a plateau that is still mostly in use today. The sequence used is gradient-echo EPI; the echo time (TE) is 40 ms. The image matrix size, defined as how many pixels each image contains, is 64 × 64. The field of view (FOV), defined as how large the imaging region is, was 24 cm. The last dimension of the image, the slice thickness, was 4 mm. These parameters are created by manipulations of the imaging gradients, the radio frequency excitation, and the receiver sampling rate. Typically, whole-brain volume coverage using a TR of 2 s is performed. Time series are typically on the order of 5–8 min in duration, and a typical experiment involves the collection of about seven time series per subject scanning session. Key determinants of functional image quality are the temporal signal-to-noise ratio, the signal change magnitude, and the amount of averaging that is performed. The last variable is generally determined by how long the subject can be comfortably kept in the scanner. Typically, researchers have about an hour of useful fMRI scanning time per subject, so they fill this hour as well as they can. For imaging of primary motor and sensory cortex, significant signal changes can be observed within a single "on–off" activation cycle lasting 30 s. Nevertheless, for cognitive function and more subtle comparisons, much more averaging is required. If one is certain of the size of the effect that he or she is looking for, as well as all variability (time point to time point, time series to time series, session to session, and subject to subject), then a power analysis may be useful for determining the necessary scanning to produce a significant result. A major obstacle to this approach is that most of these variables cannot be clearly determined. Power analyses have been performed on a wide range of studies. Multisubject studies usually settle on assessing about 12 such sessions (one per subject). Regarding hardware, a whole-brain quadrature rf coil is typically used. Around 2002, the "standard" field strength increased from 1.5T to 3T.

Beyond basic data collection, standards begin to diverge so that the domains of paradigm design and postprocessing are still evolving steadily. Nevertheless, "typical" paradigm design methods are either "boxcar," involving steady-state activation periods for 10 s or more, or more commonly, "even-related" designs enjoying the flexibility inherent to brief activation periods interspersed within the time series. For processing, SPM is the most common software (for a history of SPM, visit *www.fil.ion.ucl.ac.uk/spm/doc/history.html*), but platforms such as Brain Voyager, FSL, and AFNI are almost as ubiquitous— each having its own advantages. The most common techniques involve the use of "reference" or "regressor" functions for statistical map creation, and when multisubject data are involved, statistical maps are spatially smoothed and transformed to a standardized space for comparison or averaging.

The field of fMRI has been and is punctuated with the emergence of novel techniques, findings, and controversies. A list of 10 important developments in fMRI before 2003 is provided below to add perspective. Because limited space, neither this list nor the references associated with each topic are comprehensive.

- Parametric manipulation of brain activation demonstrated that BOLD contrast approximately followed the level of brain activation: visual system (Kwong et al., 1992), auditory system (Binder et al., 1994), and motor system (Rao et al., 1996).

- Event-related fMRI was first demonstrated (Blamire et al., 1992). Application of event-related fMRI to cognitive activation was shown (Buckner et al., 1996; McCarthy et al., 1997). Development of mixed event-related and block designs was put forward (Donaldson et al., 2002). Paradigms were demonstrated in which the activation timing of multiple brain systems timing was orthogonal, allowing multiple conditions to be cleanly extracted from a single run (Courtney et al., 1997).

- High-resolution maps were created; for spatial resolution, ocular dominance columns (Menon et al., 1997; Cheng et al., 2001) and cortical layer activation maps were created (Logothetis et al., 2002). Extraction of information at high spatial frequencies within regions of activation was demonstrated (Haxby et al., 2001), introducing the world to multivariate analysis and pattern classification in fMRI. For temporal resolution, timings from ms to hundreds of ms were extracted (Menon et al., 1998; Henson et al., 2002; Bellgowan et al., 2003).

- The development of "deconvolution" methods allowed for rapid presentation of stimuli (Dale & Buckner, 1997).

- Early BOLD contrast models were put forward (Ogawa et al., 1993; Buxton & Frank, 1997). More sophisticated models were published that more fully integrated the latest data on hemodynamic and metabolic changes (Buxton et al., 2004).

- The use of continuous variation of visual stimuli parameters as a function of time was proven a powerful method for fMRI-based retinotopy (Engel et al., 1997; Engel, 1994; DeYoe et al., 1993, 1994; Sereno et al., 1995a, 1995b, 1994).

- The development of "clustered volume" acquisition was put forth as a method to avoid scanner noise artifacts (Edmister et al., 1999).

- The findings of functionally related resting state correlations (Biswal et al., 1995) and regions that consistently show deactivation with cognitive tasks (Binder et al., 1999; Raichle et al., 2001) were described.

- Observation of the pre-undershoot in fMRI (Hennig et al., 1995; Menon et al., 1995; Hu et al., 1997) and correlation with optical imaging was reported (Malonek & Grinvald, 1996; Malonek et al., 1997).

- Simultaneous use of fMRI and direct electrophysiological recording in nonhuman primate brains during visual stimulation elucidated the relationship between fMRI and BOLD contrast (Logothetis et al., 2001a). Simultaneous electrophysiological recordings in animal models revealed a correlation between negative signal changes and decreased neuronal activity (Shmuel et al., 2002). Simultaneous electrophysiological recordings in animal models provided evidence that inhibitory input could cause an increase in cerebral blood flow (Matheiesen et al., 1998).

• Structural equation modeling was developed in the context of fMRI time series analysis (Buchel & Friston, 1998).

As mentioned, this list is only a sampling of the tremendous amount of novel work establishing fMRI as a powerful tool for investigating human brain activity. More recent, ongoing, and future innovations and issues in fMRI are described in the "Innovations" section.

Principles

Several types of physiological information can be mapped using fMRI. As described in the introduction to this chapter, this information includes baseline cerebral blood volume (Rosen et al., 1991a, 1991b), changes in blood volume (Belliveau et al., 1991; Lu et al., 2003), quantitative measures of baseline and changes in cerebral perfusion (Wong et al., 1999), changes in blood oxygenation (Ogawa et al., 1992; Kwong et al., 1992; Frahm et al., 1992; Blamire et al., 1992; Bandettini et al., 1992), resting state oxygen extraction fraction (An et al., 2001), and changes in cerebral blood oxygen consumption ($CMRO_2$) (Davis et al., 1998b; Hoge et al., 1999).

BOLD Contrast

The basic mechanism for BOLD signal changes with brain activation is described as follows (see Figure 2.3 for a schematic description). During resting state, blood oxygenation in capillaries and veins is lower than that of arteries owing to the resting state extraction of oxygen from the blood. Deoxyhemoglobin (deoxy-Hb) is paramagnetic relative to the rest of brain tissue and water, and oxyhemoglobin (oxy-Hb) has the same susceptibility as brain tissue and water. An object (in this case, a deoxy-Hb molecule or a capillary or vein containing deoxy-Hb molecules) that has a different susceptibility than its surrounding medium creates a magnetic field distortion when placed in a magnetic field. Plate 2.1 illustrates this effect. As mentioned above, water molecules ("spins") precess at a frequency that is directly proportional to the magnetic field that they are experiencing. Within a voxel, if spins are precessing at different frequencies, they rapidly become out of phase. The MRI signal is directly proportional to the coherence of spins. If they are completely out of phase, destructive addition takes place and there is no signal. If they are completely in phase, there is maximal signal. During resting state, a large enough fraction of spins are out of phase, owing to the many microscopic field distortions in each voxel, causing the MRI signal to be attenuated somewhat relative to what it would be if there were no deoxy-Hb present. During activation, blood flow increases locally so that there is an overabundance of oxygenated blood delivered to the active regions. The reason for this is still not fully understood. This causes the amount of deoxy-Hb to decrease, and therefore the magnitude of the magnetic field distortions to decrease as

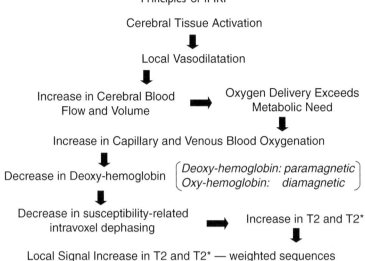

FIGURE 2.3. The cascade of neuronal, physiological, and biophysical relationships connecting neuronal activity to measured signal changes using fMRI.

well, thus increasing the coherence of spins within each voxel, leading to a signal increase of a few percent.

This signal, shown in Plate 2.2, begins to increase (to about 5% at 3T, TE of 30, and resolution of 3 mm^3) approximately 2 s after neuronal activity begins, and plateaus in the "on" state after about 7–10 s. A pre-undershoot is sometimes observed and a postundershoot is more commonly observed. These effects are likely due to transient mismatches between either blood volume (Buxton et al., 2004) or CMRO$_2$ (Lu et al., 2004) changes and flow changes. An intriguing recent theory put forth regarding the postundershoot suggests that it is due to transient microvascular constriction immediately following activation. The dynamics, location, and magnitude of the signal are highly influenced by the vasculature in each voxel. If voxels happen to capture large vessel effects, the magnitude of the signal may be large (up to an order of magnitude larger than capillary effects), the timing a bit more delayed than average (up to 4 s delayed relative to more rapid capillary effects), and the location of the signal somewhat distal (up to a centimeter) from the true region of activation. Although improvements are being made in fMRI methodology so that the effects of this variability are kept to a minimum, the problem of variable vasculature and hemodynamic coupling in fMRI nevertheless remains at all field strengths and limits the depth and range of questions that can be addressed using fMRI.

Perfusion Contrast

As mentioned in the introduction to this chapter, a technique introduced nearly simultaneously with BOLD functional MRI methods was the noninvasive method for mapping perfusion in the human brain, known as arterial spin labeling (ASL) (Detre et al., 1994; Wong et al., 1997; Ye et al., 1997; Buxton et al., 1998; Detre & Alsop, 1999; Wong, 1999; Gonzalez-At et al., 2000). The technique generally involves applying a radio frequency pulse (or continuous rf excitation) below the imaging plane (in the neck area). If there were no blood flow, the magnetization that was applied would simply decay and not influence the signal where the images were being collected. With flowing blood, the altered magnetization of the "labeled" blood affects the longitudinal magnetization (T1) in the imaging slices as it flows in and as water spins mix and exchange magnetization in the imaged brain tissue. A second set of images are obtained either with the label applied above the brain or not applied at all. The purpose of obtaining these images is to control for artifacts that can be induced by the tagging process. This second set of images is not affected in the same manner by magnetization of inflowing spins. The last step is to perform pair-wise subtraction of the two images, removing all the anatomical signal from each image, leaving behind only the effect on the signal by the label. Because of the low signal-to-noise inherent in this type of contrast, several hundred "label-minus-no label" pairs are obtained to create a map of baseline perfusion. Several perfusion image slices through the brain are shown in Figure 2.4. Here PICORE-QUIPPS II was used at 1.5T to create these images (Wong et al., 1997).

A strong determinant of perfusion contrast with this technique is the time, known as TI, between the labeling pulse and the subsequent image collection. If the TI is 200 ms, only the effects of the most rapidly flowing blood are observed (typically arteries). As the TI approaches 1 s, slower perfusing spins in and around capillaries appear. Beyond 1 s, the magnetization of the label decays significantly. A time series of these "label-minus-no label" pairs can be collected for the purpose of functional imaging of brain activation.

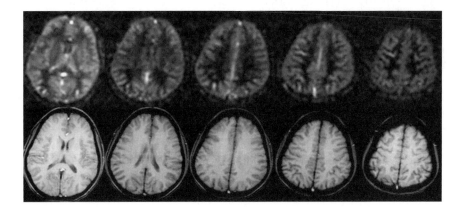

FIGURE 2.4. Top row: Perfusion images obtained completely noninvasively using arterial spin labeling (specifically, PICORE QUIPPS II, courtesy of Eric C. Wong, University of California, San Diego). Bottom row: Corresponding anatomical images.

ASL has not achieved the success of BOLD fMRI mostly because of limitations in the number of slices obtainable, temporal resolution, and decreased functional contrast to noise of the technique relative to BOLD fMRI. Nevertheless, its superior functional specificity and stability over long periods of time, along with its producing quantitative information, have made it useful for many applications where BOLD fMRI falls short (Aguirre et al., 2002).

Sensitivity

A primary struggle in the use of fMRI is to increase sensitivity. This is achieved by increasing the magnitude of the signal change or decreasing the effects of noise. This struggle has also been the impetus for imaging at ever higher field strengths. With an increase in field strength, signal-to-noise increases proportionally and both BOLD and perfusion contrast increase (BOLD, owing to greater changes in transverse relaxation, changes with activation and perfusion due to increases in T1 of blood, which allows the magnetization of the labeled blood to remain longer). The difficulty with going to higher field strength, aside from system instabilities and generally worse quality at the base of the brain due to greater effects of poor shimming, is that physiological fluctuations increase as well (Van de Moortele et al., 2002). Figure 2.5 illustrates an important point—that an increase in image signal-to-noise does not translate to an increase in temporal signal-to-noise (temporal signal-to-noise is what matters in time series analysis of fMRI data). Above a specific SNR for specific tissue compartments, the sensitivity plateaus.

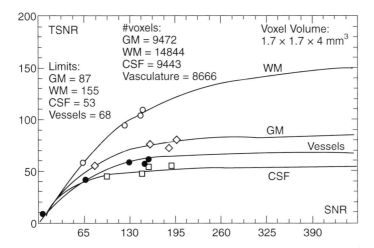

FIGURE 2.5. The relationship between temporal signal-to-noise ratio (y-axis) and image signal-to-noise ratio (x-axis) in white matter, gray matter, and cerebral spinal fluid. It is clear from these that the upper temporal signal to noise (what matters when performing time series analysis on fMRI data) reaches an upper limit around 100. This implies that it is not useful to image at a signal to noise higher than this level unless temporal filtering is performed.

Methods for removing these physiological fluctuations remain imperfect. However, a primary advantage of imaging at higher field strengths (i.e., 7T) is that the lower limit of signal-to-noise is achieved with a much smaller voxel volume, thus allowing much higher imaging resolution (down to 1 mm^3) at functional contrast levels comparable to those achieved in imaging at 3T with voxel volumes of 3 mm^3. This increase in resolution without prohibitive losses in sensitivity has likely been what has allowed imaging of ocular dominance column activation at 4T, but not at lower field strengths. Currently, successful results in imaging humans have been obtained at 7T (Vaughan et al., 2001; Ugurbil et al., 2003; Yacoub et al., 2005; Triantafyllou et al., 2005). It is certain that the number of successful, interesting, and highly relevant studies performed at 7T and even higher strengths will increase rapidly.

It should also be noted that because baseline T2* decreases as a function of field strength, the gains in sensitivity, or functional contrast, may be less than expected. Because T2* can vary considerably over space, being particularly low at the base of the brain and near susceptibility gradients, the sensitivity may not increase at all at high field strengths. Plate 2.3 shows exactly this important point. Plot A shows functional contrast at 1.5T, assuming a change in relaxation rate of $-0.8s^{-1}$ but across different T2* values (which vary with shim, etc.). Plot B shows functional contrast at 3T, assuming a doubling of the activation-induced change in relaxation rate (a reasonable assumption) also across the same baseline T2* values. The optimal contrast is obtained for TE = T2*, as shown by the peak values across TE. Plot C shows the functional contrast-to-noise across baseline T2* values for 1.5T and 3T. A baseline T2* of 40 at 1.5T will give the same optimal contrast as a baseline T2* of 20 at 3T. The bottom line is that shimming is quite important when going to high field strengths in order to keep baseline T2* values high relative to the activation-induced changes in T2*.

Radio frequency coils can also be used to increase sensitivity and resolution. The development of rf coil, pulse sequence, and receiver technology is discussed in the "Innovation" section.

Other processing steps for increasing sensitivity may include temporal and spatial smoothing. Because of the inherent temporal autocorrelation in the signal (from hemodynamics or other physiological processes), temporal smoothing is performed so that the temporal degrees of freedom may be accurately assessed. Spatial smoothing can be performed if high spatial frequency information is not desired and as a necessary prespatial normalization step (matching effective resolution with the degree of variability associated with spatial normalization techniques) for multisubject averaging and comparison. In many instances, spatial smoothing is not desired, particularly when high spatial frequency information in individual maps is compared (Haxby et al., 2001; Kriegeskorte et al., 2006; Beauchamp et al., 2004).

Once images are collected, voxel-wise time series analysis is carried out after motion correction is performed. Typically, a model function or functions are used as regressors, and the significance of the correlation of the time series data with the regressors is calculated on a voxel-wise basis. If the expected activation timing is not known, more open-ended approaches to analysis, such as independent component analysis (ICA) (Beckmann et al., 2001), are performed.

Innovation

The rate and significance of fMRI innovations, surprisingly, continue to increase. The preceding "Development" section discussed a few of the major innovations over the last 14 years; this section highlights several examples of emerging innovations that appear most promising. Those discussed below touch on imaging technology, experimental design, time series analysis, and a novel use for real-time fMRI.

Imaging Technology

A number of recent developments in acquisition hardware and imaging strategy may allow fMRI to be taken to new levels in sensitivity, resolution, and speed. A typical acquisition uses a single quadrature whole-brain rf coil feeding into one acquisition channel, and collects single-shot EPI data at 64 × 64 resolution. Recently, the ability to acquire MR data with simultaneous multiple high-bandwidth channels (Bodurka et al., 2004), feeding in from multiple rf coils, has enabled, above all, a large increase in image signal-to-noise ratio. Sensitivity is approximately proportional to the size of the rf coil used. In the past, some studies chose to sacrifice brain coverage for sensitivity by using a single "surface" rf coil for acquisition. Today, the use of multiple small rf coils covering the entire brain allows full-brain coverage and significantly higher sensitivity than one large coil.

A second use of multichannel acquisition, aside from increasing signal-to-noise, is in conjunction with a novel image acquisition/reconstruction strategy that uses the spatially distinct sensitive region of each rf coil to help spatially encode the data—with a small cost in signal-to-noise. This strategy is known as SENSE imaging (SENSitivity Encoding; de Zwart et al., 2002). By using the coil placement to aid in spatial encoding, less time is necessary for encoding the spatial information of the data. This advantage can be used in several ways. First, the readout window width can be remain the same as without SENSE, but the image resolution can be increased substantially. Second, the image resolution can remain the same, but the width of the readout window can be decreased substantially. This reduction in readout window width allows a small increase in the number of EPI slices to be collected in a TR, therefore allowing a reduction in TR for a given number of slices, more slices for a given TR (allowing thinner slices perhaps), or an increase in brain coverage for a given TR (if a shorter TR had previously limited brain coverage). Incorporating this imaging strategy at field strengths above 3T may allow robust single-shot 1 mm^3 matrix size EPI with a high enough signal-to-noise

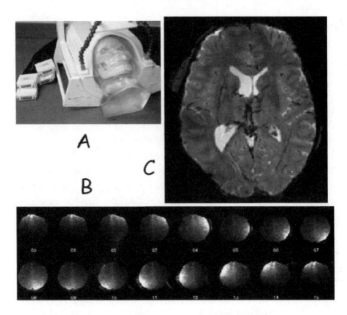

FIGURE 2.6. (A) A 16-channel RF coil system (NOVA Medical RF coil combined with NIH in-house parallel acquisition system). (B) A single-channel quadrature RF coil (GE Medical Systems). Each of the 16 small RF coils within the NOVA Medical RF coil has a distinct region of sensitivity as shown in (C). The most straightforward manner to combine these data is by simple addition after reconstruction. Figure provided courtesy of Jerzy Bodurka, Functional MRI Facility. The NOVA Medical 16-channel coil was designed by Jeff Duyn, Section on Advanced MRI, National Institute of Neurological Disorders and Stroke.

for fMRI. Figure 2.6 shows: A, a 16-channel coil setup (NOVA medical); B, a signal intensity profile for each of the 16 elements of the coil when imaging a human brain; and C, an example of a high-resolution single-shot SENSE-acquired echo-planar image (3T, 1.25 mm × 1.25 mm × 2 mm).

Free Behavior and Natural Stimuli Paradigms

A second innovation is in the context of activation paradigm design strategies. An ongoing challenge in fMRI is that of having the subject perform a task in a predictable and repeatable manner. This is not only not possible in many instances, particularly when scanning uncooperative patients, but limits the type of questions that can be addressed using fMRI. One common solution is to keep track of the responses of the subject to specific tasks, then perform post hoc data averaging based on the responses. A potentially powerful extension of this idea is to collect a continuous measure of the subject's behavior. In this manner, a natural parametric variation in the response parameters may be used to guide data analysis. Any continuous measure will suffice. The subject simply has to move a joystick or track ball or to have his or her eye position or skin conductance monitored. The subject could be following an object, determining certainty, expectation, anxiety, or subjective perception of motion, or the like. The way this data can be used is to calculate the moment-to-moment measurement and use it as a regressor in the analysis.

Related to this type of natural paradigm is the use of natural stimuli, such as having the subject view a movie. Regressors can be calculated from various salient aspects of the movie presentation such as color, motion, volume, speech, or even the interaction of continuously measured eye position with these variables. A study involving movie viewing was recently published (Hasson et al., 2004) in which a highly novel processing technique, tailored to paradigm, was used. This technique was based on the understanding that because the movie had many variables changing in an unpredictable manner, it was difficult to generate a set of reference functions for determining the similarly activated regions across subjects. Instead, the researchers played precisely the same movie sequence at least twice for each subject and across all subjects. The assumption was that a distinct, repeatable temporal pattern would be manifest. The correlation in the time series fMRI was determined across subjects rather than attempting to choose an appropriate ideal reference function and compare subsequent activation maps. This is also an effective technique to apply for the same subject across identical time series collections (Levin & Uftring, 2001), as it makes no assumption about what the data should look like—only that they show a repeatable change.

fMR-Adaptation Paradigms

Another recently developed paradigm design in fMRI of note has been named fMR-adaptation (Grill-Spector & Malach, 2001). This approach relies on the rapid adaptation and recovery properties of specific neuronal pools, and the reflection of these properties in fMRI signal, to characterize and differentiate subvoxel populations of neurons that are sensitive to subtle differences in stimulus or general paradigm properties. This type of paradigm proceeds in two stages. First, a neuronal population is adapted by repeated presentation of a single stimulus Second, a property of the stimulus is varied and the recovery from adaptation (manifested as an increase in fMRI signal) is assessed. If the signal remains adapted, it indicates that the neurons are invariant to that attribute. However, if the fMRI signal recovers from the adapted state, it implies that the neurons are sensitive to the property that was varied.

This clever approach is growing in its applications from low-level to higher-level cognition. Still, there remain several unknowns as to how to properly interpret these signal changes in the presence of variable hemodynamic effects, inhibition and excitation effects on fMRI signal changes, and unknown and likely variable adaptation dynamics as a function of stimulus timing (interstimulus interval and stimulus duration).

Real-Time fMRI Incorporating Feedback to the Subject

A technical challenge in fMRI is to perform basic analysis on data as they are being collected (Schwindack et al., 2005; Weiskopf et al., 2004; Yoo et al., 2004; DeCharms et al., 2004; Posse et al., 2003; Cohen, 2001; Smyser et al., 2001; Cox et al., 1995; Cox & Jesmanowicz, 1999). This approach is important for several reasons. A primary practical reason is to ensure data quality during the scan. This, in fact, is likely to be a necessary requirement in order for fMRI to be incorporated into daily clinical practice. A secondary reason that is just beginning to be explored is that it can allow the person scanning, or even the subject being scanned, to guide the experimental process as it is happening. A couple of truly unique twists on real-time fMRI applications have been published as well. First, it has been determined that if a measure of brain activation in specific regions activated by a cognitive task is fed back to the subject being imaged, the subject can learn, subjectively, to either increase or decrease the level of activation (Weiskopf et al., 2003). This finding offers the fascinating possibility of humans interacting directly with and through computers through simple thought process regulation. As a demonstration of this technique, the research group has trained subjects to play "pong" using mental control of a "paddle" in which the vertical location was simply proportional to the degree of activation in the controllable brain regions being activated. Using two scanners collecting data simultaneously, subjects are able to successfully play "brain pong" using subjective control of their fMRI signal changes.

A second application of this type of subjective control has been reported by DeCharms et al. (2004). In this study, patients experiencing chronic pain were instructed to reduce the fMRI signal intensity in regions that were determined in a previous experiment to be associated with pain perception. As in the brain pong experiment, the subjects were provided with feedback regarding the level of fMRI signal in these regions and were instructed to use whatever strategy they could come up with to decrease the signal. Not only did the experiment result in a subjective decrease in pain perception for most subjects, but this effect apparently lasted months after the experiment was carried out.

Classification and Machine Learning Algorithms

Although the analysis of fMRI data has evolved considerably during the past 14 years, two essentials of fMRI data analysis are nearly the same as in the initial studies. First, data are typically analyzed in terms of a subtractive methodology. Thus, two conditions, A and B, are contrasted to reveal the neural correlates associated with these conditions—that is, activations when A > B and when B > A. Second, data are typically analyzed in a univariate fashion. Although data are obtained for thousands of voxels (typically 20,000–50,000 "spatial locations"), the time series of each voxel is analyzed independently of all the other data—basically, a "massively univariate" analysis strategy.

In the past few years a growing number of studies have taken a different approach to fMRI data analysis. Instead of contrasting fMRI signals associated with two conditions, the direction of analysis is reversed in order to probe whether brain signals can be used to predict perceptual, motor, or cognitive states. In this framework, fMRI data analysis can be viewed within a standard pattern classification framework. Therefore, established statistical and machine learning techniques can be employed, such as neural networks, Bayesian networks, and support vector machines. Recently this line of research has attracted considerable attention in the neuroimaging field. By discovering distributed patterns of activation, such multivariate techniques offer the potential to go beyond the simple subtractive-univariate standard largely adopted in the field and have the potential to provide a much richer characterization of neuroimaging data.

These exciting directions that have emerged include the use of multivariate analysis (Haynes & Rees, 2005; Formisano et al., 2004; Strother et al., 2004; Cox & Savoy, 2003; Kriegeskorte et al., 2006), machine learning, and pattern classification techniques (LaConte et al., 2005; Davatzikos et al., 2005; Mitchell et al., 2004).

Early work by Haxby et al. (2001) helped pioneer this approach. It was demonstrated in this study that although spatial maps did not necessarily reveal statistically significant maps that differentiated the brain activation associated with viewing different object categories, the *pattern* of activation within the overlapping active regions corresponded well with each of the categories. In essence, this was a breakthrough in brain-mapping techniques along two avenues: (1) This was among the first methods that used spatial correlation between two halves of the time series data as a measure of the *information* contained in the activation maps, rather than using a univariate measure to map function and then compare statistically, assuming each voxel was independent, the corresponding maps, and (2) it was also among the first to turn brain mapping on its ear. Rather than determining the place in the brain that showed activation in correspondence to a stimulus, the activation map, or rather the unique voxel-wise pattern of activation, was used to provide information as to what the subject was viewing.

Since then, several articles have developed this theme. One article went so far as to call the technique "brain reading" (Cox & Savoy, 2003). In 2005, two of the more fascinating fMRI studies of the year were published in *Nature Neuroscience* (Kamitani & Tong, 2005; Haynes & Rees, 2005), both delving into the application of machine learning algorithms to characterize and use the unique and spatially distributed information (undetectable using standard univariate approaches) about the type of stimulus a subject was observing, either consciously or unconsciously. It is certain that there will be significant growth, refinement, and applications of this approach to fMRI in the very near future. Moreover, this is exactly the type of approach that will benefit significantly from high-resolution imaging.

Limitations

The limitations of fMRI in accurately assessing brain activation are fundamentally determined to be two major factors: (1) the method by which images are collected and (2) the relationship between neuronal activity and hemodynamic changes. This section describes the temporal, spatial, and interpretative limits of fMRI.

Temporal Resolution

Echo-planar images have an acquisition time of about 30 ms. Assuming an echo time of 40 ms (the center of the readout window), data acquisition ends after 55 ms. About 15 ms are usually required for gradients to be applied at the end of the sequence to eliminate remaining magnetization and for fat saturation to be applied at the beginning. The total time per plane for single-shot EPI time series collection is therefore about 65 ms, allowing for about 15 images to be collected in a second. For volume collection, typically consisting of 30 slices, a TR of 2 s is therefore required. It is also possible to collect one image (as opposed to multiple images in a volume) at a rate of 15 images per second over time.

As described, the hemodynamic response behaves like a low-pass filter for neuronal activity. At on/off frequencies of 6 s on/6 s off (0.08 Hz), BOLD responses begin to be attenuated relative to longer on/off times. At on/off frequencies of 2 s on/2 s off (0.25 Hz) the BOLD response is almost completely attenuated. Even though BOLD attenuates these rapid on/off responses, activity of very brief duration can be observed. Activity durations as low as 16 ms have been shown to cause robust BOLD signal changes, indicating that there is no apparent limit to the brevity of detectable activation. It is also heartening that when performing repeated experiments, the hemodynamic response in each voxel shows a variability on the order of 100 ms.

A desire in functional brain imaging is not only to spatially resolve activated regions but also to determine the precise timing of activation in these regions, either relative to the stimulus or to the input, and relative to each other. The temporal resolution required for this type of assessment is on the order of at least tens of milliseconds. With BOLD contrast, the latency of the hemodynamic response has a range of 4 s, due primarily to uncharacterized spatial variations in underlying hemodynamics or neurovascular coupling from voxel to voxel even within the same region of activity. If a voxel contains mostly larger venous vessels, the response is typically more delayed than if the voxel captures predominantly capillaries. This observation is only approximate. The precise reasons for latency variations are still not completely determined vary.

A number of methods have been proposed to alleviate this problem. The most direct is to try to identify larger vessels by thresholding based on percent signal change or temporal fluctuation characteristics. The accuracy of this method remains undetermined. Another solution is to use pulse sequences sensitive only to capillary effects. Arterial spin labeling techniques are more sensitive to capillaries, but the practical limitations of lower functional contrast to noise and longer interimage waiting time (due to the additionally required TI of about 1.5 s) make this unworkable for most studies. Spin–echo sequences performed at very high field strengths or with velocity-nulling gradients (both of which eliminate intravascular large vessel effects) are also sensitive to capillary effects, but the reduction in functional contrast-to-noise is a factor of about 2–4 with spin–echo (T2-weighted rather than T2*-weighted) acquisition, and an additional factor of 3 with velocity-nulling gradients to remove intravascular signal, likely rendering the contrast too low to be useful.

Another solution is to use BOLD effects, which are thought to be more related to capillaries—such as the pre-undershoot sometimes observed in fMRI. Practical applications of any kind with the pre-undershoot have proven to be difficult because of the extremely subtle magnitude and relative inconsistency, as well as the uncertain origins, of the pre-undershoot.

An alternate strategy is to focus on localized *changes* in latency and width with task timing changes. As mentioned, within a voxel, the hemodynamic response varies on the order of 100 ms over time, allowing significantly more accurate assessment if activation timing varies within a region or a voxel. For example, when using a task modulation that causes a variation in reaction time for each trial—that is, one region of the brain shows an increased width and another shows an increased delay—then it can be inferred that the region showing the width change is taking additional time to process information and the region showing the increased delay is downstream from the region showing the width change, having to wait until processing is complete in that node in order to receive any information.

Spatial Resolution

The upper in-plane resolution of standard single-shot EPI is about 2 mm^2. The use of multishot EPI (at a cost of time and stability) or more recently conceived of strategies incorporating multiple rf coils to aid in spatial encoding of data (discussed in the "Innovation" section) can allow functional image resolutions of about 1 mm^3.

As with temporal resolution limits, the spatial resolution limits are predominantly determined not by limits in acquisition but by the spatial spread of oxygenation and perfusion changes that accompany focal brain activation (Parkes et al., 2005). This "hemodynamic point spread function" has been empirically determined to be on the order of 3 mm^3 (Engel et al., 1997), but the effects of draining veins have been observed to be as distal as 1 cm from focal regions of activation identified using perfusion contrast.

The pulse sequence solutions for dealing with the variations in hemodynamics are similarly applicable as those for temporal resolution limits. In addition, spatial calibration methods have been proposed involving hypercapnia comparisons (Bandettini & Wong, 1997; Cohen et al., 2004). In spite of these limitations and limited solutions, ocular dominance column (1 mm^3) (Cheng et al., 2001; Goodyear & Menon, 2001) and cortical layer (< 0.5 mm^3) (Logothetis et al., 2002) delineations have been achieved using BOLD, perfusion-based, and blood volume-based methods. With BOLD contrast, which is thought to have the lowest resolution, columnar and layer specificity was achieved only by subtraction of activation from tasks activating interspersed yet distinct regions (i.e., columns or layers). Without this subtraction step, this resolution was not able to be obtained. An ongoing issue regarding the upper resolution of fMRI is whether or not *fine* delineation necessarily translates to *accurate* delineation—meaning that detailed activation maps may not necessarily be precisely registered with underlying function. This remains to be demonstrated.

Interpretation

Because fMRI is fundamentally based on hemodynamic changes, the accuracy with which we can interpret and essentially rely on the activation-induced signal changes to represent neuronal activity depends on how certain we are of the fidelity and consistency of the relationship between neuronal activity and hemodynamic signal changes. Although converging evidence suggest that hemodynamics are a high-fidelity and consistent marker of neuronal activity, there are several remaining unknowns.

Considerable effort has been directed toward understanding the precise relationship between fMRI signal changes and neuronal activity. Strategies for investigating this relationship have included (1) animal models and the simultaneous use of other measures of neuronal activity as via multiunit electrodes (Logothetis et al., 2001b; Matheiesen et al., 1998) or more precise measures of hemodynamic changes via optical imaging (Kennerley et al., 2005), (2) parametric modulation of magnitude or timing of activation in humans with corresponding measurement of fMRI signal changes, (3) simultaneous measures of neuronal activity (via implanted electrode or EEG) and fMRI signal changes, (4) nonsimultaneous measures of neuronal activity (MEG, EEG) and fMRI signal changes (Laufs et al., 2003), and (5) modeling of the hemodynamic response and comparing the fMRI signal changes to precise activation magnitude, timing, or pharmacological manipulations.

In summary, although fMRI is limited somewhat by scanner technology and, to a greater degree, by the unknowns regarding the spatial, temporal, and magnitude relationships between neuronal activity and hemodynamic signal changes, steady progress is being made in overcoming these limitations. A primary avenue by which the limitations of fMRI can be overcome is that involving integration with other brain activation assessment techniques.

Clinical Applications of fMRI

A primary shortcoming of fMRI is that it has not quite broken into standard, day-to-day clinical practice yet. To speculate why this might be the case, it seems that there are several reasons:

1. The signal is indirect and highly variable between subjects as well as potentially affected by medication. If a patient has any pathology that might affect the vasculature in any way, then interpretation of the patient's fMRI scan may be risky.
2. The signal, at least with BOLD contrast, mostly relies on a comparison between activation and rest. Although this may be changing as resting state fluctuations become better characterized, it is still the case. This type of requirement severely limits what fMRI can be used for, inasmuch as it requires that a patient be highly motivated and able to perform a set of tasks in the magnet.

All of these shortcomings aside, fMRI can deliver unique, highly useful information that may not only complement other types of clinical information for diagnoses of pathology and assessment of treatment, but has the potential for allowing insight into neuronal mechanisms behind the specific type of pathology. In addition, baseline information related to perfusion, potentially blood oxygenation, and resting state activity can bypass the problems of scanning subjects unable to perform tasks in a way that is useful in fMRI.

An approximate characterization of the clinical applications of fMRI involves grouping them into three categories:

1. *Directly practical.* This includes presurgical activation mapping, epileptic foci mapping, mapping of stroke extent and recovery, and mapping baseline perfusion to characterize any deficits. All of these techniques likely have the most direct and immediate applications.

2. *Characterization of differences between clinical populations.* This basically involves scanning, during a set of probe tasks, any one of a number of patient populations having neurological, psychological, behavioral, or other disorders and comparing the brain activation pattern, controlling for task performance, with a population of age-, sex-, (or other-) matched normal control subjects. The first goal is to find a difference. The second is to understand why there is a difference and to perhaps use this insight to better understand the pathology and to ultimately use the technique to help diagnose patients. Of course, because of substantial individual variability, it is far easier to determine if two large populations differ than to determine if one individual belongs to one population or another. Perhaps postprocessing techniques involving classification algorithms may help in this regard.

3. *Therapy.* As mentioned above, an interesting direction of fMRI is potentially toward biofeedback therapy. It appears, based on the one study by DeCharmes et al. (2004), that providing subjects, in real time, information about specific brain activity as measured with fMRI (so it is actually delayed by about 6–10 s) can allow them, with practice, to use it to reduce, at least in this case, chronic pain. This therapy was reported to have lasting effects—up to 6 mo.

In recent years the fMRI literature has been flooded with clinical results. In Table 2.1, I have listed some of the more highly cited and general articles dealing with each of the specific clinically related areas.

TABLE 2.1. Clinical Directions of fMRI

- *Epilepsy*: Binder et al. (1996), Desmond et al. (1995), Jack et al. (1994), Duncan (1997), Decarli et al. (1995), HertzPannier et al. (1997), Warach et al. (1996), Cuenod et al. (1995), Viondury et al. (1994), Pujol et al. (1999), Salek-Haddadi et al. (2002), Jackson et al. (1994), Detre et al. (1995)
- *Presurgical mapping*: Jack et al. (1994), Pujol et al. (1999), Nimsky et al. (1999), Fandino et al. (1999), Rosenow & Luders (2001), Michel et al. (1999), Pujol et al. (1996), Worthington et al. (1997), Bittar et al. (1999), Achten et al. (1999)
- *Stroke*: Thulborn et al. (1999), Cramer et al. (1997), Cao et al. (1998), Benson et al. (1999), Marshall et al. (2000), Hossmann & Hoehnberlage (1995), Rossini et al. (1998), Hadjikhani et al. (2001), Neumann-Haefelin et al. (2000), Beauchamp et al. (1999), Roussel et al. (1995), Cao et al. (1999), Benaron et al. (2000), Rosen et al. (2000), Barbier et al. (2001), Wu et al. (2001), Werring et al. (1998)
- *Tumor assessment*: Mueller et al. (1996), Robinson et al. (1995), Griffiths et al. (1997), Fandino et al. (1999), Stapleton et al. (1997), Kahn et al. (1996)
- *Dementia*: Grady et al. (1995), Decarli et al. (1995), Parasuraman et al. (1992), Kirchhoff et al. (2000), Viondury et al. (1994), Salerno et al. (1992), Murphy et al. (1993), Haxby et al. (1992), Grady et al. (1993)
- *Alzheimer's disease*: Bookheimer et al. (2000)
- *Schizophrenia*: Egan et al. (2001), Dierks et al. (1999), Gallagher et al. (2000), Callicott et al. (1999), Honey et al. (1999), David et al. (1996), Manoach et al. (1999, 2000), Schneider et al. (1998), Phillips et al. (1999)
- *Attention-deficit/hyperactivity disorder (ADHD)*: Mueller et al. (1996), Robinson et al. (1995), Griffiths et al. (1997), Fandino et al. (1999), Stapleton et al. (1997), Kahn et al. (1996)
- *General anxiety disorders*: Mueller et al. (1996), Robinson et al. (1995), Griffiths et al. (1997), Fandino et al. (1999), Stapleton et al. (1997), Kahn et al. (1996), Pine et al. (2002), Stein et al. (2002)
- *Autism and Asperger syndrome*: Schultz et al. (2000)
- *Dyslexia*: Eden et al. (1996), Demb et al. (1998), Habib (2000), Temple et al. (2000)
- *Pain*: Davis et al. (1995, 1997, 1998a), Peyron et al. (1999, 2000), Porro et al. (1998), Tracey et al. (2000)
- *Pain therapy*: DeCharms et al. (2004)
- *Acupuncture*: Cho et al. (1998), Hui et al. (2000), Wu et al. (1999, 2002), Siedentopf et al. (2002), Li et al. (2003)
- *Addiction*: Volkow et al. (2002)
- *Cocaine*: Garavan et al. (2000), Li et al. (2000), Gollub et al. (1998)
- *Nicotine/tobacco*: Due et al. (2002), Spinella (2005), McClernon & Gilbert (2004), Stein et al. (1998)
- *Alcohol*: Wrase et al. (2002), Streeter et al. (2002)
- *Methamphetamine*: Paulus et al. (2003)
- *Gambling*: Reuter et al. (2005), Kuhnen & Knutson (2005)
- *Heroin*: Luo et al. (2004)
- *Drug actions*: Stein (2001)

Further Information

Table 2.2 lists sources of further information on MRI and fMRI.

TABLE 2.2. Available Information about Functional MRI

MRI and fMRI basics

- *www.simplyphysics.com/MAIN.HTM*
- *defiant.ssc.uwo.ca/Jody_web/fmri4dummies.htm*

Processing software

- *afni.nimh.nih.gov/afni* (Analysis of Functional NeuroImages by Bob Cox, National Institute of Mental Health)
- *www.bic.mni.mcgill.ca/software/* (from the Brain Imaging Center at McGill University)
- *grommit.lrdc.pitt.edu/fiswidgets/* (a Java graphical user interface for a number of neuroimaging analysis packages)
- *brainmapping.loni.ucla.edu/BMD_HTML/SharedCode/SharedSoftware.html* (general analysis tools from UCLA brain imaging center)
- *www.mayo.edu/bir/Software/Analyze/Analyze.html* (from the Mayo Clinic)
- *www.brainvoyager.com/* (a commercial product from Brain Innovation: Rainer Goebel)
- *www.math.mcgill.ca/keith/fmristat/* (a set of useful Matlab programs: Keith Worsley)
- *www.fmrib.ox.ac.uk/fsl/* (a comprehensive set of analysis programs: Steve Smith, Oxford University)

Books

- *Introduction to Functional Magnetic Resonance Imaging: Principles and Techniques*, by Richard Buxton, Cambridge University Press, 2001.
- *Functional Magnetic Resonance Imaging*, by Scott A. Huettel, Allen W. Song, and Gregory McCarthy, Sinauer Associates, 2004.
- *Functional MRI: An Introduction to Methods*, edited by Peter Jezzard, Paul M. Mattthews, and Stephen M. Smith, Springer-Verlag, 2003.
- *Functional MRI*, edited by Chrit Moonen and Peter A. Bandettini, Springer-Verlag, 1999.
- *Functional MRI: Basic Principles and Clinical Applications*, edited by Scott H. Faro and Feroze B. Mohamed, Springer-Verlag, 2005.
- *Echo-Planar Imaging: Theory, Technique, and Applications*, edited by Franz Schmitt, Michael Stehling, and Robert Turner, Springer-Verlag, 1998.

Functional MRI course websites

- *www.nmr.mgh.harvard.edu/fmrivfp/*
- *www.firc.mcw.edu/course/*

Organizations

- *www.cogneurosociety.org/* (the Cognitive Neuroscience Society)
- *www.humanbrainmapping.org/* (the Organization for Human Brain Mapping)

REFERENCES

Achten, E., Jackson, G. D., Cameron, J. A., et al. (1999). Presurgical evaluation of the motor hand area with functional MR imaging in patients with tumors and dysplastic lesions. *Radiology, 210,* 529–538.

Aguirre, G. K., Detre, J. A., Zarahn, E., et al. (2002). Experimental design and the relative sensitivity of BOLD and perfusion fMRI. *NeuroImage, 15,* 488–500.

Amaro, E., Williams, S. C. R., Shergill, S. S., et al. (2002). Acoustic noise and functional magnetic resonance imaging: Current strategies and future prospects. *Journal of Magnetic Resonance Imaging, 16,* 497–510.

An, H. Y., Lin, W. L., Celik, A., et al. (2001). Quantitative measurements of cerebral metabolic rate of oxygen utilization using MRI: A volunteer study. *NMR in Biomedicine, 14,* 441–447.

Bandettini, P. A., & Wong, E. C. (1997). A hypercapnia-based normalization method for improved spatial localization of human brain activation with fMRI. *NMR in Biomedicine, 10,* 197–203.

Bandettini, P. A., Wong, E. C., Hinks, R. S., et al. (1992). Time course EPI of human brain-function during task activation. *Magnetic Resonance in Medicine, 25,* 390–397.

Barbier, E. L., Lamalle, L., & Decorps, M. (2001). Methodology of brain perfusion imaging. *Journal of Magnetic Resonance Imaging, 13,* 496–520.

Beauchamp, M. S., Argall, B. D., Bodurka, J., et al. (2004). Unraveling multisensory integration: Patchy organization within human STS multisensory cortex. *Nature Neuroscience, 7,* 1190–1192.

Beauchamp, N. J., Barker, P. B., Wang, P. Y., et al. (1999). Imaging of acute cerebral ischemia. *Radiology, 212,* 307–324.

Beckmann, C. F., Noble, J. A., & Smith, S. M. (2001). Investigating the intrinsic dimensionality of fMRI data for ICA. *NeuroImage, 13,* S76–S76.

Bellgowan, P. S. F., Saad, Z. S., & Bandettini, P. A. (2003). Understanding neural system dynamics through task modulation and measurement of functional MRI amplitude, latency, and width. *Proceedings of the National Academy of Sciences of the United States of America, 100,* 1415–1419.

Belliveau, J. W., Kennedy, D. N., McKinstry, R. C., et al. (1991). Functional mapping of the human visual cortex by magnetic resonance imaging. *Science, 254,* 716–719.

Belliveau, J. W., Kwong, K. K., Kennedy, D. N., et al. (1992). Magnetic resonance imaging mapping of brain function: Human visual cortex. *Investigative Radiology, 27,* S59–S65.

Benaron, D. A., Hintz, S. R., Villringer, A., et al. (2000). Noninvasive functional imaging of human brain using light. *Journal of Cerebral Blood Flow and Metabolism, 20,* 469–477.

Benson, R. R., FitzGerald, D. B., LeSueur, L. L., et al. (1999). Language dominance determined by whole brain functional MRI in patients with brain lesions. *Neurology, 52,* 798–809.

Binder, J. R., Frost, J. A., Hammeke, T. A., et al. (1999). Conceptual processing during the conscious resting state: A functional MRI study. *Journal of Cognitive Neuroscience, 11,* 80–93.

Binder, J. R., Rao, S. M., Hammeke, T. A., et al. (1994). Effects of stimulus rate on signal response during functional magnetic resonance imaging of auditory cortex. *Cognitive Brain Research, 2,* 31–38.

Binder, J. R., Swanson, S. J., Hammeke, T. A., et al. (1996). Determination of language dominance using functional MRI: A comparison with the Wada test. *Neurology, 46,* 978–984.

Biswal, B., Yetkin, F. Z., Haughton, V. M., et al. (1995). Functional connectivity in the motor cortex of resting human brain using echo-planar MRI. *Magnetic Resonance in Medicine, 34,* 537–541.

Bittar, R. G., Olivier, A., Sadikot, A. F., et al. (1999). Presurgical motor and somatosensory cortex mapping with functional magnetic resonance imaging and positron emission tomography. *Journal of Neurosurgery, 91,* 915–921.

Blamire, A. M., Ogawa, S., Ugurbil, K., et al. (1992). Dynamic mapping of the human visual cortex by high-speed magnetic resonance imaging. *Proceedings of the National Academy of Sciences of the United States of America, 89,* 11069–11073.

Bodurka, J., Ledden, P. J., van Gelderen, P., et al. (2004). Scalable multichannel MRI data acquisition system. *Magnetic Resonance in Medicine, 51,* 165–171.

Bookheimer, S. Y., Strojwas, M. H., Cohen, M. S., et al. (2000). Patterns of brain activation in people at risk for Alzheimer's disease. *New England Journal of Medicine, 343,* 450–456.

Bottomley, P. A., Foster, T. H., Argersinger, R. E., et al. (1984). A review of normal tissue hydrogen NMR relaxation times and relaxation mechanisms from 1–100 MHz: Dependence on tissue type, NMR frequency, temperature, species, excision, and age. *Medical Physics, 11,* 425.

Buchel, C., & Friston, K. J. (1998). Dynamic changes in effective connectivity characterized by variable parameter regression and Kalman filtering. *Human Brain Mapping, 6,* 403–408.

Buckner, R. L., Bandettini, P. A., Ocraven, K. M., et al. (1996). Detection of cortical activation during averaged single trials of a cognitive task using functional magnetic resonance imaging. *Proceedings of the National Academy of Sciences of the United States of America, 93,* 14878–14883.

Buxton, R. B., & Frank, L. R. (1997). A model for the coupling between cerebral blood flow and oxygen metabolism during neural stimulation. *Journal of Cerebral Blood Flow and Metabolism, 17,* 64–72.

Buxton, R. B., Frank, L. R., Wong, E. C., et al. (1998). A general kinetic model for quantitative perfusion imaging with arterial spin labeling. *Magnetic Resonance in Medicine, 40,* 383–396.

Buxton, R. B., Uludag, K., Dubowitz, D. J., et al. (2004). Modeling the hemodynamic response to brain activation. *NeuroImage, 23,* S220–S233.

Callicott, J. H., Mattay, V. S., Bertolino, A., et al. (1999). Physiological characteristics of capacity constraints in working memory as revealed by functional MRI. *Cerebral Cortex, 9,* 20–26.

Cao, Y., D'Olhaberriague, L., Vikingstad, E. M., et al. (1998). Pilot study of functional MRI to assess cerebral activation of motor function after poststroke hemiparesis. *Stroke, 29,* 112–122.

Cao, Y., Vikingstad, E. M., George, K. P., et al. (1999). Cortical language activation in stroke patients recovering from aphasia with functional MRI. *Stroke, 30,* 2331–2340.

Cheng, K., Waggoner, R. A., & Tanaka, K. (2001). Human ocular dominance columns as revealed by high-field functional magnetic resonance imaging. *Neuron*, *32*, 359–374.

Cho, Z. H., Chung, S. C., Jones, J. P., et al. (1998). New findings of the correlation between acupoints and corresponding brain cortices using functional MRI. *Proceedings of the National Academy of Sciences of the United States of America*, *95*, 2670–2673.

Cohen, E. R., Rostrup, E., Sidaros, K., et al. (2004). Hypercapnic normalization of BOLD fMRI: Comparison across field strengths and pulse sequences. *NeuroImage*, *23*, 613–624.

Cohen, M. S. (2001). Real-time functional magnetic resonance imaging. *Methods*, *25*, 201–220.

Courtney, S. M., Ungerleider, B. G., Keil, K., et al. (1997). Transient and sustained activity in a distributed neural system for human working memory. *Nature*, *386*, 608–611.

Cox, D. D., & Savoy, R. L. (2003). Functional magnetic resonance imaging (fMRI) "brain reading": Detecting and classifying distributed patterns of fMRI activity in human visual cortex. *NeuroImage*, *19*, 261–270.

Cox, R. W., & Jesmanowicz, A. (1999). Real-time 3D image registration for functional MRI. *Magnetic Resonance in Medicine*, *42*, 1014–1018.

Cox, R. W., Jesmanowicz, A., & Hyde, J. S. (1995). Real-time functional magnetic resonance imaging. *Magnetic Resonance in Medicine*, *33*, 230–236.

Cramer, S. C., Nelles, G., Benson, R. R., et al. (1997). A functional MRI study of subjects recovered from hemiparetic stroke. *Stroke*, *28*, 2518–2527.

Cuenod, C. A., Bookheimer, S. Y., Hertzpannier, L., et al. (1995). Functional MRI during word generation, using conventional equipment—A potential tool for language localization in the clinical environment. *Neurology*, *45*, 1821–1827.

Dale, A. M., & Buckner, R. L. (1997). Selective averaging of rapidly presented individual trials using fMRI. *Human Brain Mapping*, *5*, 329–340.

Davatzikos, C., Ruparel, K., Fan, Y., et al. (2005). Classifying spatial patterns of brain activity with machine learning methods: Application to lie detection. *NeuroImage, 28*(3), 663–668.

David, A. S., Woodruff, P. W. R., Howard, R., et al. (1996). Auditory hallucinations inhibit exogenous activation of auditory association cortex. *NeuroReport*, *7*, 932–936.

Davis, K. D., Kwan, C. L., Crawley, A. P., et al. (1998a). Functional MRI study of thalamic and cortical activations evoked by cutaneous heat, cold, and tactile stimuli. *Journal of Neurophysiology*, *80*, 1533–1546.

Davis, K. D., Taylor, S. J., Crawley, A. P., et al. (1997). Functional MRI of pain- and attention-related activations in the human cingulate cortex. *Journal of Neurophysiology*, *77*, 3370–3380.

Davis, K. D., Wood, M. L., Crawley, A. P., et al. (1995). fMRI of human somatosensory and cingulate cortex during painful electrical nerve stimulation. *NeuroReport*, *7*, 321–325.

Davis, T. L., Kwong, K. K., Weisskoff, R. M., et al. (1998b). Calibrated functional MRI: Mapping the dynamics of oxidative metabolism. *Proceedings of the National Academy of Sciences of the United States of America*, *95*, 1834–1839.

Decarli, C., Murphy, D. G. M., Tranh, M., et al. (1995). The effect of white-matter hyperintensity volume on brain structure, cognitive performance, and cerebral metabolism of glucose in 51 healthy adults. *Neurology, 45,* 2077–2084.

DeCharms, R. C., Christoff, K., Glover, G. H., et al. (2004). Learned regulation of spatially localized brain activation using real-time fMRI. *NeuroImage, 21,* 436–443.

Demb, J. B., Boynton, G. M., & Heeger, D. J. (1998). Functional magnetic resonance imaging of early visual pathways in dyslexia. *Journal of Neuroscience, 18,* 6939–6951.

Desmond, J. E., Sum, J. M., Wagner, A. D., et al. (1995). Functional MRI measurement of language lateralization in Wada-tested patients. *Brain, 118,* 1411–1419.

Detre, J. A., & Alsop, D. C. (1999). Perfusion magnetic resonance imaging with continuous arterial spin labeling: Methods and clinical applications in the central nervous system. *European Journal of Radiology, 30,* 115–124.

Detre, J. A., Sirven, J. I., Alsop, D. C., et al. (1995). Localization of subclinical ictal activity by functional magnetic resonance imaging: Correlation with invasive monitoring. *Annals of Neurology, 38,* 618–624.

Detre, J. A., Zhang, W. G., Roberts, D. A., et al. (1994). Tissue-specific perfusion imaging using arterial spin-labeling. *NMR in Biomedicine, 7,* 75–82.

DeYoe, E. A., Bandettini, P. A., Neitz, J., et al. (1994). Functional magnetic resonance imaging (fMRI) of the human brain. *Journal of Neuroscience Methods, 54,* 171–187.

DeYoe, E. A., Neitz, J., Miller, D., et al. (1993). Functional magnetic resonance imaging (fMRI) of visual cortex in human subjects using a unique video graphics stimulator. *Proceedings of the Society of Magnetic Resonance in Medicine, 12th Annual Meeting,* New York.

de Zwart, J. A., van Gelderen, P., Kellman, P., et al. (2002). Application of sensitivity-encoded echo-planar imaging for blood oxygen level-dependent functional brain imaging. *Magnetic Resonance in Medicine, 48,* 1011–1020.

Dierks, T., Linden, D. E. J., Jandl, M., et al. (1999). Activation of Heschl's gyrus during auditory hallucinations. *Neuron, 22,* 615–621.

Donaldson, D. I. (2004). Parsing brain activity with fMRI and mixed designs: What kind of a state is neuroimaging in? *Trends in Neurosciences, 27,* 442–444.

Due, D. L., Huettel, S. A., Hall, W. G., et al. (2002). Activation in mesolimbic and visuospatial neural circuits elicited by smoking cues: Evidence from functional magnetic resonance imaging. *American Journal of Psychiatry, 159,* 954–960.

Duncan, J. S. (1997). Imaging and epilepsy. *Brain, 120,* 339–377.

Eden, G. F., VanMeter, J. W., Rumsey, J. M., et al. (1996). Abnormal processing of visual motion in dyslexia revealed by functional brain imaging. *Nature, 382,* 66–69.

Edmister, W. B., Talavage, T. M., Ledden, P. J., et al. (1999). Improved auditory cortex imaging using clustered volume acquisitions. *Human Brain Mapping, 7,* 89–97.

Egan, M. F., Goldberg, T. E., Kolachana, B. S., et al. (2001). Effect of COMT Val(108/158) Met genotype on frontal lobe function and risk for schizophrenia. *Proceedings of the National Academy of Sciences of the United States of America, 98,* 6917–6922.

Engel, S. A. (1994). fMRI of human visual cortex. *Nature, 370,* 106–106.

Engel, S. A., Glover, G. H., & Wandell, B. A. (1997). Retinotopic organization in human visual cortex and the spatial precision of functional MRI. *Cerebral Cortex*, 7, 181–192.

Fandino, J., Kollias, S. S., Wieser, H. G., et al. (1999). Intraoperative validation of functional magnetic resonance imaging and cortical reorganization patterns in patients with brain tumors involving the primary motor cortex. *Journal of Neurosurgery*, 91, 238–250.

Formisano, E., Esposito, F., Di Salle, F., et al. (2004). Cortex-based independent component analysis of fMRI time series. *Magnetic Resonance Imaging*, 22, 1493–1504.

Frahm, J., Bruhn, H., Merboldt, K. D., et al. (1992). Dynamic MR imaging of human brain oxygenation during rest and photic-stimulation. *Journal of Magnetic Resonance Imaging*, 2, 501–505.

Gallagher, H. L., Happe, F., Brunswick, N., et al. (2000). Reading the mind in cartoons and stories: An fMRI study of "theory of mind" in verbal and nonverbal tasks. *Neuropsychologia*, 38, 11–21.

Garavan, H., Pankiewicz, J., Bloom, A., et al. (2000). Cue-induced cocaine craving: Neuroanatomical specificity for drug users and drug stimuli. *American Journal of Psychiatry*, 157, 1789–1798.

Garroway, A. N., Grannell, P. K., & Mansfield, P. (1974). Image formation in NMR by a selective irradiative process. *Journal of Physics C: Solid State Physics*, 7, 1457–1462.

Gollub, R. L., Breiter, H. C., Kantor, H., et al. (1998). Cocaine decreases cortical cerebral blood flow but does not obscure regional activation in functional magnetic resonance imaging in human subjects. *Journal of Cerebral Blood Flow and Metabolism*, 18, 724–734.

Gonzalez-At, J. B., Alsop, D. C., & Detre, J. A. (2000). Cerebral perfusion and arterial transit time changes during task activation determined with continuous arterial spin labeling. *Magnetic Resonance in Medicine*, 43, 739–746.

Goodyear, B. G., & Menon, R. S. (2001). Brief visual stimulation allows mapping of ocular dominance in visual cortex using fMRI. *Human Brain Mapping*, 14, 210–217.

Grady, C. L., Haxby, J. V., Horwitz, B., et al. (1993). Activation of cerebral blood flow during a visuoperceptual task in patients with Alzheimer-type dementia. *Neurobiology of Aging*, 14, 35–44.

Grady, C. L., McIntosh, A. R., Horwitz, B., et al. (1995). Age-related reductions in human recognition memory due to impaired encoding. *Science*, 269, 218–221.

Griffiths, J. R., Taylor, N. J., Howe, F. A., et al. (1997). The response of human tumors to carbogen breathing, monitored by gradient-recalled echo magnetic resonance imaging. *International Journal of Radiation Oncology Biology Physics*, 39, 697–701.

Grill-Spector, K., & Malach, R. (2001). fMR adaptation: A tool for studying the functional properties of human cortical neurons. *Acta Psychologica*, 107, 293–321.

Haacke, E. M., Brown, R. W., Thompson, M. R., et al. (1999). *Magnetic resonance imaging: Physical principles and sequence design*. New York: Wiley-Liss.

Habib, M. (2000). The neurological basis of developmental dyslexia: An overview and working hypothesis. *Brain*, 123, 2373–2399.

Hasson, U., Nir, Y., Levy, I., et al. (2004). Intersubject synchronization of cortical activity during natural vision. *Science*, 303, 1634–1640.

Haxby, J. V., Gobbini, M. I., Furey, M. L., et al. (2001). Distributed and overlapping representations of faces and objects in ventral temporal cortex. *Science, 293,* 2425–2430.

Haxby, J. V., Raffaele, K., Gillette, J., et al. (1992). Individual trajectories of cognitive decline in patients with dementia of the Alzheimer type. *Journal of Clinical and Experimental Neuropsychology, 14,* 575–592.

Haynes, J. D., & Rees, G. (2005). Predicting the orientation of invisible stimuli from activity in human primary visual cortex. *Nature Neuroscience, 8,* 686–691.

Hennig, J., Janz, C., Speck, O., et al. (1995). Functional spectroscopy of brain activation following a single light pulse: Examinations of the mechanism of the fast initial response. *International Journal of Imaging Systems and Technology, 6,* 203–208.

Henson, R. N., Price, C. J., Rugg, M. D., et al. (2002). Detecting latency differences in event-related BOLD responses: Application to words versus nonwords and initial versus repeated face presentations. *NeuroImage, 15,* 83–97.

HertzPannier, L., Gaillard, W. D., Mott, S. H., et al. (1997). Noninvasive assessment of language dominance in children and adolescents with functional MRI: A preliminary study. *Neurology, 48,* 1003–1012.

Hoge, R. D., Atkinson, J., Gill, B., et al. (1999). Linear coupling between cerebral blood flow and oxygen consumption in activated human cortex. *Proceedings of the National Academy of Sciences of the United States of America, 96,* 9403–9408.

Honey, G. D., Bullmore, E. T., Soni, W., et al. (1999). Differences in frontal cortical activation by a working memory task after substitution of risperidone for typical antipsychotic drugs in patients with schizophrenia. *Proceedings of the National Academy of Sciences of the United States of America, 96,* 13432–13437.

Hossmann, K. A., & Hoehnberlage, M. (1995). Diffusion and perfusion MR imaging of cerebral ischemia. *Cerebrovascular and Brain Metabolism Reviews, 7,* 187–217.

Hu, X. P., Le, T. H., & Ugurbil, K. (1997). Evaluation of the early response in fMRI in individual subjects using short stimulus duration. *Magnetic Resonance in Medicine, 37,* 877–884.

Hui, K. K. S., Liu, J., Makris, N., et al. (2000). Acupuncture modulates the limbic system and subcortical gray structures of the human brain: Evidence from fMRI studies in normal subjects. *Human Brain Mapping, 9,* 13–25.

Jack, C. R., Thompson, R. M., Butts, R. K., et al. (1994). Sensory-motor cortex: Correlation of presurgical mapping with functional MR imaging and invasive cortical mapping. *Radiology, 190,* 85–92.

Jackson, G. D., Connelly, A., Cross, J. H., et al. (1994). Functional magnetic-resonance imaging of focal seizures. *Neurology, 44,* 850–856.

Jezzard, P., & Balaban, R. S. (1995). Correction for geometric distortion in echo-planar images from B-0 field variations. *Magnetic Resonance in Medicine, 34,* 65–73.

Jezzard, P., Duewell, S., & Balaban, R. S. (1996). MR relaxation times in human brain: Measurement at 4T. *Radiology, 199,* 773.

Kahn, T., Schwabe, B., Bettag, M., et al. (1996). Mapping of the cortical motor hand area with functional MR imaging and MR imaging-guided laser-induced interstitial thermotherapy of brain tumors: Work in progress. *Radiology, 200,* 149–157.

Kamitani, Y., & Tong, F. (2005). Decoding the visual and subjective contents of the human brain. *Nature Neuroscience, 8,* 679–685.

Kennerley, A. J., Berwick, J., Martindale, J., et al. (2005). Concurrent fMRI and optical measures for the investigation of the hemodynamic response function. *Magnetic Resonance in Medicine, 54,* 354–365.

Kirchhoff, B. A., Wagner, A. D., Maril, A., et al. (2000). Prefrontal–temporal circuitry for episodic encoding and subsequent memory. *Journal of Neuroscience, 20,* 6173–6180.

Kriegeskorte, N., Goebel, R., & Bandettini, P. (2006). Information-based functional brain mapping. *Proceedings of the National Academy of Sciences of the United States of America, 103,* 3863.

Kuhnen, C. M., & Knutson, B. (2005). The neural basis of financial risk taking. *Neuron, 47,* 763–770.

Kwong, K. K., Belliveau, J. W., Chesler, D. A., et al. (1992). Dynamic magnetic resonance imaging of human brain activity during primary sensory stimulation. *Proceedings of the National Academy of Sciences of the United States of America, 89,* 5675–5679.

LaConte, S., Strother, S., Cherkassky, V., et al. (2005). Support vector machines for temporal classification of block design fMRI data. *NeuroImage, 26*(2), 317–329.

Laufs, H., Krakow, K., Sterzer, P., et al. (2003). Electroencephalographic signatures of attentional and cognitive default modes in spontaneous brain activity fluctuations at rest. *Proceedings of the National Academy of Sciences of the United States of America, 100,* 11053–11058.

Le Bihan, D., Urayama, S. I., Aso, T., et al. (2006). Direct and fast detection of neuronal activation in the human brain with diffusion MRI. *Proceedings of the National Academy of Sciences of the United States of America, 103,* 8263.

Li, G., Liu, H. L., Cheung, R. T. F., et al. (2003). An fMRI study comparing brain activation between word generation and electrical stimulation of language-implicated acupoints. *Human Brain Mapping, 18,* 233–238.

Li, S. J., Biswal, B., Li, Z., et al. (2000). Cocaine administration decreases functional connectivity in human primary visual and motor cortex as detected by functional MRI. *Magnetic Resonance in Medicine, 43,* 45–51.

Logothetis, N., Pauls, J., Augath, M., et al. (2001a). Neurophysiological investigation of the basis of the fMRI signal. *Nature, 412,* 150–157.

Logothetis, N. K., Merkle, H., Augath, M., et al. (2002). Ultra high-resolution fMRI in monkeys with implanted RF coils. *Neuron, 35,* 227–242.

Logothetis, N. K., Pauls, J., Augath, M., et al. (2001b). Neurophysiological investigation of the basis of the fMRI signal. *Nature, 412,* 150–157.

Lu, H. Z., Golay, X., Pekar, J. J., et al. (2004). Sustained poststimulus elevation in cerebral oxygen utilization after vascular recovery. *Journal of Cerebral Blood Flow and Metabolism, 24,* 764–770.

Lu, H. Z., Golay, X., Pekar, J. J., et al. (2003). Functional magnetic resonance imaging based on changes in vascular space occupancy. *Magnetic Resonance in Medicine, 50,* 263–274.

Luo, F., Xi, Z. X., Wu, G. H., et al. (2004). Attenuation of brain response to heroin correlates with the reinstatement of heroin-seeking in rats by fMRI. *NeuroImage, 22,* 1328–1335.

Malonek, D., Dirnagl, U., Lindauer, U., et al. (1997). Vascular imprints of neuronal activity: Relationships between the dynamics of cortical blood flow, oxygenation, and volume changes following sensory stimulation. *Proceedings of the National Academy of Sciences of the United States of America, 94,* 14826–14831.

Malonek, D., & Grinvald, A. (1996). Interactions between electrical activity and cortical microcirculation revealed by imaging spectroscopy: Implications for functional brain mapping. *Science, 272,* 551–554.

Manoach, D. S., Gollub, R. L., Benson, E. S., et al. (2000). Schizophrenic subjects show aberrant fMRI activation of dorsolateral prefrontal cortex and basal ganglia during working memory performance. *Biological Psychiatry, 48,* 99–109.

Manoach, D. S., Press, D. Z., Thangaraj, V., et al. (1999). Schizophrenic subjects activate dorsolateral prefrontal cortex during a working memory task, as measured by fMRI. *Biological Psychiatry, 45,* 1128–1137.

Mansfield, P., & Maudsley, A. A. (1977). Medical imaging by NMR. *British Journal of Radiology, 50,* 188.

Mansfield, P., Maudsley, A. A., & Baines, T. (1976). Fast scan proton density imaging by NMR. *Journal of Physics E: Scientific Instruments, 9,* 271.

Marshall, R. S., Perera, G. M., Lazar, R. M., et al. (2000). Evolution of cortical activation during recovery from corticospinal tract infarction. *Stroke, 31,* 656–661.

Matheiesen, C., Caesar, K., Akgoren, N., et al. (1998). Modification of activity-dependent increases of cerebral blood flow by excitatory synaptic activity and spikes in rat cerebellar cortex. *Journal of Physiology, 512*(2), 555–566.

McCarthy, G., Luby, M., Gore, J., et al. (1997). Infrequent events transiently activate human prefrontal and parietal cortex as measured by functional MRI. *Journal of Neurophysiology, 77,* 1630–1634.

McClernon, F. J., & Gilbert, D. G. (2004). Human functional neuroimaging in nicotine and tobacco research: Basics, background, and beyond. *Nicotine and Tobacco Research, 6,* 941–959.

Menon, R. S., Luknowsky, D. C., & Gati, J. S. (1998). Mental chronometry using latency-resolved functional MRI. *Proceedings of the National Academy of Sciences of the United States of America, 95,* 10902–10907.

Menon, R. S., Ogawa, S., Strupp, J. P., et al. (1997). Ocular dominance in human V1 demonstrated by functional magnetic resonance imaging. *Journal of Neurophysiology, 77,* 2780–2787.

Menon, R. S., Ogawa, S., & Ugurbil, K. (1995). High-temporal-resolution studies of the human primary visual cortex at 4 T:- Teasing out the oxygenation contribution in fMRI. *International Journal of Imaging Systems and Technology, 6,* 209–215.

Michel, C. M., de Peralta, R. G., Lantz, G., et al. (1999). Spatiotemporal EEG analysis and distributed source estimation in presurgical epilepsy evaluation. *Journal of Clinical Neurophysiology, 16,* 239–266.

Mitchell, D. G., & Cohen, M. (2003). *MRI Principles.* Philadelphia: Saunders.

Mitchell, T. M., Hutchinson, R., Niculescu, R. S., et al. (2004). Learning to decode cognitive states from brain images. *Machine Learning, 57,* 145–175.

Mueller, W. M., Yetkin, F. Z., Hammeke, T. A., et al. (1996). Functional magnetic resonance imaging mapping of the motor cortex in patients with cerebral tumors. *Neurosurgery, 39,* 515–520.

Murphy, D. G. M., Decarli, C. D., Daly, E., et al. (1993). Volumetric magnetic resonance imaging in men with dementia of the Alzheimer-type: Correlations with disease severity. *Biological Psychiatry, 34,* 612–621.

Neumann-Haefelin, T., Moseley, M. E., & Albers, G. W. (2000). New magnetic resonance imaging methods for cerebrovascular disease: Emerging clinical applications. *Annals of Neurology, 47,* 559–570.

Nimsky, C., Ganslandt, O., Kober, H., et al. (1999). Integration of functional magnetic resonance imaging supported by magnetoencephalography in functional neuronavigation. *Neurosurgery, 44,* 1249–1255.

Ogawa, S., Lee, T. M., Kay, A. R., et al. (1990a). Brain magnetic resonance imaging with contrast dependent on blood oxygenation. *Proceedings of the National Academy of Sciences of the United States of America, 87,* 9868–9872.

Ogawa, S., Lee, T. M., Nayak, A. S., et al. (1990b). Oxygenation-sensitive contrast in magnetic resonance image of rodent brain at high magnetic fields. *Magnetic Resonance in Medicine, 14,* 68–78.

Ogawa, S., Menon, R. S., Tank, D. W., et al. (1993). Functional brain mapping by blood oxygenation level-dependent contrast magnetic resonance imaging: A comparison of signal characteristics with a biophysical model. *Biophysical Journal, 64,* 803–812.

Ogawa, S., Tank, D. W., Menon, R., et al. (1992). Intrinsic signal changes accompanying sensory stimulation: Functional brain mapping with magnetic resonance imaging. *Proceedings of the National Academy of Sciences of the United States of America, 89,* 5951–5955.

Parasuraman, R., Greenwood, P. M., Haxby, J. V., et al. (1992). Visuospatial attention in dementia of the Alzheimer type. *Brain, 115,* 711–733.

Parkes, L. M., Schwarzbach, J. V., Bouts, A. A., et al. (2005). Quantifying the spatial resolution of the gradient echo and spin echo BOLD response at 3 tesla. *Magnetic Resonance in Medicine, 54,* 1465–1472.

Paulus, M. P., Hozack, N., Frank, L., et al. (2003). Decision making by methamphetamine-dependent subjects is associated with error-rate-independent decrease in prefrontal and parietal activation. *Biological Psychiatry, 53,* 65–74.

Peyron, R., Garcia-Larrea, L., Gregoire, M. C., et al. (1999). Haemodynamic brain responses to acute pain in humans: Sensory and attentional networks. *Brain, 122,* 1765–1779.

Peyron, R., Laurent, B., & Garcia-Larrea, L. (2000). Functional imaging of brain responses to pain. A review and meta-analysis. *Clinical Neurophysiology, 30,* 263–288.

Phillips, M. L., Williams, L., Senior, C., et al. (1999). A differential neural response to threatening and non-threatening negative facial expressions in paranoid and non-paranoid schizophrenics. *Psychiatry Research—NeuroImaging, 92,* 11–31.

Pine, D. S., Grun, J., Maguire, E. A., et al. (2002). Neurodevelopmental aspects of spatial navigation: A virtual reality fMRI study. *NeuroImage, 15,* 396–406.

Porro, C. A., Cettolo, V., Francescato, M. P., et al. (1998). Temporal and intensity coding of pain in human cortex. *Journal of Neurophysiology, 80,* 3312–3320.

Posse, S., Fitzgerald, D., Gao, K. X., et al. (2003). Real-time fMRI of temporolimbic regions detects amygdala activation during single-trial self-induced sadness. *NeuroImage, 18,* 760–768.

Pujol, J., Conesa, G., Deus, J., et al. (1996). Presurgical identification of the primary sensorimotor cortex by functional magnetic resonance imaging. *Journal of Neurosurgery, 84*, 7–13.

Pujol, J., Deus, J., Losilla, J. M., et al. (1999). Cerebral lateralization of language in normal left-handed people studied by functional MRI. *Neurology, 52*, 1038–1043.

Raichle, M. E., MacLeod, A. M., Snyder, A. Z., et al. (2001). A default mode of brain function. *Proceedings of the National Academy of Sciences of the United States of America, 98*, 676–682.

Rao, S. M., Bandettini, P. A., Binder, J. R., et al. (1996). Relationship between finger movement rate and functional magnetic resonance signal change in human primary motor cortex. *Journal of Cerebral Blood Flow and Metabolism, 16*, 1250–1254.

Reuter, J., Raedler, T., Rose, M., et al. (2005). Pathological gambling is linked to reduced activation of the mesolimbic reward system. *Nature Neuroscience, 8*, 147–148.

Robinson, S. P., Howe, F. A., & Griffiths, J. R. (1995). Noninvasive monitoring of carbogen-induced changes in tumor blood flow and oxygenation by functional magnetic resonance imaging. *International Journal of Radiation Oncology Biology Physics, 33*, 855–859.

Rosen, B. R., Belliveau, J. W., Aronen, H. J., et al. (1991a). Susceptibility contrast imaging of cerebral blood volume: Human experience. *Magnetic Resonance in Medicine, 22*, 293–299.

Rosen, B. R., Belliveau, J. W., Buchbinder, B. R., et al. (1991b). Contrast agents and cerebral hemodynamics. *Magnetic Resonance in Medicine, 19*, 285–292.

Rosen, H. J., Petersen, S. E., Linenweber, M. R., et al. (2000). Neural correlates of recovery from aphasia after damage to left inferior frontal cortex. *Neurology, 55*, 1883–1894.

Rosenow, F., & Luders, H. (2001). Presurgical evaluation of epilepsy. *Brain, 124*, 1683–1700.

Rossini, P. M., Caltagirone, C., Castriota-Scanderbeg, A., et al. (1998). Hand motor cortical area reorganization in stroke: A study with fMRI, MEG and TCS maps. *NeuroReport, 9*, 2141–2146.

Roussel, S. A., Vanbruggen, N., King, M. D., et al. (1995). Identification of collaterally perfused areas following focal cerebral ischemia in the rat by comparison of gradient-echo and diffusion-weighted MRI. *Journal of Cerebral Blood Flow and Metabolism, 15*, 578–586.

Salek-Haddadi, A., Merschhemke, M., Lemieux, L., et al. (2002). Simultaneous EEG-correlated ictal fMRI. *NeuroImage, 16*, 32–40.

Salerno, J. A., Murphy, D. G. M., Horwitz, B., et al. (1992). Brain atrophy in hypertension: A volumetric magnetic resonance imaging study. *Hypertension, 20*, 340–348.

Schmitt, F., Stehling, M. K., & Turner, R. (Eds.). (1998). *Echo-planar imaging: Theory, technique, and application*. Berlin: Springer-Verlag.

Schneider, F., Weiss, U., Kessler, C., et al. (1998). Differential amygdala activation in schizophrenia during sadness. *Schizophrenia Research, 34*, 133–142.

Schultz, R. T., Gauthier, I., Klin, A., et al. (2000). Abnormal ventral temporal cortical activity during face discrimination among individuals with autism and Asperger syndrome. *Archives of General Psychiatry, 57*, 331–340.

Schwindack, C., Siminotto, E., Meyer, M., et al. (2005). Real-time functional magnetic resonance imaging (rt-fMRI) in patients with brain tumours: Preliminary findings using motor and language paradigms. *British Journal of Neurosurgery, 19*, 25–32.

Seifritz, E., Di Salle, F., Esposito, F., et al. (2006). Enhancing BOLD response in the auditory system by neurophysiologically tuned fMRI sequence. *NeuroImage, 29*, 1013.

Sereno, M. I., Dale, A. M., Reppas, J. B., et al. (1995a). Borders of multiple visual areas in humans revealed by functional magnetic resonance imaging. *Science, 268*, 889–893.

Sereno, M. I., Dale, A. M., Reppas, J. R., et al. (1995b). Functional MRI reveals borders of multiple visual areas in humans. *Science, 268*, 889–893.

Sereno, M. I., McDonald, C. T., & Allman, J. M. (1994). Analysis of retinotopic maps in extrastriate cortex. *Cerebral Cortex, 4*, 601–620.

Shmuel, A., Yacoub, E., Pfeuffer, J., et al. (2002). Sustained negative BOLD, blood flow and oxygen consumption response and its coupling to the positive response in the human brain. *Neuron, 36*, 1195–1210.

Siedentopf, C. M., Golaszewski, S. M., Mottaghy, F. M., et al. (2002). Functional magnetic resonance imaging detects activation of the visual association cortex during laser acupuncture of the foot in humans. *Neuroscience Letters, 327*, 53–56.

Smyser, C., Grabowski, T. J., Frank, R. J., et al. (2001). Real-time multiple linear regression for fMRI supported by time-aware acquisition and processing. *Magnetic Resonance in Medicine, 45*, 289–298.

Spinella, M. (2005). Compulsive behavior in tobacco users. *Addictive Behaviors, 30*, 183–186.

Stapleton, S. R., Kiriakopoulos, E., Mikulis, D., et al. (1997). Combined utility of functional MRI, cortical mapping, and frameless stereotaxy in the resection of lesions in eloquent areas of brain in children. *Pediatric Neurosurgery, 26*, 68–82.

Stark, D. D., & Bradley, W. G. (1999). *Magnetic resonance imaging.* New York: Mosby.

Stehling, M. K., Turner, R., & Mansfield, P. (1991). Echo-planar imaging: Magnetic resonance imaging in a fraction of a second. *Science, 254*, 43–50.

Stein, E. A. (2001). fMRI: A new tool for the in vivo localization of drug actions in the brain. *Journal of Analytical Toxicology, 25*, 419–424.

Stein, E. A., Pankiewicz, J., Harsch, H. H., et al. (1998). Nicotine-induced limbic cortical activation in the human brain: A functional MRI study. *American Journal of Psychiatry, 155*, 1009–1015.

Stein, M. B., Goldin, P. R., Sareen, J., et al. (2002). Increased amygdala activation to angry and contemptuous faces in generalized social phobia. *Archives of General Psychiatry, 59*, 1027–1034.

Streeter, C. C., Gulliver, S. B., Baker, E., et al. (2002). Videotaped cue for urge to drink alcohol. *Alcoholism—Clinical and Experimental Research, 26*, 627–634.

Strother, S., La Conte, S., Hansen, L. K., et al. (2004). Optimizing the fMRI data-processing pipeline using prediction and reproducibility performance metrics: I. A preliminary group analysis. *NeuroImage, 23*, S196–S207.

Temple, E., Poldrack, R. A., Protopapas, A., et al. (2000). Disruption of the neural response to rapid acoustic stimuli in dyslexia: Evidence from functional MRI.

Proceedings of the National Academy of Sciences of the United States of America, 97, 13907–13912.

Thulborn, K. R., Carpenter, P. A., & Just, M. A. (1999). Plasticity of language-related brain function during recovery from stroke. *Stroke*, 30, 749–754.

Tracey, I., Becerra, L., Chang, I., et al. (2000). Noxious hot and cold stimulation produce common patterns of brain activation in humans: A functional magnetic resonance imaging study. *Neuroscience Letters*, 288, 159–162.

Triantafyllou, C., Hoge, R. D., Krueger, G., et al. (2005). Comparison of physiological noise at 1.5 T, 3 T and 7 T and optimization of fMRI acquisition parameters. *NeuroImage*, 26, 243–250.

Turner, R., Lebihan, D., Moonen, C. T. W., et al. (1991). Echo-planar time course MRI of cat brain oxygenation changes. *Magnetic Resonance in Medicine*, 22, 159–166.

Ugurbil, K., Adriany, G., Andersen, P., et al. (2003). Ultrahigh field magnetic resonance imaging and spectroscopy. *Magnetic Resonance Imaging*, 21, 1263–1281.

Van de Moortele, P. F., Pfeuffer, J., Glover, G. H., et al. (2002). Respiration-induced B-0 fluctuations and their spatial distribution in the human brain at 7 tesla. *Magnetic Resonance in Medicine*, 47, 888–895.

Vaughan, J. T., Garwood, M., Collins, C. M., et al. (2001). 7T vs. 4T: RF power, homogeneity, and signal-to-noise comparison in head images. *Magnetic Resonance in Medicine*, 46, 24–30.

Viondury, J., Meyerhoff, D. J., Cozzone, P. J., et al. (1994). What might be the impact on neurology of the analysis of brain metabolism by in-vivo magnetic resonance spectroscopy. *Journal of Neurology*, 241, 354–371.

Volkow, N. D., Fowler, J. S., Wang, G. J., et al. (2002). Role of dopamine, the frontal cortex and memory circuits in drug addiction: Insight from imaging studies. *Neurobiology of Learning and Memory*, 78, 610–624.

Warach, S., Ives, J. R., Schlaug, G., et al. (1996). EEG-triggered echo-planar functional MRI in epilepsy. *Neurology*, 47, 89–93.

Weiskopf, N., Scharnowski, F., Veit, R., et al. (2004). Self-regulation of the local bold signal and its behavioral consequences: A real-time fMRI study. *Psychophysiology*, 41, S28–S28.

Weiskopf, N., Veit, R., Erb, M., et al. (2003). Physiological self-regulation of regional brain activity using real-time functional magnetic resonance imaging (fMRI): Methodology and exemplary data. *NeuroImage*, 19, 577–586.

Werring, D. J., Clark, C. A., Barker, G. J., et al. (1998). The structural and functional mechanisms of motor recovery: Complementary use of diffusion tensor and functional magnetic resonance imaging in a traumatic injury of the internal capsule. *Journal of Neurology, Neurosurgery and Psychiatry*, 65, 863–869.

Williams, D. S., Detre, J. A., Leigh, J. S., et al. (1992). Magnetic resonance imaging of perfusion using spin-inversion of arterial water. *Proceedings of the National Academy of Sciences of the United States of America*, 89, 212–216.

Wong, E. C. (1999). Potential and pitfalls of arterial spin labelling-based perfusion imaging techniques for functional MRI. In C. T. W. Moonen & P. A. Bandettini (Eds.), *Functional MRI*. Berlin: Springer.

Wong, E. C., Bandettini, P. A., & Hyde, J. S. (1992). Echo-planar imaging of the human brain using a three axis local gradient coil. *Proceedings of the Society of Magnetic Resonance in Medicine, 11th Annual Meeting*, Berlin.

Wong, E. C., Buxton, R. B., & Frank, L. R. (1997). Implementation of quantitative perfusion imaging techniques for functional brain mapping using pulsed arterial spin labeling. *NMR in Biomedicine, 10*, 237–249.

Wong, E. C., Buxton, R. B., & Frank, L. R. (1999). Quantitative perfusion imaging using arterial spin labeling. *Neuroimaging Clinics of North America, 9*, 333–342.

Worthington, C., Vincent, D. J., Bryant, A. E., et al. (1997). Comparison of functional magnetic resonance imaging for language localization and intracarotid speech amytal testing in presurgical evaluation for intractable epilepsy: Preliminary results. *Stereotactic and Functional Neurosurgery, 69*, 197–201.

Wrase, J., Grusser, S. M., Klein, S., et al. (2002). Development of alcohol-associated cues and cue-induced brain activation in alcoholics. *European Psychiatry, 17*, 287–291.

Wu, M. T., Hsieh, J. C., Xiong, J., et al. (1999). Central nervous pathway for acupuncture stimulation: Localization of processing with functional MR imaging of the brain: Preliminary experience. *Radiology, 212*, 133–141.

Wu, M. T., Sheen, J. M., Chuang, K. H. S., et al. (2002). Neuronal specificity of acupuncture response: A fMRI study with electroacupuncture. *NeuroImage, 16*, 1028–1037.

Wu, O., Koroshetz, W. J., Ostergaard, L., et al. (2001). Predicting tissue outcome in acute human cerebral ischemia using combined diffusion- and perfusion-weighted MR imaging. *Stroke, 32*, 933–942.

Yablonskiy, D. A., Ackerman, J. H., & Raichle, M. E. (2000a). Coupling between changes in human brain temperature and oxidative metabolism during prolonged visual stimulation. *Proceedings of the National Academy of Sciences of the United States of America, 97*, 9819–9819.

Yablonskiy, D. A., Ackerman, J. J. H., & Raichle, M. E. (2000b). Coupling between changes in human brain temperature and oxidative metabolism during prolonged visual stimulation. *Proceedings of the National Academy of Sciences of the United States of America, 97*, 7603–7608.

Yacoub, E., Van De Moortele, P. F., Shmuel, A., et al. (2005). Signal and noise characteristics of Hahn SE and GE BOLD fMRI at 7 T in humans. *NeuroImage, 24*, 738–750.

Ye, F. Q., Smith, A. M., Yang, Y. H., et al. (1997). Quantitation of regional cerebral blood flow increases during motor activation: A steady-state arterial spin tagging study. *NeuroImage, 6*, 104–112.

Yoo, S. S., Fairneny, T., Chen, N. K., et al. (2004). Brain–computer interface using fMRI: Spatial navigation by thoughts. *NeuroReport, 15*, 1591–1595.

CHAPTER 3

Principles of Electroencephalography and Magnetoencephalography

Anto Bagic
Susumu Sato

This chapter provides a brief overview of history of electroencephalographic (EEG) and magnetoelectroencephalographic (MEG) signal processing, methods, and basic and clinical research applications. Although EEG is a classic and well-established functional method for examining brain activity with an extensive history of both research and clinical application, MEG is a relatively novel method. The temporospatial resolution offered by MEG surpasses that of all other functional techniques (Plate 3.1A). Because of this, MEG holds significant promise as a method in both basic and clinical sciences. The following review focuses primarily on the general description of EEG and MEG methods and how they may be combined in order to examine brain mechanisms. Finally, an overview of the prominent clinical and scientific applications for using MEG and EEG is provided. These applications focus on the use of novel electrophysiological methods in presurgical planning and to advance the understanding of psychopathology and cognitive deficit.

Brief History of EEG and MEG

Electroencephalography

The first attempt to study electrical activity of the brain is credited to a British physician, Richard Caton (1842–1926) (Brazier, 1961), who studied electrical properties of the exposed brains of rabbits and monkeys. His two cardinal reports appeared in the *British Medical Journal* in 1875 and 1877 (Caton, 1875, 1877). By placing two electrodes on the surface of the brain or, alternatively, via one electrode on the cortex and one on the skull and using a galvanometer and beam of light for visualization (Caton, 1877), he demonstrated that "currents of varying direction pass through the amplifier" (Brazier, 1961). This landmark work represented the discovery of basic EEG constituents (Niedermeyer, 2005).

During the late 1920s, EEG enjoyed relatively widespread research exploration, and in 1929, Hans Berger, a German psychiatrist, was the first to report observing and recording the alpha rhythm from human brain (Niedermeyer, 2005). Berger's work was significantly confounded by the limited technology of his day, but by using a string galvanometer in his instrumentation, he laid the foundation for later EEG work. Initially, Berger used a one-channel bipolar EEG recording that included one electrode placed on the frontal and one on the occipital part of the patient's scalp, an EKG channel, and a time marker. His initial recordings included a few minutes of brain activity recorded, containing the alpha rhythm intermixed with some faster beta activity, on photographic paper. With this early work as the foundation, EEG became the standard in clinical diagnostics of brain disorders from the mid-1930s through the mid-1970s, and research applying EEG to examine cerebral functioning became widespread (Niedermeyer, 2005). With the emergence of structural imaging in the mid-1970s, the clinical application of EEG diminished and became restricted in its use to specific areas of neurology for examining epilepsy, sleep disorders, encephalopathy, and brain injury (Quinonez, 1998). In the past decade, EEG research methods have advanced to include an increasing number of electrodes, resulting in increased spatial resolution for examining neural activity. Today, EEG continues to make important contributions to scientific discovery and clinical practice.

Magnetoencephalography

The foundation for examining human neural activity based on using its magnetic manifestations was initiated in 1968 when an MIT physicist, David Cohen, reported observations of human alpha activity using a single MEG sensor and recording it within a multilayer magnetically shielded chamber (Cohen, 1968). Incidentally, Cohen would later contribute seminal work to the development of the field of biomagnetism (Cohen, 1972; Cohen & Halgren, 2003). However, it was not until the 1980s when four New York University researchers, Williamson, Kaufman, Romani, and Okada, were credited with establishing the theory, principles, and usefulness of MEG in studying cerebral functioning (Okada et al., 1982, 1984; Romani et al., 1982; Williamson & Kaufman, 1987).

In a series of experiments in the 1980s and 1990s, Okada and his coworkers made critical contributions to the understanding of the physiological origin of neuromagnetic signals and provided empirical support for theoretical assumptions used in EEG and MEG data interpretation (Okada, 2003). Using a single-channel MEG system, Okada and colleagues performed the first measurements of the magnetic fields generated by dendritic input from an *in vitro* turtle cerebellum preparation (Okada et al., 1987). In these studies, they confirmed that a measured magnetic field had two extrema orthogonal to the electric current flow and they correctly predicted the strength of the magnetic field generated by a 2–4 mm² area of active neuronal tissue (Okada & Nicholson, 1988a, 1988b). In subsequent studies using the same model they demonstrated magnetic field distribution, confirmed that magnetic signal is generated by the sources positioned in parallel ("tangential") to the bath surface (Purkinje cells) and were also able to confirm the presumed relationship between the orientation of a given signal source and corresponding magnetic fields (Okada et al., 1989). After their further improving *in vitro* understanding of the underlying processes and corresponding magnetic fields using hippocampal guinea pig slices and a high-resolution MEG system (Okada et al., 1994, 1997; Okada, Xu, 1996; Wu & Okada, 1998), it was critical to confirm these *in vitro* findings in an *in vivo* model. To do so, Okada and colleagues used MEG and EEG concurrently in their piglet brain model in order to test the cardinal assumptions used to interpret integrative MEG and EEG data (Okada et al., 1999b). This important series of studies revealed critical information about MEG and EEG signal sources. The signal from each of these techniques provides complementary information about the signal sources, with EEG picking up signals generated in gyri and sulci, and MEG mostly signals from sulci (Okada et al., 1999a, 1999b).

Since that time, validation of MEG has resulted in greater scientific and clinical application. Three companies (4-D NeuroImaging [San Diego, California], VSM MedTech Ltd. [Vancouver, Canada], and Elekta Neuromag Oy [Helsinki, Finland]) now manufacture commercial MEG equipment. As of April 2006, there were between 90 and 100 MEG installations worldwide. Although Japan has about one-third of the world's MEG systems, the United States hosts 30 functional installations at this point, and about 20 of these are the systems of the latest generation.

Methods in EEG and MEG

Despite the recent advances in structural and functional neuroimaging techniques such as functional magnetic resonance imaging (fMRI) and positron emission tomography (PET), EEG and MEG continue to maintain important methodological advantages. For example, in contrast to the fMRI signal, which measures the delayed hemodynamic response associated with neural firing, EEG and MEG represent direct measurements of neural activity (Table 3.1). Because of this, EEG and MEG provide unparalleled temporal resolution on the order of milliseconds. Scalp-recorded EEG has been used extensively in research, clinical neurophysiology, and practice, but its spatial resolution

TABLE 3.1. Comparative Summary of the Key Features of MEG and EEG

Feature	MEG	EEG
Reference dependence	Free	Dependent
Sources of signal	Tangential (mostly)	Radial > > > Tangential
Distortion by the intervening tissues	No	Significant
Necessary active cortex	Probably < 1 cm^2; < 4–5 cm^2	~6 cm^2 (scalp)
Temporal resolution	Milliseconds	10s–100s ms (scalp); ms (iEEG)
Spatial resolution	Millimeters	10s mm (scalp); mm (iEEG)
Number of sensors	100 to > 500	Up to 128
Electrode placement	No	Yes
Environment	Critical (shielded room)	(Relatively) unimportant
Duration of recording	Limited	Unlimited
Data analysis	Laborious, source based	Simpler, mostly visual
Mobility	Fixed within a shielded room	Portable/mobile
Equipment cost	$2–3 million	$20,000–40,000
Reimbursement	$Several thousand	$10s (routine)–1,000s (vEEG, iEEG)

Note. iEEG, invasive EEG; vEEG, video EEG. Data from Vrba and Robinson (2001), Barkley (2004), and Baumgartner (2004).

remains poor because the electrical signal generated by synchronized neural activity is attenuated and distorted by intervening tissue such as the cerebrospinal fluid (CSF), dura, skull, and scalp. The combination of insulating properties of the skull and conduction properties of the scalp has a major role in this. One method for improving spatial resolution of EEG is the use of *invasive monitoring* that includes a placement of subdural and/or depth electrodes for more direct recording of spontaneous or evoked neural activity (Spencer et al., 1997). However, the poor spatial resolution of *scalp EEG* and risks associated with *invasive EEG* necessitated the search for an alternative method providing the temporal resolution afforded by EEG while improving its spatial resolution. Like EEG, MEG directly measures neural activity, but spatial resolution is improved because the signal is not distorted by intervening tissue (Okada et al., 1999b). In addition, during routine EEG interpretation the examiner performs a mental reconstruction of the recorded signal from the electrodes and deduces the location of its underlying source. MEG data analysis requires computations of signals from hundreds of sensors and integration of all signals while adhering to restrictions placed on the data by the model of the source and conductor. This algorithm calculates the most probable localization of the source meeting these requirements and superimposes the results on to a computer-reconstructed (3D) volumetric MRI. This process of co-registering MRI and MEG data is termed "magnetic source imaging" (MSI), and it provides a spatial resolution measured in millimeters. An important caveat to understanding the contribution made by MEG to examining electrophysiological data is that the magnetic signal decays very quickly as it travels from the origin (approximately $1/r^2$ to $1/r^3$, depending on which field component is measured, where r is the distance from the source). Therefore, although MEG has improved temporal and spatial resolution as compared with noninvasive EEG, because of the cancellation effects by symmetry and the rapid magnetic signal decay it is not yet a reliable method for measuring neural activity generated in deep brain structures. Furthermore, the MEG signal is distorted by competing biological (within the brain and body) and external (from the earth, electrical equipment, moving magnetic objects) magnetic fields, whereas the EEG signal is not affected by these influences. For these reasons, MEG has been used in a complementary fashion with EEG to improve spatial resolution for surface structures while maintaining excellent temporal resolution (Rose et al., 1987).

EEG and MEG Signal Sources

The EEG signal represents an *extracellular* field potential produced by summated postsynaptic activity (i.e., excitatory and inhibitory postsynaptic potentials) of the cortical pyramidal cells (Buzsáki et al., 2003). In order to detect an EEG "spike" (a sharply contoured EEG waveform lasting 20–70 ms) while recording over the intact scalp, a synchronous firing of a 6 cm^2 cortical area is necessary (Cooper et al., 1965). In contrast, the MEG signal is thought to represent dominantly the magnetic field corresponding to the *intracellular* electrical activity. The reasons for this are complex cancellation effects of various magnetic components produced by the extracellular electrical activity and head geometry (Williamson & Kaufman, 1987).

To better understand the mechanics leading to the detectable EEG and/or MEG signals on the scalp (EEG) or outside of the skull (MEG), a basic law of physics that determines the orthogonal relationship between electrical currents and their corresponding magnetic fields is helpful to consider. This law is the "right-hand rule" of physics, and it illustrates the fundamental mutual relationship between electric currents and magnetic fields using a linear conductor (Figures 3.1A and B). According to the right-hand rule of physics, if one grasps a conductor by encircling the fingers around it, while pointing the thumb in the direction of its current, then the direction of the fingers illustrates the direction of the magnetic vector field (Figure 3.1B). In Figure 3.1, the primary sources of the EEG and MEG signals are the same—synchronously moving charged electrical particles that constitute the basic neural processes and their corresponding extracellular (EEG) and intracellular (MEG) electrical currents and corresponding fields. If neuronal sources—synchronously firing assemblies of mutually parallel neuronal cells—are con-

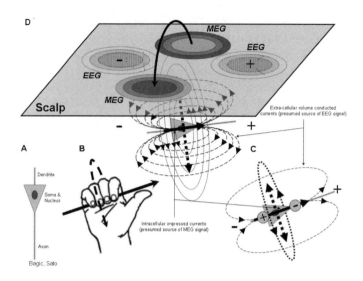

FIGURE 3.1. The relationship between EEG and MEG signals (based on Vrba & Robinson, 2001). (A) Simplified representation of a neuronal cell with its key anatomical elements. (B) The right-hand rule of physics: If the hand is wrapped around a conductor (in this case, a neuronal cell represented by the thick solid line) with the extended thumb parallel to it representing the direction of the electrical current flow (thick solid arrow), then the fingers point in the direction of the corresponding magnetic field (thick broken arrow) in the orthogonal plane. (C) Depiction of the electrical and magnetic fields as applied on a neuronal cell symbolically representing tens of thousands of (nearly) simultaneously activated neuronal cells oriented in the same direction necessary to cause extracranially detectable magnetic signal. (D) Simplified representation of the electrical current (thick solid arrow), corresponding electrical field (broken thin line), and orthogonally positioned (broken thick arrow) magnetic field (dotted thin line), along with their respective surface manifestation as seen by EEG electrodes (EEG –, EEG +) and magnetic sensors (thick curved arrow from MEG outflow to MEG inflow).

ceptualized as a linear conductor, this law describes how EEG and MEG detect the same primary ionic currents from orthogonal positions and explains how the source orientation determines its "visibility" in each modality (outlined below).

   There are important differences in the anatomical sources of the signals for EEG and MEG (Plate 3.2). In EEG, the source of the signal emanates from parallel assemblies of pyramidal cells that are arranged radially and, to a somewhat lesser extent, tangentially to the skull surface. Cell assemblies along the crest of a cortical gyrus are considered radial within the sphere approximating the shape of the cranium and represent about 30% of the cortex cell assemblies (Plate 3.2A). Cell assemblies within the wall of a sulcus are considered "tangential" sources and constitute 70% of the cortex (Plate 3.2B). This is an anatomical approximation that is extended to the physiology assuming that pyramidal cells and their dendrites are evenly distributed along the cortex. Whereas EEG measures sources from both radial and tangential orientations (but predominantly from radial sources), MEG favors the tangential sources. Magnetic fields created by tangential sources (parallel to the skull surface) spread outside of the skull toward sensors. In contrast, magnetic fields generated by radial sources do not spread outward toward sensors (Nunez, 1995). Because the extracellular currents (presumed source of EEG signal; Figures 3.1C and 3.1D) are distributed throughout the volume of tissues in which the active neuron is contained (a phenomenon known as volume conduction), they can be recorded from the brain using EEG electrodes that are "seeing" the potential at its location with respect to a distant "indifferent" electrode placed in a relatively inactive area (Holsheimer & Feenstra, 1977). In sum, EEG and MEG quantify the same neuronal processes from two orthogonal positions, and their measurements are therefore most informative when they are combined during data acquisition and analysis.

Instrumentation and Recording Techniques of EEG and MEG

EEG measures electrical brain activity via electrodes placed on the scalp, on the surface of the brain (Plate 3.1C), or at specific sites in the neural tissue ("invasive EEG"; Plate 3.1C). Two EEG electrodes create one EEG channel, and the difference in the signal between the two electrodes provides information about extracellular field potentials (Cooper et al., 1980). In noninvasive EEG, electrodes may be applied to the scalp individually or as a part of an electrode cap, where electrodes are preattached (Le et al., 1998). In clinical cases, such as epilepsy, encephalopathy, or coma, electrode montages (predefined sets of mutually connected electrodes) are well standardized. In research settings, routine applications include 20 or more electrodes, and some experimental procedures may include up to 128 electrodes. Moreover, additional electrodes and alternative settings for recording data (Misulis, 1989), or even special instruments such as microelectrodes (Vanhatalo et al., 2003; Worrell et al., 2004), may be used, depending on the experimental question. Advances in digital technology have made it possible to accommodate an increasing number of channels and amount of data (Van Cott & Brenner, 1998).

Duration of EEG data collection can vary dramatically. Typically, EEG is recorded with the person in the supine position for only 30 min ("routine EEG"), but data can be collected over the course of a day to examine brain function during normal daily activity ("24-h EEG" or "ambulatory EEG"), or even for a few weeks in hospital settings ("video-EEG monitoring" performed in an epilepsy monitoring unit; EMU). For a more extensive review of EEG methods, see Gevin and Remond (1987), and for applications relevant to clinical disorders such as epilepsy, see Delgado-Escueta et al. (1986).

As noted, MEG records very weak magnetic fields of the brain, which are on the order of picotesla (10^{-12} tesla) to femtotesla (10^{-15} tesla), or roughly $1/10^9$–$1/10^6$ of the earth's magnetic field (Nakaya & Mori, 1992). In order to measure the minute magnetic fields produced by intracellular currents, MEG makes use of a device called the superconducting quantum interference device (SQUID; Silver & Zimmerman, 1965). The superconducting condition (Kammerling Onnes, 1911) requires a state where there is no resistance to the flow of electrical current (Josephson, 1962). This state can be attained by cooling down the alloy containing metal niobium (Nb, atomic number 41) to a temperature of liquid helium (4.2°K; –269°C, –484°F) (Clarke, 1993). SQUIDs are very sensitive to a number of sources of environmental noise, and these signals are significantly stronger than the biological signals to be measured. Thus, the elimination of signal contamination by environmental noise is essential and is achieved by using a magnetically shielded room (Cohen et al., 2002; Zimmerman & Silver, 1964). The shielded room used in MEG is a multilayered structure built from an alloy called "mu metal," which provides a low-reluctance path for surrounding environmental magnetic fields. Some modern shielded rooms include additional electronic components for "active shielding" (Yumoto, 2000).

A SQUID is attached to a coil or combination of coils, often referred to as flux transformers. If a coil has a simple circular or square configuration, it is considered a magnetometer—a sensor that is sensitive to the near and far magnetic fields. When a coil configuration includes two loops connected in series but wound in opposite directions, the sensor is called a gradiometer. If the loops are next to each other in a horizontal plane, the sensor is called a planar gradiometer, and if the coils are one above the other, the sensor is called an axial gradiometer. Whereas magnetometers measure an "absolute" magnetic flux (fT), gradiometers measure a magnetic "gradient" in fT/cm. An MEG sensor may be a combination of round coils of 15–20 mm in diameter (in VSM systems; Fife et al., 2002; Vrba & Robinson, 2001) or in the form of an integrated "triple sensor" that includes a magnetometer and two planar gradiometers (in Elekta Neuromag systems), arranged together in a helmet-shaped distribution (Nenonen et al., 2004). In practice, the performance of any MEG system is dependent on the number of sensors, their mutual arrangements, helmet geometry, associated electronics, and analytical algorithms. Although rare systems with fewer than 100 sensors are still in use, the latest models of whole-head MEG systems have 248 (4D-Neuromaging), 275 (VSM-CTF), or 306 (Elekta Neuromag, Figure 3.2) sensors. By increasing the number of sensors, spatial resolution is often improved. It should be noted that current mathematical modeling studies suggest that the current technology and the number of sensors applied may have reached a "practical plateau" in the relationship between the number of sensors and spatial resolution (Nenonen et al., 2004). This implies that further expansion in the number of sensors much beyond 300 would not necessarily provide a practical advan-

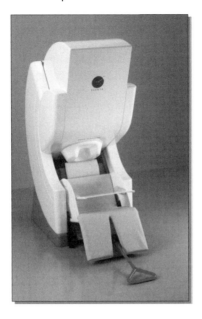

FIGURE 3.2. An example of a modern MEG system positioned for seated recording. The latest generation of Elekta Neuromag MEG system (Vectorview 306 channels with a 128-EEG channels module, Elekta Neuromag Oy, Helsinki, Finland). Like all modern systems, this one can be positioned for recording in seated (shown) or supine position. Photo kindly provided by Elekta Neuromag.

tage. Even so, there are early indications that the next generation of MEG systems may have a 500-channel capability (Della Penna et al., 2004).

The Inverse Problem in EEG and MEG

The goal of EEG and MEG is to localize intracranial signal sources and to monitor their activity based on activity recorded extracranially. However, multiple neural sources or source combinations may produce similar or even identical potentials (observed with EEG) or magnetic fields (observed with MEG). Thus, the source of the neural activity is difficult to determine because more than one source configuration could account for the observed activity. This is known as the *inverse problem* of electroencephalography and magnetoencephalography, or a problem without a unique solution. Thus when EEG or MEG is used to examine neural processes, the electrical potential or magnetic field detected outside the brain will give only an estimate for the source of the signal (Vrba & Robinson, 2001; Williamson & Kaufman 1987) (Plate 3.3).

To limit the number of possible solutions for determining the source of neural activity, assumptions must be made about the signal source and its surroundings (in this case, the head). Before solving the inverse problem, one has to solve the forward problem (Hämäläinen & Sarvas, 1989; Hämäläinen et al., 1992). This implies calculating expected output of the gradiometers assuming activity of a certain region of cortex. For this purpose, the head has routinely been modeled as a plain sphere. However, continued efforts are being made to use the true shape of the cranium as a realistic model to improve localization and anatomical correlation (Rose et al., 1987). Specifically, an inverse solution can be achieved by modeling the source as a single point with two extrema. This single point is called an equivalent current dipole (ECD, or simply "dipole") and may be conceptualized as a "center of gravity" for a given active region. Ultimately, the exact locations of these dipoles in the head are calculated and are marked on a reconstructed 3D MRI image, which is known as "source localization." This modeling simplification makes very complex computations feasible. Through an iterative process, an algorithm computes best-matching dipole location and calculates a measure called "goodness of fit" that tells how well the dipole model accounts for the measured MEG and EEG data. As previously stated, the ECD is used most frequently as the source model, and a simple sphere as the head model. Because a singular point (i.e., the ECD) cannot accurately represent the complex arrangements of neural inputs and a simple sphere (i.e., the model for the head) is far from a realistic representation of the outer shape of the human brain, there are several assumptions made in order to accommodate these significant discrepancies. These assumptions vary, depending on unique physiological parameters, as well as the source and head model implemented. The most common assumption is that a focal brain activity can be modeled by a single source represented as focal point (ECD) generated within a simple sphere that approximates the brain. When testing the models, any computed sources of signals not meeting these requirements are rejected. Because neural sources are frequently too complex to be explained by a single ECD, attempts are made to use models with multiple dipoles (Barth et al., 1984). The methods described here for improving an inverse solution originated in the EEG literature but have been successfully applied to MEG data analysis. (For a more comprehensive review of the inverse methods, see Darvas et al., 2004, and Faugeras et al., 2004).

There are other methods that do not rely on an explicit model of the neural sources, instead employing spatial filters such as beam formers. One such method is synthetic aperture magnetometry (SAM), recently developed by Robinson and Vrba (1998). Unlike the ECD model, SAM takes into account the temporospatial relationship between various characteristics of recorded activity (e.g., "sharpness") and provides visualization of their statistical distribution. SAM is more appropriate for assessing general regions of neural activity or for determining laterality of brain activation, and may be useful for research questions that do not require detailed localization or those that involve wide or multiregional activity. In these cases, SAM is preferred because it is potentially capable of revealing the involvement of different brain regions instead of providing only the "center of gravity" (Plate 3.3G). A more recent and perhaps more powerful beam former method called DICS (dynamic imaging of coherent sources; Gross et al., 2001) is getting increasing popularity. A group of analytical methods that try to explain the measured data without a priori knowledge about the number, locations, and strength of the potential underlying sources is known as minimum norm estimates (MNE; Hämäläinen & Ilmoniemi, 1994; Sekihara & Scholz, 1995). While the conceptual details of these methods are beyond the scope of this chapter, it is important to bring them into readers' attention, since they are very powerful research tools: LORETA (low-resolution electromagnetic tomography; Pascual-Marqui et al., 1994), MCE (minimum current estimate; Uutela et al., 1998), dSPM (dynamic statistical parametric mapping; Dale et al., 2000), LAURA (local auto regressive average; Grave de Peralta Menendez et al., 2001; Lantz et al., 2001); EPIFOCUS (Grave de Peralta Menendez et al., 2001; Lantz et al., 2001), and sLORETA (standardized low-resolution brain electromagnetic tomography; Pascual-Marqui, 2002).

As discussed above, MEG may not be able to localize deeper signal sources because of cancellation and rapid decay of magnetic field strength, whereas EEG can provide information about activity in deeper brain structures. For example, results from a recent simulation modeling study suggested that EEG is superior for localizing mesial temporal signal sources, whereas MEG is ideal for localizing frontal (and generally neocortical) sources (de Munck et al., 2004). Again, improved source localization supports the complementary nature of these two applications (Baillet et al., 1999). The key differences between EEG and MEG are summarized in Table 3.1.

High-Frequency EEG and MEG Signals

Conventionally, any frequency range above 70 Hz is ignored or filtered when using EEG. However, recent literature suggests that several high-frequency oscillations (HFOs), up to 200, 300, and even 800 Hz, may have physiological significance (Bragin et al., 1999; Buzsaki, 1989, 1996; Buzsaki et al., 1992; Curio, 2002; Curio et al., 1994; Engel et al., 2003; Grenier et al., 2001, 2003; Lisman & Idiart, 1995; Llinas, 1988). Spontaneous 200-Hz HFOs were convincingly demonstrated for the first time in the electrophysiological recordings performed by Buzsaki et al. (1992), and, using MEG, Curio and coworkers (1994) presented the first noninvasive recording of HFOs associated with somatosensory evoked potentials. Since that time, a series of invasive electrophysiological EEG studies in humans has demonstrated fast oscillations of up to 800 Hz frequencies (Bragin et al., 1999, 2002; Engel et al., 2003; Fisher et al., 1992; Grenier et al., 2003; Ponomarenko et al., 2003; Staba et al., 2002; Worrell et al., 2004). These high-frequency signals have been referred to as gamma ripples or fast ripples. Some recent work has linked a frequency range of 20–120 Hz with visual processing (Munk & Neuenschwander, 2000), a frequency of ~200 Hz with memory function (Draguhn et al., 2000), and ~600 Hz with somatosensory evoked potentials (Curio, 2000) and localization-related epilepsy (Bragin et al., 2002).

To date, the physiological role of HFOs has been implicated in learning (Lisman & Idiart, 1995; Llinas, 1988), memory consolidation (Bragin et al., 1999; Buzsaki, 1989, 1996; Grenier et al., 2001), and somatosensory evoked potentials (Curio, 2000). Recent invasive work has revealed a potentially important association between HFOs and seizures in cases of epilepsy (Bragin et al., 1999, 2002; Engel et al., 2003; Fisher et al., 1992; Grenier et al., 2003; Ponomarenko et al., 2003; Staba et al., 2002, Worrell et al., 2004). Fast ripples may represent a new marker of epileptogenesis once their acquisition is optimized and their correlation with epileptogenesis established (Engel et al., 2003). Thus, there have been important advances in the understanding of higher-frequency electrophysiological responses, and MEG and EEG provide the opportunity to fully characterize their role in cognitive, motor, and sensory functioning.

Applications of EEG and MEG in Medicine and Clinical Research

The application of MEG in clinical research has increased dramatically over the last several years (Halgreen et al., 2004). In fact, MEG is at times chosen over EEG to answer selected clinical research questions, but the cost of equipment and its operation (a modern MEG system is at least 50 times more expensive than most expensive EEG equipment) make its use almost prohibitive for small institutions. Because of its unparalleled spatiotemporal resolution, MEG holds significant promise for clinical interventions. An increasing number of health insurers are reimbursing for the use of MEG during seizure localization procedures and for presurgical brain mapping. Even so, widespread application of MEG in clinical diagnostics and interventions has yet to be firmly established. Common MEG applications are listed in Table 3.2 (see also Plate 3.3).

Presurgical Planning

EEG is an essential tool in the evaluation of epilepsy, particularly when recorded simultaneously with video in the setting of long-term monitoring over several days or weeks (known as video EEG; *v-EEG*). In these cases, patient behavior during seizures is correlated with concomitant EEG activity, referred to as "electroclinical correlation," providing important information to aid in localizing the source of eleptiform activity and in defining the epileptic syndrome. When surface electrode recording fails to localize the seizure origin, direct recording from the brain surface or within the brain substance

**TABLE 3.2. General Summary of MEG
Research and Clinical Applications**

MEG research applications

Spontaneous MEG brain activity
Cognitive processes
    Language
    Memory
    Sensory processing
    Other cognitive processes
Evoked magnetic fields
    Somatosensory
    Auditory
    Visual
Epilepsy
Cortical plasticity
Movement physiology
Pain
Psychiatric and cognitive disorders
    Schizophrenia
    Depression
    Anxiety
    Dementia
Traumatic brain injury
High-frequency signals
DC MEG
Fetal MEG (fMEG)
Magnetocardiography (MCG)[a]

MEG clinical applications[b]

Epilepsy
Presurgical functional brain mapping (PFBM)

Note. Based in part on Halgreen et al. (2004).
[a] MCG is a part of the biomagnetism, but not MEG
method per se.
[b] At this point (August 2006), epilepsy and PFBM are
the only approved clinical applications.

using subdural or depth electrodes (*invasive monitoring*) may be used (Engel, 1993). Separately, long-term video EEG monitoring has been used to monitor unconscious patients in neurointensive care units. In these clinical settings, video EEG serves to detect clinically unrecognizable seizures (nonconvulsive *status epilepticus*) and may be used to monitor recovery from coma (Jordan, 1999; Vespa et al., 1999; Young & Campbell, 1999, Mizrahi & Lesser, 2003). Video EEG is indispensable when invasive electrode placement is required for seizure localization (Spencer et al., 1997; Sperling & Shewmon, 1997).

    Quantitative EEG is a method whereby EEG data are digitally processed and quantified using various mathematical functions according to the features of interest (frequencies, amplitudes, fields, etc.). Subsequently, this form of

EEG analysis can provide corresponding topographic maps (e.g., power in various frequency bands, voltage maps), thus providing additional means for studying brain function (Nuwer, 1998). For instance, frequency spectral mapping, or spatial distribution of the signal frequency, may be useful to evaluate patients with cerebrovascular diseases and dementia (Nuwer, 1997, 1998).

A recent review by Michel et al. (2004) describes the various methods of EEG source localization. EEG source localization of epileptiform discharges has been examined by Scherg et al. (1999), who revealed that the identification of the cortical generators of the earliest phase of interictal spikes is most plausible when combining the temporal evolution of EEG scalp topography, multiple coexisting sources, and the information from localization and orientation of ECD sources.

An important methodology used to facilitate seizure focus localization and surgical treatment of epilepsy is *intraoperative electrocorticography*. In intraoperative electrocorticography, EEG data are acquired directly from the brain surface during epilepsy surgery. These EEG data are used to confirm the existence of interictal epileptiform discharges and to aid in the presurgical localization of the discharging focus. Electrocorticography can also assist in the mapping of functional anatomy by monitoring their responses upon electrical stimulation of a particular brain area in patients who are alert during surgery (Chatrian, 2003). Of note, *long-term invasive monitoring* using subdural and/or depth electrodes is a routine clinical application as well and offers an opportunity to examine the EEG signal over a long period and outside the operating room. This procedure provides an opportunity for data collection at time of seizure onset in order to localize seizure onset zones (Spencer et al., 1997). Furthermore, this method of EEG monitoring allows for functional-anatomical mapping to localize eloquent cortex (vital brain centers; Spencer et al., 1997).

A number of recent studies have validated the use of MEG in the surgical treatment of epilepsy, and it has been clinically approved for seizure localization and presurgical planning in epilepsy. Work by Wheless et al. (1999) studied 58 patients with refractory partial epilepsy and found the MEG dipole localization method to be a promising presurgical diagnostic technique. When combined with positron emission tomography (PET), MEG can provide additional information about the location of epileptogenic zones (Lamusuo et al., 1999). Recently, MEG has been used to guide the placement of subdural electrodes and to differentiate between patients with mesial and lateral temporal seizure onsets (Pataraia et al., 2002). When an MEG study is performed during a seizure, it is called an *ictal MEG*, which is an important method for seizure assessment when invasive studies are contraindicated (Eliashiv et al., 2002). In a study of 455 patients, the largest compiled cohort published thus far (Stefan et al., 2003), MEG provided otherwise unavailable information in 35% of the patients and "crucial localizing information" in 10%. MEG has been reported to be most useful in presurgical planning for those patients with either a partially localizing or nonlocalizing seizure focus (Pataraia et al.,

2004). In 40% of these cases, additional data about the nature of the seizures were acquired with MEG. For more details about MEG applications in epilepsy, the reader is referred to one of the recent comprehensive reviews (Barkley, 2004; Barkley & Baumgartner, 2003; Baumgartner, 2004; Knowlton & Shih, 2004).

MEG has proven very useful for brain mapping of primary motor and somatosensory cortical areas (Plate 3.3H). For example, Hari and Kaukoranta (1985) were the first to study the somatosensory cortex using MEG, and Morioka et al. (1995) provided the first investigations of motor evoked potentials using MEG. When combined with magnetic resonance (MR) images, MEG data from the sensorimotor cortex has been incorporated into an intraoperative neuronavigational system that informs neurosurgical strategies (Ganslandt et al., 1999). Several groups have worked to establish MEG algorithms for standardization of noninvasive brain mapping in surgical cases (Baumgartner et al., 1991; Hari, 1991; Lopes da Silva et al., 1991; Sato & Smith, 1985, Castillo et al., 2004). These efforts aim to maximize the information available in regard to functional neuroanatomy for presurgical planning.

Important work has applied MEG to examine separate areas of sensory functioning. Using MEG, the somatosensory homunculus has been detailed (Nakamura et al., 1998), gustatory evoked magnetic fields have been examined (Saito et al., 1998), and the somatosensory, auditory, and visual evoked magnetic fields have been studied in patients with brain diseases (Nakasato & Yoshimoto, 2000). This body of work subsequently led to a comprehensive MEG protocol for studying evoked responses (Castillo et al., 2004).

In sum, MEG is becoming an increasingly popular noninvasive method for brain mapping in patients with epilepsy, cerebral tumors, or other brain disorders. MEG applications have simplified presurgical planning and are beginning to replace invasive procedures for brain mapping of primary motor and language areas. By integrating MEG brain mapping data with a neurosurgical navigational system, clinical investigators are working to improve accuracy and minimize invasiveness of the neurosurgical procedures (Ganslandt et al., 1999; Jannin et al., 2002).

Assessment of the Functional Integrity of the Neural Axis Using Evoked Potentials Recorded by EEG

Routine evoked potentials relevant to clinical evaluation include somatosensory, visual, and brainstem auditory evoked potentials (Chiappa, 1997). *Somatosensory evoked potentials* (SSEPs) have been used routinely in clinical settings to evaluate sensory pathways by stimulating the median and posterior tibial nerves. SSEPs are a very helpful clinical tool for quick, noninvasive assessment of the integrity of the posterior columns of the spinal cord that conduct vibration and position senses from the peripheral stimulated nerves (most frequently, the median nerve on the arm and tibial on the leg) to the cortex. Considering that this is a critical white matter tract that spans the entire neural axis, information about its integrity is often critical to assess and a variety of symptomatologies may occur due to lesions anywhere along its path. The components of somatosensory evoked potentials have been the target of intensive research (Mauguiere, 2000; Restuccia, 2000; Sonoo, 2000; Yamada, 2000). Separately, *visual evoked potentials* (VEPs) provide an opportunity to evaluate the status of the optic nerve and are recorded from the occipital lobe. Responses are evoked by stimulating each eye with shifting checkerboard patterns or strobe flashes. For evaluation of the postchiasmatic pathway, half of the visual field needs to be stimulated (Epstein, 2003). The latency and amplitude of P100 (100 ms after stimulation) are measured most frequently and may be used clinically to diagnose optic nerve injury secondary to inflammation, trauma, or tumors. *Auditory evoked potentials* (AEPs) examine the latency in the response to the stimulus and can be divided into short-latency (≤ 10 ms), middle-latency (10–50 ms) and long-latency (≥ 50 ms) responses (Spehlmann, 1985). The short-latency response, or the *brainstem auditory evoked potential* (BAEP), is the response of primary interest in clinical practice. BAEPs have been used extensively to evaluate hearing in infants because the same level of "cooperation" required by standard audiometric methods is not required (Celesia & Brigell, 1993). Middle- and long-latency potentials are typically the focus of research examining basic auditory processing

Clinical Research Applications of MEG

The usefulness MEG to study cortical plasticity was first investigated by Weiss et al. (1997). Rossini and colleagues (1998) used MEG successfully in studying the reorganization of the sensory hand areas following a unilateral hemispheric lesion in humans, and Ramachandran and Hirstein (1998) proposed its use in elucidating the mechanisms responsible for "phantom limb syndrome," Druschky et al. (2002) in studying poststroke cortical reorganization, and Cornelissen et al. (2003) in studying adult brain plasticity seen following anomia treatment. Ishibashi et al. (2002) successfully employed MEG to asses the severity of the cortical lamination defects in hemimegalencephaly. Kujala et al. (2003) studied plastic cortical changes induced by patients' learning to communicate with nonspeech sounds, and Osaki et al. (2004) studied the cortical processing of tactile language in a deaf–blind subject. Taken together, these studies demonstrate the rapidly developing array of applications for using MEG to elucidate functional recovery mechanisms in cases of brain injury and disease.

MEG has also been applied to the investigation of psychiatric disorders. Specifically, MEG measurement of the spontaneous brain activity in schizophrenia was initiated almost a decade ago (Canive et al., 1996; Hajek et al., 1997). Subsequently, MEG has been used to examine the role of slow wave activity in schizophrenia (Fehr et al., 2001) and the influence of medications on patients with schizophrenia (Canive et al., 1998; Sperling et al., 1999). Ishii and colleagues examined increases in theta rhythm in the left superior temporal cortex as evidence for a source of auditory hallucinations in individuals diagnosed with schizophrenia (Ishii et al., 2000). Separately, the use of electroconvulsive shock therapy to treat depression has been examined in a few studies using MEG (Heikman et al., 2001; Sperling et al., 2000). Results indicate that efficient ECT treatment is associated with increases in MEG theta activity (3–7 Hz) in the frontal cortex (Heikman et al., 2001). Other examiners have noted increases in the slow activity (0–7 Hz) in the frontal and temporal regions of patients with depression after electroconvulsive therapy (ECT) and decreased the fast activity (12.5–30 Hz) in the temporal and parietal regions (Sperling et al., 2000).

A potentially important clinical research application of MEG has been the examination of fetal development. Fetal MEG auditory evoked fields from 27 pregnant, healthy women (third trimester of an uncomplicated pregnancy) revealed reproducible results across subjects and shows promise for using fetal MEG to assess prenatal development (Schneider et al., 2001). Recent advances have demonstrated that fetal MEG can be used to examine the development of the fetal auditory responses. Such responses provide both early indicators of potential auditory abnormalities and some insights into the nature of underlying abnormalities (Holst et al., 2005; Draganova et al., 2005). Finally, recent work demonstrated that fetal MEG can be used to follow development of the visual system as early as 28 wk gestation (Eswaran et al., 2004). The use of MEG in examining a variety of clinical disorders has proliferated greatly over the past decade (Makela et al., 2006; Bieier et al., 2006). The superior spatiotemporal resolution provided by MEG and its noninvasiveness (Plate 3.1A) make it extraordinarily useful in the identification and characterization of a wide array of neurological abnormalities

Concluding Remarks

The goal of this chapter was to provide a brief overview of the theory and principles of EEG and MEG and their experimental and clinical applications. These two most potent functional techniques measure electric (EEG) and magnetic (MEG) manifestations of the same cellular events. Although "head-to-head" comparisons of EEG and MEG have proven methodologically challenging, it does appear that their identical use provides comparable temporal and spatial resolution. Ultimately, the simplicity and versatility of EEG, and the temporal and spatial resolution of routine MEG, provide more information combined than either of these methods individually. The most important example of this is in the clinical examination of epileptic foci in patients with epilepsy. The superior temporal and spatial resolution that can be attained noninvasively using MEG is improving the invasive application of EEG (by guiding subdural EEG electrode placement), the accuracy and outcome of surgical interventions (by providing very accurate functional maps for intraoperative neuronavigation), and may even replace invasive methods in some cases (by providing the same or better data noninvasively). EEG and MEG continue to provide clinicians, as well as basic and applied researchers, with invaluable tools to examine real-time neural processes. With the integration of other imaging techniques (e.g., magnetic resonance imaging; MRI), multimodal imaging is now providing researchers with previously unattainable spatial resolution. Such advancements now allow for more detailed and sophisticated analysis of phenomena in both the basic and applied neurosciences. Although many important research questions about human brain function can be answered by appropriately used EEG, MEG is an ideal method for studying neural processes that require the combination of superb temporal resolution with high spatial resolution.

REFERENCES

Baillet, S., Garnero, L., Marin, G., et al. (1999). Combined MEG and EEG source imaging by minimization of mutual information. *IEEE Transactions on Biomedical Engineering, 46*, 522–534.

Barkley, G. L. (2004). Controversies in neurophysiology. MEG is superior to EEG in localization of interictal epileptiform activity: Pro. *Clinical Neurophysiology, 115*, 1001–1009.

Barkley, G. L., & Baumgartner, C. (2003). MEG and EEG in epilepsy. *Journal of Clinical Neurophysiology, 20*, 163–178.

Barth, D. S., Sutherling, W., Engle, J., Jr., et al. (1984). Neuromagnetic evidence of spatially distributed sources underlying epileptiform spikes in the human brain. *Science, 223*, 293–296.

Baumgartner, C. (2004). Controversies in clinical neurophysiology. MEG is superior to EEG in the localization of interictal epileptiform activity: Con. *Clinical Neurophysiology, 115*, 1010–1020.

Baumgartner, C., Doppelbauer, A., Deecke, L., et al. (1991). Neuromagnetic investigation of somatotopy of human hand somatosensory cortex. *Experimental Brain Research, 87*, 641–648.

Bragin, A., Engel, J., Jr., Wilson, C. L., et al. (1999). High-frequency oscillations in human brain. *Hippocampus, 9*, 137–42.

Bragin, A., Wilson, C. L., Staba, R. J., et al. (2002). Interictal high-frequency oscillations (80–500 Hz) in the human epileptic brain: Entorhinal cortex. *Annals of Neurology, 52*, 407–415.

Brazier, M. A. B. (1961). *A history of the electrical activity of the brain. The first half-century*. London: Pitman.

Buzsáki, G. (1989). Two-stage model of memory trace formation: A role for "noisy" brain states. *Neuroscience, 31*, 551–570.

Buzsáki, G. (1996). The hippocampo-neocortical dialogue. *Cerebral Cortex, 6*, 81–92.

Buzsáki, G., Horvath, Z., Urioste, R., et al. (1992). High-frequency network oscillation in the hippocampus. *Science, 25*, 1025–1027.

Buzsáki, G., Traub, R. D., & Pedley, T. A. (2003). The cellular basis of EEG activity. In J. S. Ebersole & T. A. Pedley (Eds.), *Current practice of clinical electroencephalography* (3rd ed., pp. 1–11). Philadelphia: Lippincott Williams & Wilkins.

Canive, J. M., Lewine, J. D., Edgar, J. C., et al. (1996). Magnetoencephalographic assessment of spontaneous brain activity in schizophrenia. *Psychopharmacology Bulletin, 32,* 741–50.

Canive, J. M., Lewine, J. D., Edgar, J. C., et al. (1998). Spontaneous brain magnetic activity in schizophrenia patients treated with aripiprazole. *Psychopharmacology Bulletin, 34,* 101–105.

Castillo, E. M., Simos, P. G., Wheless, J. W., et al. (2004). Integrating sensory and motor mapping in a comprehensive MEG protocol: Clinical validity and replicability. *NeuroImage, 21,* 973–983.

Caton, R. (1875). The electrical currents of the brain. *British Medical Journal, 2,* 278.

Caton, R. (1877). Interim report on investigations of the electric currents of the brain. *British Medical Journal* (Suppl. 50), 62–65.

Celesia, G. G., & Brigell, M. (1993). Auditory evoked potentials. In E. Niedermeyer & F. Lopes da Silva (Eds.), *Electroencephalography: Basic principles, clinical applications, and related fields* (3rd ed., pp. 937–956). Baltimore: Williams & Wilkins.

Chatrian, G. E. (2003). Intraoperative electrocorticography. In J. S. Ebersole & T. A. Pedley (Eds.), *Current practice of clinical electroencephalography* (3rd ed., pp. 681–712). Philadelphia: Lippincott Williams & Wilkins.

Chiappa, K. (1997). *Evoked potentials in clinical medicine* (3rd ed.). Philadelphia: Lippincott-Raven.

Clarke, J. (1993). SQUIDs: Theory and practice. In H. Weinstock & R. W. Ralston (Eds.), *The new superconducting electronics* (pp. 123–180). Dordrecht, The Netherlands: Kluwer.

Cohen, D. (1968). Magnetoencephalography: Evidence of magnetic fields produced by alpha-rhythm currents. *Science, 161,* 784–786.

Cohen, D. (1972). Magnetoencephalography: Detection of the brain's electrical activity with a superconducting magnetometer. *Science, 175,* 664–666.

Cohen, D., & Halgren, E. (2003). Magnetoencephalography (Neuromagnetism). In D. Cohen & E. Halgreen (Eds.), *Encyclopedia of neuroscience* (3rd ed., pp. 1–7). Philadelphia: Elsevier.

Cohen, D., Schläpfer, U., Ahlfors, S., et al. New six-layer magnetically-shielded room for MEG. *Biomag2002 Proceedings of the 13th International Conference on Biomagnetism.* Available online at *biomag2002.uni-jena.de/show_proceedings.html*

Cooper, R., Osselton, J. W., Shaw, J. (1980). *EEG technology.* London: Butterworths.

Cooper, R., Winter, A. L., Crow, H. J., et al. (1965). Comparison of subcortical, cortical and scalp activity using chronically indwelling electrodes in man. *Electroencephalography and Clinical Neurophysiology, 18,* 217–228.

Cornelissen, K., Laine, M., Tarkiainen, A., et al. (2003). Adult brain plasticity elicited by anomia treatment. *Journal of Cognitive Neuroscience, 15,* 444–461.

Curio, G. (2000). Linking 600-Hz "spikelike" EEG/MEG wavelets ("sigma-bursts") to cellular substrates: Concepts and caveats. *Journal of Clinical Neurophysiology, 17,* 377–396.

Curio, G., Mackert, B. M., Burghoff, M., et al. (1994). Localization of evoked neuromagnetic 600 Hz activity in the cerebral somatosensory system. *Electroencephalography and Clinical Neurophysiology, 91,* 483–487.

Dale, A. M., Liu, A. K., Fischl, B. R., et al. (2000). Dynamic statistical parametric mapping: Combining fMRI and MEG for high-resolution imaging of cortical activity. *Neuron, 26,* 55–67.

Darvas, F., Pantazis, D., Kucukaltun-Yildirim, E., et al. (2004). Mapping human brain function with MEG and EEG: Methods and validation. *NeuroImage, 23*(S1), S289–S299.

Delgado-Escueta, A. V., Ward, A. A., Woodburyg, D. M., et al. (Eds.). (1986). Basic mechanisms of the epilepsies, molecular and cellular approaches. *Advances in Neurology, 44,* 3–55.

Della Penna, S., Del Gratta, C., Cianflone, F., et al. (2004). A 500 channel MEG system. In E. Halgreen, S. Ahlfors, M. Hämäläinen, & D. Cohen (Eds.), *Proceedings of the 14th International Conference on Biomagnetism* (pp. 619–620). Boston.

de Munck, J. C., de Jongh, A., & Ossenblok, P. (2004). Differences in MEG/EEG epileptic spike yields explained by regional differences in signal to noise ratios. In E. Halgreen, S. Ahlfors, M. Hämäläinen, & D. Cohen (Eds.), *Biomag 2004. Proceedings of the 14th International Conference on Biomagnetism* (p. 746). Boston: Biomag.

Draganova, R., Eswaran, H., Murphy, P., et al. (2005). Sound frequency change detection in fetuses and newborns: A magnetoencephalographic study. *NeuroImage, 28,* 354–361.

Draguhn, A., Traub, R., Bibbig, A., et al. (2000). Ripple (~200-Hz) oscillations in temporal structures. *Journal of Clinical Neurophysiology, 17,* 361–376.

Druschky, K., Kaltenhauser, M., Hummel, C., et al. (2002). Post-apoplectic reorganization of cortical areas processing passive movement and tactile stimulation: A neuromagnetic case study. *Neuroreport, 13,* 2581–2586.

Eliashiv, D. S., Elsas, S. M., Squires, K., et al. (2002). Ictal magnetic source imaging as a localizing tool in partial epilepsy. *Neurology, 59,* 1600–1610.

Engel, J., Jr. (Ed.). (1993). *Surgical treatment of the epilepsies* (2nd ed.). New York: Raven Press.

Engel, J., Jr., Wilson, C., & Bragin, A. (2003). Advances in understanding the process of epileptogenesis based on patient material: What can the patient tell us? *Epilepsia, 44,* 60–71.

Epstein, C. M. (2003). Visual evoked potentials. In J. S. Ebersole & T. A. Pedley (Eds.), *Current practice of clinical electroencephalography* (3rd ed., pp. 833–863). Philadelphia: Lippincott Williams & Wilkins.

Eswaran, H., Lowery, C. L., Wilson, J. D., et al. (2004). Functional development of the visual system in human fetus using magnetoencephalography. *Experimental Neurology,190S1,* S52–S58.

Faugeras, O., Adde, G., Charpiat, G., et al. (2004). Variational, geometric, and statistical methods for modeling brain anatomy and function. *NeuroImage, 23*(S1), S46–S55.

Fehr, T., Kissler, J., Moratti, S., et al. (2001). Source distribution of neuromagnetic slow waves and MEG-delta activity in schizophrenic patients. *Biological Psychiatry, 50,* 108–116.

Fife, A. A., Vrba, J., Robinson, S. E., et al. (2002). A 275 channel whole-cortex MEG system. *Biomag2002 Proceedings.* Available online at *biomag2002.uni-jena.de/ show_proceedings.html*

Fisher, R. S., Webber, W. R., Lesser, R. P., et al. (1992). High-frequency EEG activity at the start of seizures. *Journal of Clinical Neurophysiology, 9,* 441–448.

Ganslandt, O., Fahlbusch, R., Nimsky, C., et al. (1999). Functional neuronavigation with magnetoencephalography: Outcome in 50 patients with lesions around the motor cortex. *Journal of Neurosurgery, 91,* 73–79.

Gevin, A. S., & Remond, A. (1987). *Handbook of electroencephalography and clinical neurophysiology: Vol. 1. Methods of analysis of brain electrical and magnetic signals* (Rev. series). New York: Elsevier.

Grave de Peralta Menendez, R., Gonzalez Andino, S., Lantz, G., et al. (2001). Noninvasive localization of electromagnetic epileptic activity. I. Method descriptions and simulations. *Brain Topography, 14*(2), 131–137.

Grenier, F., Timofeev, I., & Steriade, M. (2001). Focal synchronization of ripples (80–200 Hz) in neocortex and their neuronal correlates. *Journal of Neurophysiology, 86,* 1884–1898.

Grenier, F., Timofeev, I., & Steriade, M. (2003). Neocortical very fast oscillations (ripples, 80–200 Hz) during seizures: Intracellular correlates. *Journal of Neurophysiology, 89,* 841–852.

Gross, J., Kujala, J., Hämäläinen, M. S., et al. (2001). Dynamic imaging of coherent sources: Studying neural interactions in the human brain. *Proceedings of the National Academy of Sciences of the United States of America, 98*(2), 694–699.

Hajek, M., Boehle, C., Huonker, R., et al. (1997). Abnormalities of auditory evoked magnetic fields in the right hemisphere of schizophrenic females. *Schizophrenia Research, 24,* 329–332.

Halgreen, E., Ahlfors, S., Hämäläinen, M., et al. (Eds.). (2004). *Proceedings of the 14th International Conference on Biomagnetism.* Boston: Biomag 2004.

Hämäläinen, M. S., Hari, R., Ilmoniemi, R. J., et al. (1993). Magnetoencephalography: Theory, instrumentation, and applications to noninvasive studies of the working human brain. *Reviews of Modern Physics, 65,* 413–497.

Hämäläinen, M. S., & Ilmoniemi, R. J. (1994). Interpreting magnetic fields of the brain: Minimum norm estimates. *Medical and Biological Engineering and Computing, 32*(1), 35–42.

Hämäläinen, M. S., & Sarvas, J. I. (1989). Realistic conductivity geometry model of the human head for interoperation of neuromagnetic data. *IEEE Transactions on Bio-Medical Engineering, 36,* 165–171.

Hari, R. (1991). On brain's magnetic responses to sensory stimuli. *Journal of Clinical Neurophysiology, 8,* 157–169.

Hari, R., & Kaukoranta, E. (1985). Neuromagnetic studies of somatosensory system: Principles and examples. *Progress in Neurobiology, 24,* 233–256.

Heikman, P., Salmelin, R., Makela, J. P., et al. (2001). Relation between frontal 3–7 Hz MEG activity and the efficacy of ECT in major depression. *Journal of ECT, 17,* 136–40.

Holsheimer, J., & Feenstra, B. W. (1977). Volume conduction and EEG measurements within the brain: A quantitative approach to the influence of electrical spread on the linear relationship of activity measured at different locations. *Electroencephalography and Clinical Neurophysiology, 43,* 52–58.

Holst, M., Eswaran, H., Lowery, C., et al. (2005). Development of auditory evoked fields in human fetuses and newborns: A longitudinal MEG study. *Clinical Neurophysiology, 116,* 1949–1955.

Ishibashi, H., Simos, P. G., Wheless, J. E., et al. (2002). Somatosensory evoked magnetic fields in hemimegalencephaly. *Neurological Research*, *24*, 459–462.

Ishii, R., Shinosaki, K., Ikejiri, Y., et al. (2000). Theta rhythm increases in left superior temporal cortex during auditory hallucinations in schizophrenia: A case report. *NeuroReport*, *11*, 3283–3287.

Jannin, P., Morandi, X., Fleig, O. J., et al. (2002). Integration of sulcal and functional information for multimodal neuronavigation. *Journal of Neurosurgery*, *96*, 713–723.

Jordan, K. G. (1999). Continuous EEG monitoring in the neuroscience intensive care unit and emergency department. *Journal of Clinical Neurophysiology*, *16*, 14–39.

Josephson, B. D. (1962). Possible new effects in superconductive tunneling. *Physics Letters*, *1*, 251–253.

Kammerling Onnes, H. (1911). *Community physics laboratory* (Nos. 119, 120, 122).

Kammerling Onnes, H. (1911). Zero resistance! Mercury SC transition. *Community Physics Laboratory*, *12*, 120.

Knowlton, R. C., & Shih, J. (2004). Magnetoencephalography in epilepsy. *Epilepsia*, *45*, 61–71.

Kujala, A., Huotilainen, M., Uther, M., et al. (2003). Plastic cortical changes induced by learning to communicate with non-speech sounds. *NeuroReport*, *14*, 1683–1687.

Kujala, J., Pammer, K., Cornelissen, P., et al. (2006). Phase coupling in a cerebro-cerebellar network at 8-13 Hz during reading. *Cerebral Cortex*. PMID: 16926241.

Lamusuo, S., Forss, N., Ruottinen, H. M., et al. (1999). [18F]FDG-PET and whole scalp MEG localization of epileptogenic cortex. *Epilepsia*, *40*, 921–930.

Lantz, G., Spinelli, L., Menendez, R. G., et al. (2001). Localization of distributed sources and comparison with functional MRI. *Epileptic Disorders* [Special Issue], 45–58.

Le, J., Lu, M., Pellouchoud, E., et al. (1998). A rapid method for determining standard 10/10 electrode positions for high resolution EEG studies. *Electroencephalography and Clinical Neurophysiology*, *106*, 554–558.

Lisman, J. E., & Idiart, M. A. (1995). Storage of 7 +/- 2 short-term memories in oscillatory subcycles. *Science*, *267*, 1512–1515.

Llinas, R. R. (1988). The intrinsic electrophysiological properties of mammalian neurons: Insights into central nervous system function. *Science*, *242*, 1654–1664.

Lopes da Silva, F. H., Wieringa, H. J., & Peters, M. J. (1991). Source localization of EEG versus MEG: Empirical comparison using visually evoked responses and theoretical considerations. *Brain Topography*, *4*, 133–142.

Makela, J. P., Forss, N., Jaaskelainen, J., et al. (2006). Magnetoencephalography in neurosurgery. *Neurosurgery*, *59*(3), 493–510.

Mauguiere, F. (2000). Anatomic origin of the cervical N13 potential evoked by upper extremity stimulation. *Journal of Clinical Neurophysiology*, *17*, 236–245.

Michel, C. M., Murray, M. M., Lantz, G., et al. (2004). EEG source imaging. *Clinical Neurophysiology*, *115*, 2195–2222.

Misulis, K. E. (1989). Basic electronics for clinical neurophysiology. *Journal of Clinical Neurophysiology*, *6*, 41–74.

Mizrahi, E. M., & Lesser, R. P. (2003). Video-electroencephalographic monitoring. In J. S. Ebersole & T. A. Pedley (Eds.), *Current practice of clinical electroencephalography* (3rd ed., pp. 588–609). Philadelphia: Lippincott Williams & Wilkins.

Morioka, T., Yamamoto, T., Mizushima, A., et al. (1995). Comparison of magneto-encephalography, functional MRI, and motor evoked potentials in the localization of the sensory-motor cortex. *Neurology Research, 17*, 361–367.

Munk, M. H. J., & Neuenschwander, S. (2000). High-frequency oscillations (20 to 120 Hz) and their role in visual processing. *Journal of Clinical Neurophysiology, 17*, 341–360.

Nakamura, A., Yamada, T., Goto, A., et al. (1998). Somatosensory homunculus as drawn by MEG. *NeuroImage, 7*, 377–386.

Nakasato, N., & Yoshimoto, T. (2000). Somatosensory, auditory, and visual evoked magnetic fields in patients with brain diseases. *Journal of Clinical Neurophysiology, 17*, 201–211.

Nakaya, Y., & Mori, H. (1992). Magnetocardiography. *Clinical Physiology of Physiological Measurements, 13*, 191–229.

Nenonen, J., Kajola, M., Simola, J., et al. (2004). Total information of multichannel MEG sensor arrays. *Proceedings of the 14th International Conference on Biomagnetism*, Boston: Biomag 2004.

Niedermeyer, E. (2005). Historical aspects. In E. Niedermeyer & F. Lopes da Silva (Eds.), *Electroencephalography: Basic principles, clinical applications, and related fields* (5th ed., pp. 1–15). Baltimore: Lippincott Williams & Wilkins.

Nunez, P. L. (1995). Quantitative states of neocortex. In P. L. Nunez (Ed.), *Neocortical dynamics and human EEG rhythms* (pp. 3–67). New York: Oxford University Press.

Nuwer, M. R. (1998). Assessing digital and quantitative EEG in clinical settings. *Journal of Clinical Neurophysiology, 15*, 458–463.

Nuwer, M. R. (1997). Assessment of digital EEG, quantitative EEG, and EEG brain mapping: Report of the American Academy of Neurology and the American Clinical Neurophysiology Society. *Neurology, 49*, 227–292.

Okada, Y. C. (2003). Toward understanding the physiological origins of neuro-magnetic signals. In L. Zhong-Lin & L Kaufman (Eds.), *Magnetic source imaging of the human brain* (1st ed., pp. 43–76.), Mahwah, NJ: Erlbaum.

Okada, Y., Lahteenmaki, A., & Xu, C. (1999a). Comparison of MEG and EEG on the basis of somatic evoked responses elicited by stimulation of the snout in the juvenile swine. *Clinical Neurophysiology, 110*, 214–229.

Okada, Y. C., Lahteenmaki, A., & Xu, C. (1999b). Experimental analysis of distortion of MEG signals by the skull. *Electroencephalography and Clinical Neurophysiology, 110*, 230–238.

Okada, Y. C., Lauritzen, M., & Nicholson, C. (1987). Magnetic field associated with neural activities in an isolated cerebellum. *Brain Research, 412*, 151–155.

Okada, Y. C., & Nicholson C. (1988a). Currents underlying the magnetic evoked field in the cerebellum. In I. Atsumi, M. Kotani, S. Ueno, T. Katila, & S. J. Williamson (Eds.), *Biomagnetism '87* (pp. 198–201). Tokyo: Tokyo Denki University Press.

Okada, Y. C., & Nicholson, C. (1988b). Magnetic evoked field associated with transcortical currents in turtle cerebellum. *Biophysical Journal, 53*, 723–731.

Okada, Y. C., Nicholson, C., & Llinás, R. (1989). Magnetoencephalography (MEG) as a new tool for non-invasive realtime analysis of normal and abnormal brain activity in humans. In D. Ottoson & W. Rostene (Eds.), *Visualization of brain functions* (pp. 245–266). New York: Stockton Press.

Okada, Y. C., Shah, B., & Huang, J. C. (1994). Ferromagnetic high-permeability alloy alone can provide sufficient low-frequency and eddy-current shieldings for biomagnetic measurements. *IEEE Transactions on Biomedical Engineering, 41,* 688–697.

Okada, Y. C., Tanenbaum, R., Williamson, S. J., et al. (1984). Somatotopic organization of the human somatosensory cortex revealed by neuromagnetic measurements. *Experimental Brain Research, 56,* 197–205.

Okada, Y. C., Williamson, S. J., & Kaufman L. (1982). Magnetic field of the human sensorimotor cortex. *International Journal of Neuroscience 17,* 33–38.

Okada, Y. C., Wu, J., & Kyuhou, S. (1997). Genesis of MEG signals in a mammalian CNS structure. *Electroencephalography and Clinical Neurophysiology 103,* 474–485.

Okada, Y. C., & Xu, C. (1996). Single-epoch neuromagnetic signals during epileptiform activities in guinea pig longitudinal CA3 slices. *Neuroscience Letters, 211,* 155–158.

Osaki, Y., Doi, K., Takasawa, M., et al. (2004). Cortical processing of tactile language in a postlingually deaf–blind subject. *NeuroReport, 15,* 287–291.

Parviainen, T., Helenius, P., Poskiparta E., et al. (2006). Cortical sequence of word perception in beginning readers. *Journal of Neuroscience, 26*(22), 6052–6061.

Pascual-Marqui, R. D. (2002). Standardized low-resolution brain electromagnetic tomography (sLORETA): Technical details. *Methods and Findings in Experimental and Clinical Pharmacology, 24*(Suppl. D), 5–12.

Pascual-Marqui, R. D., Michel, C. M., & Lehmann, D. (1994). Low-resolution electromagnetic tomography: A new method for localizing electrical activity in the brain. *International Journal of Psychophysiology, 18*(1), 49–65.

Pataraia, E., Baumgartner, C., Lindinger, G., et al. (2002). Magnetoencephalography in presurgical epilepsy evaluation. *Neurosurgical Review, 25,* 141–159.

Pataraia, E., Simos, P. G., Castillo, E. M., et al. (2004). Does magnetoencephalography add to scalp video-EEG as a diagnostic tool in epilepsy surgery? *Neurology, 62,* 943–948.

Ponomarenko, A. A., Lin, J. S., Selbach, O., et al. (2003). Temporal pattern of hippocampal high-frequency oscillations during sleep after stimulant-evoked waking. *Neuroscience, 121,* 759–769.

Quinonez, D. (1998). Common applications of electrophysiology (EEG) in the past and today: The technologist's view. *Electroencephalography and Clinical Neurophysiology, 106,* 108–112.

Ramachandran, V. S., & Hirstein, W. (1998). The perception of phantom limbs. The D. O. Hebb lecture. *Brain, 121,* 1603–1630.

Restuccia, D. (2000). Anatomic origin of P13 and P14 scalp far-field potentials. *Journal of Clinical Neurophysiology, 17,* 246–257.

Robinson, S. E., & Vrba, J. (1998). Functional neuroimaging by synthetic aperture magnetometry (SAM). In *Proceedings of the 11th International Conference on Biomagnetism* (pp. 302–305). Sendai, Japan: Biomag 98.

Romani, G. L., Williamson, S. J., & Kaufman, L. (1982). Biomagnetic instrumentation. *Review of Scientific Instrumentation, 53,* 1815–1845.

Rose, D. F., Smith, P. D., & Sato, S. (1987). Magnetoencephalography and epilepsy research. *Science, 238,* 329–335.

Rossini, P. M., Tecchio, F., Pizzella, V., et al. (1998). On the reorganization of sensory hand areas after mono-hemispheric lesion: A functional (MEG)/anatomical (MRI) integrative study. *Brain Research, 782,* 153–166.

Saito, S., Endo, H., Kobayakawa, T., et al. (1998). Temporal process from receptors to higher brain in taste detection studied by gustatory-evoked magnetic fields and reaction times. *Annals of the New York Academy of Sciences, 855,* 493–497.

Salmelin, R. (2007). Clinical neurophysiology of language: The MEG approach. *Clinical Neurophysiology, 118*(2), 237–254.

Salmelin, R., & Kujala, J. (2006). Neural representation of language: Activation versus long-range connectivity. *Trends in Cognitive Sciences, 10*(11), 519–525.

Sato, S., & Smith, P. D. (1985). Magnetoencephalography. *Journal of Clinical Neurophysiology, 2,* 173–192.

Scherg, M., Bast, T., & Berg, P. (1999). Multiple source analysis of interictal spikes: Goals, requirements, and clinical value. *Journal of Clinical Neurophysiology, 16,* 214–224.

Schneider, U., Schleussner, E., Haueisen, J., et al. (2001). Signal analysis of auditory evoked cortical fields in fetal magnetoencephalography. *Brain Topography, 14,* 69–80.

Sekihara, K., & Scholz, B. (1995). Average-intensity reconstruction and Wiener reconstruction of bioelectric current distribution based on its estimated covariance matrix. *IEEE Transactions on Bio-Medical Engineering, 42*(2), 149–157.

Silver, A. H., & Zimmerman, J. E. (1965). Quantum transitions and loss in multiply connected superconductors. *Physical Review Letters, 15,* 888–891.

Sonoo, M. (2000). Anatomic origin and clinical application of the widespread N18 potential in median nerve somatosensory evoked potentials. *Journal of Clinical Neurophysiology, 17,* 258–268.

Spencer, S, S., Sperling, M. R., & Shewmon, D. A. (1997). Intracranial electrodes. In J. Engel Jr. & T. A. Pedley (Eds.), *Epilepsy: A comprehensive textbook* (pp. 1719–1747). Philadelphia: Lippincott-Raven.

Sperling, M. R., & Shewmon, D. A. (1997). General principles for presurgical evaluation. In J. Engel Jr. & T. A. Pedley (Eds.), *Epilepsy: A comprehensive textbook* (pp. 1697–1705). Philadelphia: Lippincott-Raven.

Sperling, W., Martus, P., & Alschbach, M. (2000). Evaluation of neuronal effects of electroconvulsive therapy by magnetoencephalography (MEG). *Progress in Neuro-Psychopharmacology and Biological Psychiatry, 24,* 1339–1354.

Sperling, W., Vieth, J., Martus, M., et al. (1999). Spontaneous slow and fast MEG activity in male schizophrenics treated with clozapine. *Psychopharmacology, 142,* 375–382.

Staba, R. J., Wilson, C. L., Bragin, A., et al. (2002). Quantitative analysis of high-frequency oscillations (80–500 Hz) recorded in human epileptic hippocampus and entorhinal cortex. *Journal of Neurophysiology, 88,* 1743–1752.

Stefan, H., Hummel, C., Scheler, G., et al. (2003). Magnetic brain source imaging of focal epileptic activity: A synopsis of 455 cases. *Brain, 126,* 2396–2405.

Uutela, K., Hämäläinen, M., & Salmelin, R. (1998). Global optimization in the localization of neuromagnetic sources. *IEEE Transactions on Bio-Medical Engineering, 45*(6), 716–723.

Van Cott, A., & Brenner, R. (1998). Technical advantages of digital EEG. *Journal of Clinical Neurophysiology, 15,* 464–475.

Vanhatalo, S., Holmes, M. D., Tallgren, P., et al. (2003). Very slow EEG responses lateralize temporal lobe seizures: An evaluation of non-invasive DC-EEG. *Neurology, 60,* 1098–1104.

Vespa, P. M., Nenow, V., & Nuwer, M. R. (1999). Continuous EEG monitoring in the intensive care unit: Early findings and clinical efficacy. *Journal of Clinical Neurophysiology*, *16*, 1–13.

Vihla, M., Laine, M., & Salmelin, R. (2006). Cortical dynamics of visual/semantic vs. phonological analysis in picture confrontation. *NeuroImage*, *33*(2), 732–738.

Vrba, J., & Robinson, S. E. (2001). Signal processing in magnetoencephalography. *Methods*, *25*, 249–271.

Weiss, T., Miltner, W., Rosburg, T., et al. (1997). Reliability of dipole localization for the movement-evoked field component MEF I. *International Journal of Neuroscience*, *91*, 123–132.

Wheless, J. W., Willmore, L. J., Breier, J. I., et al. (1999). A comparison of magnetoencephalography, MRI, and V-EEG in patients evaluated for epilepsy. *Epilepsia*, *40*, 931–941,

Williamson, S. J., & Kaufman, L. (1987). Analysis of neuromagnetic signals: Methods of analysis of brain electrical and magnetic signals. In A. S. Gevins & A. Remond (Eds.), *EEG handbook* (Rev. series, Vol. 1, pp. 405–448). Amsterdam: Elsevier Science.

Worrell, G. A., Parish, L., Cranstoun, S. D., et al. (2004). High-frequency oscillations and seizure generation in neocortical epilepsy. *Brain*, *127*, 1496–1506.

Wu, J., & Okada, Y. C. (1998). Physiological bases of the synchronized population spikes and slow wave of the magnetic field generated by a guinea-pig longitudinal CA3 slice preparation. *Electroencephalography and Clinical Neurophysiology*, *107*, 361–373.

Yamada, T. (2000). Neuroanatomic substrates of lower extremity somatosensory evoked potentials. *Journal of Clinical Neurophysiology*, *17*, 269–279.

Young, B. G., & Campbell, V. C. (1999). EEG monitoring in the intensive care unit: Pitfalls and caveats. *Journal of Clinical Neurophysiology*, *16*, 40–45.

Yumoto, M. (2000). Recent advances of MEG. *Rinsho Byori*, *48*, 38–41.

Zimmerman, J. E., & Silver, A. H. (1964). Quantum effects in type II superconductors. *Physics Letters*, *10*, 47–48.

PART II

NEUROIMAGING METHODS

CHAPTER 4

Considerations for the Application of BOLD Functional Magnetic Resonance Imaging to Neurologically Impaired Populations

Adam Gazzaley
Mark D'Esposito

Over the past decade, functional magnetic resonance imaging (fMRI) has developed into a powerful method for studying physiology in the functioning human brain. Although its predominant use has been by neuroscientists to examine the neural basis of cognitive and behavioral processes, it is more frequently being used to study patients with neurological disease. Its widespread availability, noninvasiveness, high spatiotemporal resolution, and reasonable cost, especially when compared with positron emission tomography (PET) scanning, have all contributed to its increasing popularity. In addition, fMRI has earned a strong reputation over the last 10 years by reproducing and extending many important neurophysiological findings, which have previously been the domain of experimental animal research. Thus, with mounting confidence, a diverse group of investigators, including neurologists, neuropsychologists, and psychiatrists have begun to apply this technology to study neurologically impaired populations. The motivation of these researchers is to use fMRI to gain insight into the neural mechanisms and/or associated neural alterations of neurological diseases. Another motivation for clinical researchers is to develop fMRI as a clinical tool that can serve as a diagnostic measure and aid in treatment planning.

Most fMRI studies directed at achieving these goals are based on experimental designs pioneered by cognitive neuroscientists, using behavioral tasks to probe neural function with the blood-oxygen-level-dependent (BOLD) signal as a dependent measure (Ogawa et al., 1990). A common approach to studying neurologically impaired populations has been to compare the BOLD signal of a group of patients to a group of healthy age-matched controls performing a task believed to tap into a cognitive process compromised by the disease. Although the BOLD signal arises from the vasculature and is not a direct marker of neural activity, almost all conclusions generated from these studies equate changes in BOLD signal magnitude and anatomical distribution to changes in neural activity. Thus, it is assumed that differences in the pattern of fMRI activity between healthy and neurologically impaired patients are due to neural and not vascular differences between these groups.

It is important to be aware of the many potential differences between patient and control populations aside from neural differences, which when unrecognized and uncontrolled may obscure the interpretation of BOLD signal alterations as being reflective of neural alterations. Examples include differences in cognitive performance, strategy used to accomplish a task, influence of neural activity on hemodynamic properties of surrounding vasculature (e.g., neurovascular coupling), medication usage, and sensory abilities. Although investigators do occasionally comment on such confounds within the discussion in an article, awareness of these issues and consideration during the design phase of an experiment is of tremendous importance. With careful planning of subject recruitment, screening, experimental design, and analysis, more meaningful interpretations of fMRI data from neurologically impaired populations can be obtained. In this chapter, we discuss some of the important differences between patient populations and control groups that may affect the design and interpretation of fMRI studies. We also offer several options for addressing these issues when planning an fMRI experiment.

Pathophysiological Factors

Many fMRI studies comparing populations rely on the assumption that differences in BOLD signals between the populations reflect differences in neural activity. The reason that this interpretation is not always a reasonable one is that *the BOLD signal is an indirect measure of neural activity* that depends on the blood-flow-mediated relationship between neural activity and the concentration of deoxyhemoglobin within the surrounding microvasculature. When a neural event occurs anywhere in the brain, there is a local blood flow increase (Leniger-Follert & Hossmann, 1979) that results in a decrease in the concentration of paramagnetic deoxygenated hemoglobin in the microvasculature surrounding the activated region (Malonek & Grinvald, 1996). This local increase in the ratio of nonparamagnetic oxygenated hemoglobin to paramagnetic deoxygenated hemoglobin (Thulborn et al., 1982; Turner et al., 1991) results in the detection of an increase in the BOLD signal (Ogawa et al., 1992). Neural activity drives the change in this ratio by influencing several

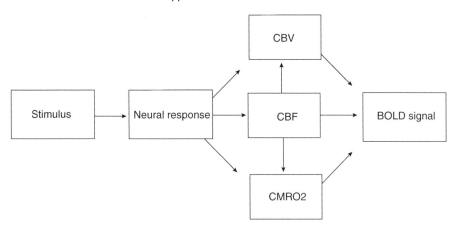

FIGURE 4.1. Schematic illustration of the transformation stages of stimulus-elicited neural activity to a hemodynamic response resulting in a BOLD signal.

factors, including cerebral blood flow (CBF), blood volume (CBV), and blood oxygen consumption (CMRO₂) (Buxton & Frank, 1997; see Figure 4.1). The still incompletely characterized process by which neural activity influences the hemodynamic properties of the surrounding vasculature is referred to as *neurovascular coupling.*

When assessing BOLD signal levels and making conclusions regarding the magnitude and localization of neural activity, numerous assumptions are made regarding neurovascular coupling (behavioral stimulus → neural activity → hemodynamic response [HRF] → BOLD signal), as well as the regional variability of the metabolic and vascular factors that influence the BOLD signal. The impact of these factors is further amplified when comparing different populations. This concern is especially relevant to populations in which structural changes in cerebral vasculature, such as local vascular compromise or diffuse vascular disease, can alter vascular responsiveness to neural activity. For example, a vascular disparity occurring in the absence of a difference in neural activity may alter neurovascular coupling and modify a component of the hemodynamic response to neural activity, such as CBF. This in turn will alter the influx of oxyhemoglobin into the region, thus affecting the BOLD signal and leading to a potential misinterpretation of a signal change as reflecting a difference in neural activity.

Alterations in Neurovascular Coupling

Because most fMRI studies are performed in healthy young individuals, little attention has been focused on the effects of changes in the cerebrovascular system on the BOLD signal (D'Esposito et al., 2003). However, direct comparisons of the BOLD signal between populations rely heavily on the assump-

TABLE 4.1. Potential Mechanisms Causing Altered Neurovascular Coupling

- Chronic cerebral ischemia.
- Chronic cereberal vasodilatation secondary to carotid stenosis.
- Astrocytic proliferation due to neural injury causing gliosis.
- Developmental changes in expression of neurotransmitter receptors on astrocytes.
- Effects of medications.
- Abnormal reduction or enhancement of specific neurotransmitter systems such as glutamate, acetylcholine, or GABA.

tion of comparable neurovascular coupling. Alterations in the cerebrovascular dynamics of many different etiologies, such as atherosclerosis or changes in vascular reactivity, may affect neurovascular coupling (see Table 4.1). In addition, alterations in the levels of any of the mediators of the neurovascular response, including neurotransmitters, are important to consider (see Table 4.2). This issue affects the study of almost all neurological disorders, such as stroke, trauma, migraine, and neurodegenerative disease, as well as the process of normal aging.

For example, many published fMRI studies have sought to identify changes in the neural substrate of cognitive function that occur with normal aging (Gazzaley & D'Esposito, 2003; Grady, 2000). These studies often directly compare changes in BOLD signal intensity across age groups by relying on the assumption of age-equivalent coupling of neural activity to the BOLD signal. However, there is empirical evidence suggesting that this general assumption may not hold true. One way to test this assumption is to study the spatial and temporal characteristics of the BOLD hemodynamic response function (HRF) during a stimulation that is expected to result in equivalent neural activity in young and old subjects, such as a simple motor task (Buckner et al., 2000; D'Esposito et al., 1999; Hesselmann et al., 2001; Mattay et al., 2002; Taoka et al., 1998) or a simple visual stimulation task (Buckner et al., 2000; Huettel et al., 2001; Ross et al., 1997). If there are changes in the HRF in response to a task that is assumed to induce no age-

TABLE 4.2. Alterations in Vascular Dynamics Observed in Normal Aging and in Neurological Disease

- Ultrastructural changes in cerebral vessels due to atherosclerosis.
- Increased tortuosity of cerebral vessels.
- Changes in collateral circulation after recanalization of occluded cerebral vessels.
- Reduction in resting cerebral blood flow.
- Changes in vascular reactivity.
- Lowered resting cerebral metabolic rate of oxygen consumption.

related change in neural activity, then these changes can be attributed to an alteration in another contributor to the HRF, such as a change in CBF or neurovascular coupling. We compared the HRF characteristics in the sensorimotor cortex of young and older subjects in response to a simple motor reaction-time task (D'Esposito et al., 1999). The provisional assumption was made that there was identical neural activity between the two populations, based on physiological findings of equivalent movement-related electrical potentials in subjects under similar conditions (Cunnington et al., 1997). Thus, we presumed that any changes observed in the BOLD fMRI signal between young and older individuals in motor cortex would not be due to neural activity changes in normal aging. Several important similarities and differences were observed between age groups. Although there was no significant difference in the shape of the HRF curve or peak amplitude of the signal, we found a significantly decreased signal-to-noise ratio in the BOLD signal in older individuals as compared with young individuals. This was attributed to a greater level of noise in the signal from older subjects. We also observed a decrease in the spatial extent of the BOLD signal in older individuals, as compared with younger individuals, in the sensorimotor cortex (i.e., the median number of suprathreshold voxels). These findings suggest that there is some property of the coupling between neural activity and the BOLD signal that changes with age.

What is the source of these BOLD changes that occur with age? Extensive research on the aging neurovascular system has revealed that it undergoes significant changes in multiple domains on a continuum throughout the human lifespan, probably as early as the fourth decade (Farkas & Luiten, 2001). These changes affect the vascular ultrastructure (Fang, 1976), the resting CBF (Bentourkia et al., 2000; Schultz et al., 1999), the vascular responsiveness of the vessels (Yamamoto et al., 1980), and the cerebral metabolic rate of oxygen consumption (Takada et al., 1992; Yamaguchi et al., 1986). Aging is also frequently associated with comorbidities such as diabetes, hypertension, and hyperlipidemia, all of which may affect the BOLD signal by altering CBF and neurovascular coupling (Claus et al., 1998). Any one of these age-related differences in the vascular system, or conditions that affect the vascular system, could conceivably produce activity-independent differences in the BOLD fMRI signal, greatly affecting the interpretation of results from such studies (Gazzaley & D'Esposito, 2004).

The notion that vascular differences between individuals may affect the BOLD signal is especially of concern when considering patient populations with known vascular disease, such as stroke. A recent fMRI study addressed the issue of the influence of vascular factors on the BOLD signal in a symptomatic stroke population (Pineiro et al., 2002). The investigators analyzed the time course of the BOLD HRF in the sensorimotor cortex of patients with an isolated subcortical lacunar stroke as compared with a group of age-matched controls. They found a decrease in the rate of rise and the maximal BOLD HRF to a finger- or hand-tapping task in both the sensorimotor cortex of the hemisphere affected by the stroke and the unaffected hemisphere. These investigators suggested that given the widespread changes of these BOLD signal differences, the change was unlikely a direct consequence of the subcortical lacunar stroke on neural activity.

Another recent fMRI study concluded that severe extracranial carotid stenosis in a patient, without MRI evidence of an infarct, led to neurovascular uncoupling that presented as a paradoxical negative BOLD signal response during a motor task (Rother et al., 2002) Furthermore, this negative BOLD response occurred in only the affected hemisphere and correlated with a severely impaired hemodynamic response to hypercapnia isolated to that hemisphere. Given that there was no reason to suspect an abnormality in neural activity in this patient with normal motor performance, the finding was interpreted as a local activity-driven increase in deoxyhemoglobin, secondary to oxygen consumption in the absence of an accompanying increase in CBF. Although this is a rather extreme example of the effect of impaired autoregulation on the BOLD response, it serves as an important illustration that extracranial vascular disease can impair this process and alter the BOLD response.

There are several possible approaches when designing fMRI studies that could limit the confounds of alterations in neurovascular coupling on the BOLD signal. One straightforward option is careful selection and characterization of all subjects being studied in order to reduce variance between study groups. Investigators who include subjects with potential vascular pathology in their studies should carefully assess the status of their neurovascular systems, as well as secondary factors in their subjects (i.e., comorbidities and medications). To date, most fMRI studies have not collected images with appropriate pulse sequences to detect clinically silent white matter lesions (i.e., T2 weighted sequences, optimally fluid-attenuated inversion recovery [FLAIR]). Moreover, the routine screening typically performed for most fMRI studies may miss symptoms consistent with vascular pathology. Not infrequently, a subject is unaware of having vascular risk factors or ever experiencing neurological symptoms. Investigators performing fMRI studies of patients with vascular pathology may also consider employing Doppler ultrasound or magnetic resonance angiography (MRA) to evaluate extracranial vasculature for the presence of significant occlusion.

In addition to obtaining a detailed characterization of the study population, there are several approaches to both experimental design and statistical analysis of fMRI data that can help address this confound.

Testing for Group × Task Interactions

Instead of testing for a main effect between groups on a particular behavioral task, a safer approach is to assess group × task interactions. That is, test for relative differences in the BOLD signal within a region of interest between two different tasks rather than directly comparing the signal between groups on a single task. The goal here is not to identify overall differences in levels of neural activation between populations (i.e., main effect), but rather a relative difference between the populations on the two tasks (i.e., age × condition interaction). For example, this was done in an fMRI study comparing the BOLD signal in young and older adults on a memory task (Mitchell et al., 2000). The investigators did not attempt to identify "overall differences in levels of neural activation between young and older adults (i.e., main effect of age), but rather in the relative performance of young and older adults on working memory trials that required combining different types of information together (i.e., object and spatial features) versus working memory trials that required remembering only a single feature (i.e., an age × condition interaction)" (p. 198). Thus, this analysis was designed to identify areas that were differentially active between young and older adults in the memory combination condition relative to the memory for single features conditions. The results revealed that the BOLD signal associated with the combination condition relative to the single feature condition was increased only in the young group and not in the older group. Because a study design of this nature employs an internal control (i.e., within-group comparisons), these results are more likely to reflect population differences in neural activity between tasks rather than hemodynamic differences.

It is important to note, however, that in some instances the finding of a main effect of age can be interpretable. For example, Logan et al. (2002) formed direct comparisons between BOLD signal levels from a young and an older study group in a memory paradigm. They found that there was a main effect of age in decreasing the BOLD signal amplitude in certain frontal regions. Such an effect is often interpreted as underrecruitment of neural systems. As already mentioned, a decreased age-related BOLD signal could be due to an age-related decrease in neurovascular reactivity or a decrease in the baseline CBF, and not a decrease in neural activity. However, Logan et al. also identified new areas of significant BOLD activity in older subjects that were not present in young adults, as well as regions that did not seem to change from the young adult baseline. The finding that some brain regions exhibit decreased age-related activity, some increased age-related activity, and some no change between older and young groups is unlikely to be accounted for by a global change in neurovascular coupling in the aging brain. In addition, the finding of recruitment of brain regions in older individuals that are not recruited in younger individuals during a particular cognitive task cannot likely be accounted for by age-related changes in neurovascular coupling.

Testing for Brain–Behavior Relationships

Correlating changes in the BOLD signal with behavioral measures (e.g., accuracy or reaction times) will increase the likelihood that observed group differences are true correlates of changes in neural activity. For example, Rypma and D'Esposito (2000) found that better behavioral performance was associated with less prefrontal cortex activation in young individuals and increased prefrontal cortex activation in older individuals.

Statistical and Methodological Approaches

Rypma and D'Esposito (2000) also investigated age-related differences in prefrontal neural activity with random-effects tests of age differences using the mean parameter estimates (i.e., the beta values derived from the least-squares solution of a linear model of the dependent data) that characterized the BOLD fMRI signal during each task period. Unlike the common procedure, these parameter estimates were not scaled by the error term, which would typically be used to obtain *t*-statistics for each voxel, and were thus less affected by the potential confound of BOLD fMRI signal intrinsic noise differences between the groups that was mentioned above (D'Esposito et al., 1999). Moreover, multivariate statistical techniques such as coherence (Sun et al., 2004) and beta-series correlation analysis (Gazzaley et al., 2004; Rissman et al., 2004) are also useful approaches to consider inasmuch as they are not as sensitive to regional differences in the HRF.

Attempts can be made to quantify differences in vascular reactivity and hemodynamic response for all subjects in order to establish baseline measures to normalize the BOLD signal. For example, in addition to the experimental task, each subject could perform sensorimotor and/or visual tasks to characterize regional HRFs (Aguirre et al., 1998; Handwerker et al., 2004). Other approaches, such as assessing the BOLD response to breath holding (i.e., increasing CO_2 concentration leads to a neural activity-independent increase in the BOLD signal) are also potentially useful in estimating differences in vascular reactivity between groups (Riecker et al., 2003). Estimates of vascular reactivity independent of neural activity could provide a means of calibrating the BOLD signal between subject groups.

Finally, combining electrical measures such as event-related potentials, which assess neural activity more directly but lack adequate spatial resolution, with fMRI measurement may add converging evidence that a given change in BOLD activity is related to neural rather than neurovascular changes. However, such combined data are rarely conclusive inasmuch as (1) given multiple foci of BOLD activations (across space) and multiple electrical components (across time), it may be difficult to determine which BOLD signal foci are correlated with a given electrical component, and (2) it remains to be determined which electrical events captured on the scalp are correlated with changes in blood flow (Arthurs & Boniface, 2002; Lauritzen & Gold, 2003; Logothetis, 2003; see Ogawa et al., 2000, for recent discussion of the brain electrical events that lead to a BOLD response).

Behavioral and Cognitive Factors

A patient with a neurological disorder exhibiting a deficit in sensorimotor, behavioral, or cognitive function differs from a healthy individual at many levels. The neural basis for these differences may be the very essence of what is being studied when fMRI is used as a tool. However, comparing brain–

behavior relationships between two distinct populations of subjects presents the researcher with several significant challenges in designing and interpreting fMRI experiments.

Participants in studies that assess cognitive abilities invariably exhibit a range of performance on any experimental task, unless the task is so easy that performance is at ceiling. If the overall group performance is reasonably high, this is usually not detrimental for a study focused on a single population. In fact, slight variation in normal performance can be a used as an effective correlate with neural activity measures. For example, a correlation between activity in specific brain regions and how accurate the subject is on a working memory task can provide insight into the neural mechanisms underlying memory function (Curtis et al., 2004; Rypma & D'Esposito, 2000). However, a serious confound is introduced when there is a significant discrepancy in performance levels between two populations whose BOLD levels are being compared (Murphy & Garavan, 2004). Trials that are associated with incorrect responses are likely to have been processed differently than trials associated with correct responses. If both correct and incorrect responses are considered together, as they are for the majority of fMRI experiments, noise is introduced into the signal of interest. Thus, differences in neural activity between populations may merely be the result of differences in error rate between the groups and not indicative of a neural difference induced by the condition being studied. It also becomes impossible to determine whether neural differences are the result of poor task performance in one group of subjects or whether the performance deficit is a consequence of an alteration in neural processing in the impaired group (Price & Friston, 1999).

Thus, unlike neuropsychological experiments where the goal is to identify performance deficits in patients as compared with age- and education-matched control subjects, fMRI studies are often designed with the goal of having patients adequately perform the task. This should involve careful piloting experiments prior to scanning, ideally in a mock scanner, because there are reasons for performance differences between populations aside from those related to a direct impact of the disease state. The MRI scanner, as compared with a standard behavioral testing room, is less than ideal for conducting most cognitive neuroscience experiments. Experiments are performed with the patient in the awkward position of lying on his or her back, often requiring the subject to visualize the presentation of stimuli through a mirror in an acoustically noisy environment. Moreover, many individuals develop some degree of claustrophobia because of the small bore of the MRI scanner and find it difficult to remain motionless for the long duration of time that is required for most experiments (e.g., usually 60–90 m). Some populations, such as patients with memory and attention deficits, may be differentially encumbered by these practical constraints. Thus, it is important to consider the population being studied in the setting of the scanner environment when designing a task.

In this regard, it is also important to consider task design, as several options exist for designing fMRI experiments (Aguirre & D'Esposito, 1999).

The prototypical fMRI experimental design, known as a blocked design, consists of behavioral tasks presented in blocks of trials alternating over the course of a scanning session, with the BOLD signals compared between the tasks. This design has advantages for patient studies, such as increased statistical power that compensates somewhat for the limited number of patients available for such studies. It can also be preferable at a behavioral level because it prevents frequent shifting between different behavioral conditions, which can be difficult for older individuals and patients. However, block designs have the disadvantage of relying on the assumptions of cognitive subtraction, which may not always be valid (Zarahn et al., 1999). It also is necessary of equate task performance between groups to make valid comparisons.

Another class of experimental design, known as event-related fMRI, attempts to detect changes associated with individual trials, as opposed to the larger unit of time comprising a block of trials (Rosen et al., 1998; Zarahn et al., 1997). Each individual trial may be composed of one behavioral "event," such as the presentation of a single stimulus (e.g., a face or object to be perceived), or several behavioral events such as in the delayed-response task, (i.e., an item to be remembered, a delay period, and a motor response). An event-related design has the distinct advantage for a population comparison of permitting the independent analysis of correct and incorrect trials. Unlike a block design, in which this is not possible, an event-related design allows the investigator to tolerate differences in the overall accuracy between study groups, because analysis of only the correct trials effectively matches performance (Murphy & Garavan, 2004). It is important to note that although performance is not required to be precisely matched in this design, it is important to be convinced that the correct trials are not merely a reflection of correct guesses and that there are enough correct trials to generate sufficient analytical power.

Another option for addressing the issue of differences in cognitive performance is to include a large number of subjects in the study and then subdivide the study group based on task performance or an independent neuropsychological measure (Cabeza et al., 2002; Daselaar et al., 2003). For example, Cabeza et al. (2002) used fMRI to assess prefrontal activity in younger adults, low-performing older adults, and high-performing older adults on a memory task. Low-performing older adults recruited right prefrontal regions, as did young adults, but high-performing older adults engaged prefrontal regions bilaterally. The investigators concluded that low-performing older adults recruited a network similar to that recruited by young adults but used it inefficiently, whereas high-performing older adults counteracted age-related neural decline through a plastic reorganization of neurocognitive networks.

A further option is to study a patient population without using a cognitive task at all. There is a growing body of literature on fMRI experiments studying the resting-state network or default mode of brain function that occurs when a participant is resting quietly and not performing a task (Greicius et al., 2003; Hampson et al., 2002). This approach has already been applied to study Alzheimer's disease (AD) (Greicius et al., 2004). It was found that patients with AD showed decreased resting-state activity in the posterior cingulate and hippocampus, suggesting that disrupted connectivity between these two regions accounts for the posterior cingulate hypometabolism commonly detected in PET studies of early AD.

Another related approach has been to use BOLD fMRI to assess correlates of basal metabolism, such as in studies evaluating alterations in the metabolism of the hippocampal subregions in patients with AD (Small et al., 1999) and healthy older subjects (Small et al., 2002). With this approach, it was found that two hippocampal subregions—the subiculum and the dentate gyrus—decline normally with age, whereas the entorhinal cortex declines pathologically. These applications of BOLD fMRI may be a reasonable option in severely compromised patient populations that cannot adequately perform cognitive tasks. Of course, these approaches do not provide the ability to draw conclusions about brain–behavior relationships.

As already discussed, fMRI studies of neurologically impaired patient populations often attempt to assess activity alterations in the brain during the performance of a cognitive task. However, it is clear that the cognitive strategy assumed by the participants in order to accomplish a task can vary between individuals, and the particular strategy chosen will influence brain activity (Burbaud et al., 2000; Iaria et al., 2003; Speer et al., 2003). Thus, it can be difficult to interpret whether observed activity alterations are the result of modified neural implementation secondary to pathology or alternative cognitive strategies adopted by the patient group. Unfortunately, it is not possible to dissociate these options based solely on the functional neuroimaging data. If the goal of the experiment is to evaluate alterations in brain activity that are the result of neural, rather than strategic, differences between the study groups, efforts must be made to constrain the types of strategies that can be employed in a given cognitive task by optimizing the task design and by explicit instructions that are given to the subjects prior to performing the task. However, this is challenging, as it is difficult to exert perfect control over a subject's strategy, even with a well-designed task, and to demonstrate conclusively that an alternative strategy was being engaged inasmuch as there may be no reliable measure. Nevertheless, care should be taken to provide detailed descriptions of the task requirements to all subjects and the task should be designed to constrain the cognitive strategy employed. When possible, measures of cognitive strategy should be implemented, such as eye tracking (Gitelman et al., 2000) and postexperiment testing/questionnaires (Gazzaley et al., 2005).

Subject Factors

Although in most fMRI studies of patient populations some basic subject matching is done by finding a group of control subjects who are matched in age and education, there are characteristics of patient populations that are often not matched. Some of these are discussed below.

Medications

A further consideration, aside from the presence and influence of pathological processes, is that most patients are prescribed medications for the prevention or treatment of these conditions. Few studies strictly screen subjects for the use of all medications, including estrogen replacement therapy and common nonprescription drugs such as nonsteroidal anti-inflammatory drugs (e.g., aspirin) that inhibit the cycloxygenase pathway of arachidonic acid and may alter neurovascular coupling and thus the BOLD signal, independent of the pathological influence. There are few studies that have investigated the effect of medications on CBF (Bednar & Gross, 1999; Miller et al., 1997; Nobler et al., 2002) or the BOLD signal (Neele et al., 2001; Pariente et al., 2001). The necessity to increase our understanding of the effects of medications, such as aspirin and hypertensive and hyperlipidemic medications, on the BOLD signal will be ever greater as groups of patients with neurovascular disease are studied.

In addition, we need to be cognizant of the potential effects on the BOLD signal of frequently used substances such as caffeine and nicotine. Little is known about these substances, which may have independent vascular or neural effects (Jacobsen et al., 2002; Laurienti et al., 2002; Mulderink et al., 2002; Stein et al., 1998). Caffeine, even at moderate doses, is a cerebral vasoconstrictor that can decrease the resting CBF by 20–30% (Cameron et al., 1990) and the BOLD baseline signal by 4.4%. This can result in an exaggerated task-induced BOLD response because of the larger difference between the resting and active states (Mulderink et al., 2002). Complicating the picture is the observation that the caffeine-related increased BOLD signal response is not uniform across the visual and motor cortices and not of comparable magnitude in all subjects (Laurienti et al., 2002).

Peripheral Sensory Abilities

In our eagerness to explore differences in brain function, alterations in peripheral sensory systems are often ignored. If a subject is performing a cognitive task in the scanner involving auditory or visual stimulation, it is important to ensure that hearing and vision are either normal or corrected to avoid this becoming another confound when comparing two groups. For example, visual changes are common in normal aging and may confound interpretations of changes in occipital cortex activity that occurs with age. MRI-compatible glasses are available and should be worn by all subjects with the need for visual correction during a visual fMRI experiment.

Methodological Factors

Studies of patient populations must also consider the impact of anatomical differences in the brains of the study groups on data analysis and interpretation. Populations that are particularly susceptible to these influences include oncology patients and those with neurodegenerative disease, and stroke. The presence of atrophy and brain lesions results in several analysis considerations, perhaps the most salient of which is the impact on automated algorithms that are frequently used to spatially normalize patient brains to a standard template. This is used to facilitate comparisons of functional data within groups and across populations. However, in the presence of a focal lesion, standard automated algorithms can produce distortion when attempting to reduce mismatch at the site of the lesion. Recently developed masking tools to exclude the area of lesion from normalization should be considered when normalizing brains with focal lesions (Brett et al., 2001).

There is a similar issue when attempting to normalize brains with extensive atrophy since standard templates are generated from young, healthy brains. Although the impact of normalizing an atrophic brain to a normal template with fMRI has not been fully assessed, concern has been raised by an evaluation of normalization of PET imaging data (Ishii et al., 2001). There has also been the recent development of a merged young-and-old adult template specifically created to serve as a normalization template in aging and dementia studies (Buckner et al., 2004). Buckner et al. determined that the Atlas Scaling Factor, automatically generated to match each brain to the atlas target, was only minimally biased in older adults with dementia with marked atrophy and yielded measurements of head size correction equivalent to those derived by manual methods (Buckner et al., 2004). It is also important to realize that region of interest (ROI) analysis in native space (i.e., prior to spatial normalization) may still be the safest alternative to analyze data from older adults and patients with dementia.

Conclusions

The use of functional neuroimaging has the potential to revolutionize our understanding of alterations in neural activity associated with neurological disease. Moreover, it has great potential as a clinical tool that may be helpful in diagnosis and treatment planning. Its high spatial resolution, coupled with its ability to assess correlates of neural activity while subjects are performing cognitive tasks, make its role invaluable. However, as emphasized in this chapter, caution must be exercised to avoid misinterpreting the results of BOLD fMRI studies. The BOLD signal is usually a fairly direct reflection of the influence of neural activity on CBF, and therefore changes in resting CBF or neurovascular coupling may influence our ability to attribute BOLD signal changes to alterations in neural activity (D'Esposito et al., 2003). Aside from vascular alterations in patients that alter neurovascular coupling, differences in performance, cognitive strategy, medication, sensory abilities, and anatomy must all be considered. Until new imaging methods are developed to more closely link the measured signal to neural activity, care must be taken at all levels of study design, analysis, and interpretation to maximize our ability to contribute valuable and accurate insights to the literature on neurological disease.

REFERENCES

Aguirre, G. K., & D'Esposito, M. (1999). Experimental design for brain fMRI. In C. T. W. Moonen & P. A. Bandettini (Eds.), *Functional MRI* (pp. 369–380). Berlin: Springer-Verlag.

Aguirre, G. K., Zarahn, E., & D'Esposito, M. (1998). The variability of human BOLD hemodynamic responses. *NeuroImage, 8*(4), 360–369.

Arthurs, O. J., & Boniface, S. (2002). How well do we understand the neural origins of the fMRI BOLD signal? *Trends in Neurosciences, 25*(1), 27–31.

Bednar, M. M., & Gross, C. E. (1999). Aspirin reduces experimental cerebral blood flow in vivo. *Neurological Research, 21*(5), 488–490.

Bentourkia, M., Bol, A., Ivanoiu, A., et al. (2000). Comparison of regional cerebral blood flow and glucose metabolism in the normal brain: Effect of aging. *Journal of the Neurological Sciences, 181*(1–2), 19–28.

Brett, M., Leff, A. P., Rorden, C., et al. J. (2001). Spatial normalization of brain images with focal lesions using cost function masking. *NeuroImage, 14*(2), 486–500.

Buckner, R. L., Head, D., Parker, J., et al. (2004). A unified approach for morphometric and functional data analysis in young, old, and demented adults using automated atlas-based head size normalization: Reliability and validation against manual measurement of total intracranial volume. *NeuroImage, 23*(2), 724–738.

Buckner, R. L., Snyder, A. Z., Sanders, A. L., et al. (2000). Functional brain imaging of young, nondemented, and demented older adults. *Journal of Cognitive Neuroscience, 12*(Suppl. 2), 24–34.

Burbaud, P., Camus, O., Guehl, D., et al. (2000). Influence of cognitive strategies on the pattern of cortical activation during mental subtraction: A functional imaging study in human subjects. *Neuroscience Letters, 287*(1), 76–80.

Buxton, R. (2002). The physiological basis of the BOLD effect. In R. Buxton (Ed.), *Introduction to functional magnetic resonance imaging: Principles and techniques* (pp. 408–412). Cambridge, UK: Cambridge University Press.

Buxton, R. B., & Frank, L. R. (1997). A model for the coupling between cerebral blood flow and oxygen metabolism during neural stimulation. *Journal of Cerebral Blood Flow and Metabolism, 17*(1), 64–72.

Cabeza, R., Anderson, N. D., Locantore, J. K., et al. (2002). Aging gracefully: Compensatory brain activity in high-performing older adults. *NeuroImage, 17*(3), 1394–1402.

Cameron, O. G., Modell, J. G., & Hariharan, M. (1990). Caffeine and human cerebral blood flow: A positron emission tomography study. *Life Sciences, 47*(13), 1141–1146.

Claus, J. J., Breteler, M. M., Hasan, D., et al. (1998). Regional cerebral blood flow and cerebrovascular risk factors in the elderly population. *Neurobiology of Aging, 19*(1), 57–64.

Cunnington, R., Iansek, R., Johnson, K. A., et al. (1997). Movement-related potentials in Parkinson's disease: Motor imagery and movement preparation. *Brain, 120*(Pt. 8), 1339–1353.

Curtis, C. E., Rao, V. Y., & D'Esposito, M. (2004). Maintenance of spatial and motor codes during oculomotor delayed response tasks. *Journal of Neuroscience*, 24(16), 3944–3952.

Daselaar, S. M., Veltman, D. J., Rombouts, S. A., et al. (2003). Neuroanatomical correlates of episodic encoding and retrieval in young and elderly subjects. *Brain*, 126(Pt. 1), 43–56.

D'Esposito, M., Deouell, L. Y., & Gazzaley, A. (2003). Alterations in the BOLD fMRI signal with ageing and disease: A challenge for neuroimaging. *Nature Reviews Neuroscience*, 4(11), 863–872.

D'Esposito, M., Zarahn, E., Aguirre, G. K., et al. (1999). The effect of normal aging on the coupling of neural activity to the bold hemodynamic response. *NeuroImage*, 10(1), 6–14.

Fang, H. C. H. (1976). Observations on aging characteristics of cerebral blood vessels, macroscopic and microscopic features. In S. Gerson & R. D. Terry (Eds.), *Neurobiology of Aging*. New York: Raven.

Farkas, E., & Luiten, P. G. (2001). Cerebral microvascular pathology in aging and Alzheimer's disease. *Progress in Neurobiology*, 64(6), 575–611.

Gazzaley, A., Cooney, J., McEvoy, L. K., et al. (2005). Top-down enhancement and suppression of the magnitude and speed of neural activity. *Journal of Cognitive Neuroscience*, 17(3), 1–11.

Gazzaley, A., & D'Esposito, M. (2003). The contribution of functional brain imaging to our understanding of cognitive aging. *Science of Aging Knowledge Environment*. Available online at *sageke.sciencemag.org/cgi/content/full/sageke;2003/4/?*

Gazzaley, A., & D'Esposito, M. (2004). BOLD functional MRI and cognitive aging. In R. Cabeza, L. Nyberg, & D. Park (Eds.), *Cognitive neuroscience of aging: Linking cognitive and cerebral aging* (pp. 107–131). New York: Oxford University Press.

Gazzaley, A., Rissman, J., & D'Esposito, M. (2004). Functional connectivity during working memory maintenance. *Cognitive, Affective and Behavioral Neuroscience*, 4(4), 580–599.

Gitelman, D. R., Parrish, T. B., LaBar, K. S., et al. (2000). Real-time monitoring of eye movements using infrared video-oculography during functional magnetic resonance imaging of the frontal eye fields. *NeuroImage*, 11(1), 58–65.

Grady, C. L. (2000). Functional brain imaging and age-related changes in cognition. *Biological Psychology*, 54(1–3), 259–281.

Greicius, M. D., Krasnow, B., Reiss, A. L., et al. (2003). Functional connectivity in the resting brain: A network analysis of the default mode hypothesis. *Proceedings of the National Academy of Sciences of the United States of America*, 100(1), 253–258.

Greicius, M. D., Srivastava, G., Reiss, A. L., et al. (2004). Default-mode network activity distinguishes Alzheimer's disease from healthy aging: Evidence from functional MRI. *Proceedings of the National Academy of Sciences of the United States of America*, 101(13), 4637–4642.

Hampson, M., Peterson, B. S., Skudlarski, P., et al. (2002). Detection of functional connectivity using temporal correlations in MR images. *Human Brain Mapping*, 15(4), 247–262.

Handwerker, D. A., Ollinger, J. M., & D'Esposito, M. (2004). Variation of BOLD hemodynamic responses across subjects and brain regions and their effects on statistical analyses. *NeuroImage*, 21(4), 1639–1651.

Hesselmann, V., Zaro Weber, O., Wedekind, C., et al. (2001). Age related signal decrease in functional magnetic resonance imaging during motor stimulation in humans. *Neuroscience Letters, 308*(3), 141–144.

Huettel, S. A., Singerman, J. D., & McCarthy, G. (2001). The effects of aging upon the hemodynamic response measured by functional MRI. *NeuroImage, 13*(1), 161–175.

Iaria, G., Petrides, M., Dagher, A., et al. (2003). Cognitive strategies dependent on the hippocampus and caudate nucleus in human navigation: Variability and change with practice. *Journal of Neuroscience, 23*(13), 5945–5952.

Ishii, K., Willoch, F., Minoshima, S., et al. (2001). Statistical brain mapping of 18F-FDG PET in Alzheimer's disease: Validation of anatomic standardization for atrophied brains. *Journal of Nuclear Medicine, 42*(4), 548–557.

Jacobsen, L. K., Gore, J. C., Skudlarski, P., et al. (2002). Impact of intravenous nicotine on BOLD signal response to photic stimulation. *Magnetic Resonance Imaging, 20*(2), 141–145.

Laurienti, P. J., Field, A. S., Burdette, J. H., et al. (2002). Dietary caffeine consumption modulates fMRI measures. *NeuroImage, 17*(2), 751–757.

Lauritzen, M., & Gold, L. (2003). Brain function and neurophysiological correlates of signals used in functional neuroimaging. *Journal of Neuroscience, 23*(10), 3972–3980.

Leniger-Follert, E., & Hossmann, K. A. (1979). Simultaneous measurements of microflow and evoked potentials in the somatomotor cortex of the cat brain during specific sensory activation. *Pflugers Archiv European Journal of Physiology, 380*, 85–89.

Logan, J. M., Sanders, A. L., Snyder, A. Z., et al. (2002). Under-recruitment and nonselective recruitment: Dissociable neural mechanisms associated with aging. *Neuron, 33*(5), 827–840.

Logothetis, N. K. (2003). The underpinnings of the BOLD functional magnetic resonance imaging signal. *Journal of Neuroscience, 23*(10), 3963–3971.

Malonek, D., & Grinvald, A. (1996). Interactions between electrical activity and cortical microcirculation revealed by imaging spectroscopy: Implications for functional brain mapping. *Science, 272*, 551–554.

Mattay, V. S., Fera, F., Tessitore, A., et al. (2002). Neurophysiological correlates of age-related changes in human motor function. *Neurology, 58*(4), 630–635.

Miller, D. D., Andreasen, N. C., O'Leary, D. S., et al. (1997). Effect of antipsychotics on regional cerebral blood flow measured with positron emission tomography. *Neuropsychopharmacology, 17*(4), 230–240.

Mitchell, K. J., Johnson, M. K., Raye, C. L., et al. (2000). fMRI evidence of age-related hippocampal dysfunction in feature binding in working memory. *Brain Research: Brain Research Reviews, 10*(1–2), 197–206.

Mulderink, T. A., Gitelman, D. R., Mesulam, M. M., et al. (2002). On the use of caffeine as a contrast booster for BOLD fMRI studies. *NeuroImage, 15*(1), 37–44.

Murphy, K., & Garavan, H. (2004). Artifactual fMRI group and condition differences driven by performance confounds. *NeuroImage, 21*(1), 219–228.

Neele, S. J., Rombouts, S. A., Bierlaagh, M. A., et al. (2001). Raloxifene affects brain activation patterns in postmenopausal women during visual encoding. *Journal of Clinical Endocrinology and Metabolism, 86*(3), 1422–1424.

Nobler, M. S., Olvet, K. R., & Sackeim, H. A. (2002). Effects of medications on cerebral blood flow in late-life depression. *Current Psychiatry Reports, 4*(1), 51–58.

Ogawa, S., Lee, T.-M., Stepnoski, R., et al. (2000). An approach to probe some neural systems interaction by functional MRI at neural time scale down to milliseconds. *Proceedings of the National Academy of Sciences of the United States of America, 97*(20), 11026–11031.

Ogawa, S., Lee, T. M., Kay, A. R., et al. (1990). Brain magnetic resonance imaging with contrast dependent on blood oxygenation. *Proceedings of the National Academy of Sciences of the United States of America, 87*(24), 9868–9872.

Ogawa, S., Tank, D. W., Menon, R., et al. (1992). Intrinsic signal changes accompanying sensory stimulation: Functional brain mapping using MRI. *Proceedings of the National Academy of Sciences of the United States of America, 89,* 5951–5955.

Pariente, J., Loubinoux, I., Carel, C., et al. (2001). Fluoxetine modulates motor performance and cerebral activation of patients recovering from stroke. *Annals of Neurology, 50*(6), 718–729.

Pineiro, R., Pendlebury, S., Johansen-Berg, H., et al. (2002). Altered hemodynamic responses in patients after subcortical stroke measured by functional MRI. *Stroke, 33*(1), 103–109.

Price, C. J., & Friston, K. J. (1999). Scanning patients with tasks they can perform. *Human Brain Mapping, 8*(2–3), 102–108.

Riecker, A., Grodd, W., Klose, U., et al. (2003). Relation between regional functional MRI activation and vascular reactivity to carbon dioxide during normal aging. *Journal of Cerebral Blood Flow and Metabolism, 23*(5), 565–573.

Rissman, J., Gazzaley, A., & D'Esposito, M. (2004). Measuring functional connectivity during distinct stages of a cognitive task. *NeuroImage, 23*(2), 752–763.

Rosen, B. R., Buckner, R. L., & Dale, A. M. (1998). Event-related functional MRI: Past, present, and future. *Proceedings of the National Academy of Sciences of the United States of America, 95*(3), 773–780.

Ross, M. H., Yurgelun-Todd, D. A., Renshaw, P. F., et al. (1997). Age-related reduction in functional MRI response to photic stimulation. *Neurology, 48*(1), 173–176.

Rother, J., Knab, R., Hamzei, F., et al. (2002). Negative dip in BOLD fMRI is caused by blood flow–oxygen consumption uncoupling in humans. *NeuroImage, 15*(1), 98–102.

Rypma, B., & D'Esposito, M. (2000). Isolating the neural mechanisms of age-related changes in human working memory. *Nature Neuroscience, 3*(5), 509–515.

Schultz, S. K., O'Leary, D. S., Boles Ponto, L. L., et al. (1999). Age-related changes in regional cerebral blood flow among young to mid-life adults. *NeuroReport, 10*(12), 2493–2496.

Small, S. A., Perera, G. M., DeLaPaz, R., et al. (1999). Differential regional dysfunction of the hippocampal formation among elderly with memory decline and Alzheimer's disease. *Annals of Neurology, 45*(4), 466–472.

Small, S. A., Tsai, W. Y., DeLaPaz, R., et al. (2002). Imaging hippocampal function across the human life span: Is memory decline normal or not? *Annals of Neurology, 51*(3), 290–295.

Speer, N. K., Jacoby, L. L., & Braver, T. S. (2003). Strategy-dependent changes in memory: Effects on behavior and brain activity. *Cognitive, Affective and Behavioral Neuroscience, 3*(3), 155–167.

Stein, E. A., Pankiewicz, J., Harsch, H. H., et al. (1998). Nicotine-induced limbic cortical activation in the human brain: A functional MRI study. *American Journal of Psychiatry, 155*(8), 1009–1015.

Sun, F. T., Miller, L. M., & D'Esposito, M. (2004). Measuring interregional functional connectivity using coherence and partial coherence analyses of fMRI data. *NeuroImage, 21*(2), 647–658.

Takada, H., Nagata, K., Hirata, Y., et al. (1992). Age-related decline of cerebral oxygen metabolism in normal population detected with positron emission tomography. *Neurological Research, 14*(Suppl. 2), 128–131.

Taoka, T., Iwasaki, S., Uchida, H., et al. (1998). Age correlation of the time lag in signal change on EPI-fMRI. *Journal of Computer Assisted Tomography, 22*(4), 514–517.

Thulborn, K. R., Waterton, J. C., Matthews, P. M., et al. (1982). Oxygenation dependence of the transverse relaxation time of water protons in whole blood at high field. *Biochimica et Biophysica Acta, 714(2), 265–270.*

Turner, R., Le Bihan, D., Moonen, C. T., et al. (1991). Echo-planar time course MRI of cat brain oxygenation changes. Magnetic Resonance in Medicine, *22(1), 159–166.*

Yamaguchi, T., Kanno, I., Uemura, K., et al. (1986). Reduction in regional cerebral metabolic rate of oxygen during human aging. *Stroke, 17*(6), 1220–1228.

Yamamoto, M., Meyer, J. S., Sakai, F., et al. (1980). Aging and cerebral vasodilator responses to hypercarbia: Responses in normal aging and in persons with risk factors for stroke. *Archives of Neurology, 37*(8), 489–496.

Zarahn, E., Aguirre, G., & D'Esposito, M. (1997). A trial-based experimental design for fMRI. *NeuroImage, 6*(2), 122–138.

Zarahn, E., Aguirre, G. K., & D'Esposito, M. (1999). Temporal isolation of the neural correlates of spatial mnemonic processing with fMRI. *Brain Research: Brain Research Reviews, 7*(3), 255–268.

CHAPTER 5

Network Analysis of the Human Brain

APPLICATIONS TO UNDERSTANDING NORMAL
AND ABNORMAL NEURAL SYSTEM OPERATIONS

Anthony R. McIntosh
Cheryl L. Grady

One of the current challenges in neuroscience is to understand how brain operations give rise to mental phenomena ranging from sensation and perception to memory and attention. We now know a great deal about how the brain functions in basic sensory and motor systems. For higher mental functions, there has been a long scientific battle as to whether such functions are localizable. A dominant assumption in neuroscience is that certain parts of the brain have unique roles in mental function. This idea of one region/one function comes from early studies that showed some remarkable cognitive deficits following lesions in specific parts of the brain. Up until the last 15–20 years, the tools available to neuroscientists have allowed them to examine only small parts of the brain at a time, the findings from such examinations reinforcing the notion of discrete functions in specific brain regions.

Modern neuroimaging tools allow us to measure how the *entire* brain reacts as people perform different mental operations. We are finding that many more brain areas "light up" when someone pays attention, thinks, and remembers than we would have expected based on the results from lesion studies. However, many researchers in the field, who continue to focus on one or two critical brain regions, overlook this new information.

The brain is made up of individual elements, ranging from neurons to ensembles. These elements are connected, so their *individual actions* can be combined through their *interactions*. The combined responses of small groups of cells give interacting brain areas a rich response repertoire, from simple sensation to consciousness and reason. When neuroimaging data are examined in terms of brain interactions, it is observed that many regions cooperate in our thought processes. Emerging neurobiological theories emphasize the combined actions of interacting brain elements (cells to ensembles to regions) as the link between the brain and human mental function (McIntosh, 2000a, 2000b).

From a network perspective, anything that affects the integrity of a specific brain region necessarily influences the operation of the entire network or networks in which this region participates. Behavioral deficits following damage, or arising from disease processes, may thus reflect either the abnormal operation of a damaged network or the formation of a completely different network with a new behavioral repertoire. Thus, much can be learned about brain dysfunction, as well as normal function, by examining network operations in cases where mental functions are compromised by damage or disease.

If it is the case that normal brain function and dysfunction result from the action of distributed networks, then analytic approaches tuned to such dynamics would best capture these actions. The focus of this chapter is to review a few of the applications of network analysis to normal aging and dementia to illustrate how such an application has helped develop a comprehensive appreciation for how networks change in an attempt to adapt to damage or deterioration. We review some of the basic methods our group has used for network analysis and present the underlying theory for the application and the development of a new perspective that serves to unite the understanding of brain function and dysfunction within one framework.

Theoretical Basis of Network Analysis and the Tools

Network analysis as applied to neuroimaging can be considered as a collection of analytic methods (e.g., interregional correlations/covariances or the corresponding measure in the frequency domain such as coherence) that attempt to measure the interdependency among brain areas during different cognitive states. The driving assumption behind the use of these approaches is that the covariances/correlations of activity are measures of neural interactions. Neural interactions refer, in a general sense, to influences that different elements in the nervous system have on each other via synaptic communication (the term "elements" refers to any constituent of the nervous system, either a single neuron or collections thereof). Traditional approaches to the understanding of neural interactions have focused on systematic variation in activity with some manipulated parameter. However, activity changes in one neural element usually result from a change in the influence of other connected elements, so focusing on activity in one area will miss the change in afferent influence. Furthermore, it is logically possible for the influences on an element to change without an appreciable change in measured activity. The simplest example is the case in which an afferent influence switches from one source to another, without a change in the strength of the influence. For example, in the feedforward network depicted in Figure 5.1, region C may show similar activity patterns when effective connections from either A or B are strong. Monitoring regional activity alone would not be able to differentiate the source of the effects, but measures of the relation of activity between elements (i.e., paths *v* vs. *w*) would be able to.

The measurement of neural interactions in neuroimaging has developed under two general approaches. The first emphasizes pairwise interactions, often in terms of correlations or covariances. The second incorporates additional information, such as anatomical connections, and considers an interaction of several neural elements simultaneously to explicitly quantify the effect one element has on another. These two approaches are known as *functional* and *effective connectivity*, respectively. Both terms were introduced in the context of electrophysiological recordings from multiple cells (Aertsen et al., 1987) and have been used in reference to neuroimaging data (Friston et al., 1993; Friston, 1994; Horwitz & Braun, 2004). Two methods that are discussed here typify the use of covariance tools in the analysis of neuroimaging data: partial least squares (PLS), which can be used to assess functional connectivity (McIntosh et al., 1996a, 2004), and covariance structural equation modeling (CSEM), which estimates effective connectivity (McIntosh & Gonzalez-Lima, 1991, 1994). Both methods have been used in other scientific disciplines and are discussed here as they pertain to neuroimaging. The present focus is on how to use these methods to ask specific questions about the functional organization of the nervous system.

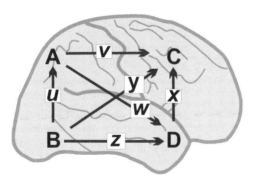

FIGURE 5.1. Hypothetical anatomical network linking four cortical regions. The labels on the connections, *u, v, w, x, y, z*, correspond to the estimated path coefficients, which represent the effective connections between regions. Region C may show similar activity between two conditions despite have different patterns of effective connections. For instance, the activity in C would be the same if the effect through path *v* is high and *y* is zero, or if the effect in *v* is zero and *y* is high. Such a change in effective connection is accessible only through analysis covariances of activity between regions.

Although the majority of studies of network interactions have focused on the young healthy brain, there are tremendous gains to be had in studying these operations in other age groups and patient populations. From a developmental perspective, the fact that brain structure changes across the entire life-span has obvious implications for network operations. As we discuss below, even in cases where overt behavior does not show an age-related change there may be quite different sets of regional activity and interactivity between age groups. In clinical populations, the network reorganization may be even more dramatic, depending on the source of pathology. In cases of brain damage, network reorganization is likely to be seen both in terms of primary response to damage (degeneration, diaschisis) and in terms of secondary responses as the networks reconfigure in an attempt to adapt to the insult (compensatory mechanisms). The interesting implication is that some of the behavioral deficits may reflect the secondary response. It is likely that a similar reorganization also occurs in degenerative disorders, although over a more protracted length of time. Finally, mental disorders will affect the integrity of network operations. Although we do not discuss applications to mental disorders here, there are several examples in the literature (Jennings et al., 1998; Welchew et al., 2002; Seminowicz et al., 2004).

Definitions

Covariances used in multivariate analyses can identify the dominant functional and/or effective connections during the performance of a cognitive or behavioral operation. In the context of neuroimaging, *functional connectivity* indicates that two regions show some non-zero correlation of activity, but does not specify how this correlation comes about, whereas *effective connectivity* indicates the direct effect one region has on another, usually explicitly accounting for mutual or intervening influences. Linear regression methods sometimes appear to lie in a gray area between functional and effective connectivity. For example, the method to estimate psychophysiological interactions (PPIs; Friston et al., 1997) in the statistical parametric mapping (SPM) package is used to assess task-dependent changes in the degree that one region—Y—predicts/explains the activity of another—X (McIntosh & Gonzalez-Lima, 1994). However, the PPI approach provides the same statistical result that would be obtained if the roles of X and Y were reversed. Thus, the PPI method is most similar to an estimate of functional connectivity, specifically task-dependent changes in functional connectivity.

Major Steps in Network Analysis

The progression from data collection to the final stage of a network analysis depends, largely, on the question one asks of the data. Assuming that a comprehensive analysis is planned, the steps can be outlined as follows:

1. *Perform activation analysis.* This step is the usual first step in any image analysis. It is a reasonable assumption that regions showing similar activity changes between tasks may also be part of the same functional network (although this is not a certainty; Stephan, 2004). Although the typical mode of activation analysis uses a univariate approach, multivariate approaches may be preferable when one is attempting to identify cohesive networks. The primary reason for this is that in the case where there are dependencies among measured (dependent) variables, multivariate approaches will have greater sensitivity because they explicitly make use of these correlations (Lukic et al., 2002).

2. *Relate brain activity to behavioral measures.* Although the most common approach in neuroimaging is activation analysis, there are a growing number of people who are relating activity patterns either to performance measured during the experiment or to demographic measures. In the former instance, the brain–behavior analysis may be considered as completing a "causal chain," in the sense that the activation analysis would be most sensitive to the input side of the chain and behavior analysis to the output. Combining brain–behavior analysis with activation analysis can be seen as getting the most comprehensive coverage of most, if not all, regions that are part of the functional network for a given task. Finally, relating the patterns of functional or effective connectivity provides an anchor for interpretation in that they act to confirm that the patterns of interactivity actually "make a difference" in performance.

3. *Analyze functional connectivity.* Once the candidate nodes are collected, the pattern of interactions can be used to examine functional connectivity. Probably the simplest approach to this is the calculation of pairwise correlations/covariances. Functional connectivity estimates can be compared across tasks or groups to define dependencies on this dimension.

4 *Analyze effective connectivity.* Functional connectivity can be easily assessed across any number of regions of interest, but effective connectivity requires a more focused approach wherein a subsection of regions identified in the previous steps are considered for models that are more detailed.

We do not suggest that all of the network analysis steps listed above must be carried across to every dataset. Obviously, the choice of analysis—functional or effective connectivity—depends on the particular question one has about the data. Functional connectivity analyses are likely satisfactory when the goal is in the exploratory/explanatory mode. For example, if a peculiar activation pattern is noted in one group, assessment of the functional connectivity of that region with the rest of the brain may help explain the peculiarity in terms of a difference in the pattern of interactions in that group relative to controls. However, if the question is phrased in terms of directed influences, then analysis of effective connectivity is needed. For example, if the question is whether top-down influences from prefrontal to temporal cortices vary between groups, an analysis like CSEM must be performed to distinguish top-down from bottom-up effects.

Partial Least Squares

Partial least squares (PLS) is a multivariate tool that can be used to describe the relation between a set of exogenous measures, like experimental design or behavioral measures, and a set of functional brain images (McIntosh et al., 1996a; McIntosh & Lobaugh, 2004). What results from a PLS analysis are sets of images that may be interpreted as nodes of neural systems representing some experimental effect or relating to some behavior measure. The same analytic tool can be used to explore whether a part of the brain, represented by an image voxel, shows any task-related changes in its relation to the rest of the brain.

A highly idealized graphical description of the PLS procedure used to analyze changes in regional correlation (functional connectivity) is presented in Figure 5.2. In panel A of Figure 5.2, activity from a particular seed voxel (middle right of the image) is correlated with the activity from the rest of the image in three tasks. This produces a correlational map for each task depicting areas that are correlated with the seed voxel.

When interpreting the correlation maps, a researcher would usually identify where the maps differ across three tasks. For example, in Figure 5.2A the seed voxel shows an opposite pattern of correlations with posterior areas in tasks 2 and 3 and correlates with its contralateral homologue in task 1 only. Common correlations across the three tasks are in contralateral prefrontal regions and, of course, with the seed voxel with itself. The advantage of using PLS to do this type of analysis is that one can extract both commonalities and differences in the correlation maps from multiple task conditions. The PLS analysis of the correlation maps, or seed PLS, operates on the three correlation maps together and, through singular value decomposition (SVD), provides sets of mutually orthogonal latent variable (LV) pairs. One element of the pair contains numerical weights for each task, creating a profile that depicts either a common correlation pattern or a task-related difference (i.e., a contrast).[1] The other element of the LV pair identifies the parts of the image that show the profile across tasks and can be displayed in image space. Because it is derived from SVD, it is called it a *singular image*. Within the singular image are numerical weights for each voxel, and their variation across the image shows which areas are maximally expressed on the particular LV. The weights for both the singular image and the task profile are called *saliences*. In reference to Figure 5.2B, the singular image from the first LV shows positive saliences at the location of the seed voxel (middle right of the image) and negative saliences at the contralateral prefrontal voxel. In the bar graph below the singular image, the saliences across tasks are equal, so the first LV is the com-

---

[1] Another way to think about this is to consider an experiment with only two tasks and thus only two correlation maps. The sum of these two maps (or average) represents areas of common correlation, and a subtraction of the two maps identifies differences in correlations (McIntosh & Gonzalez-Lima, 1998). This is essentially what occurs in PLS, and whether a singular image depicts common correlations or differences would be identified in the task profiles.

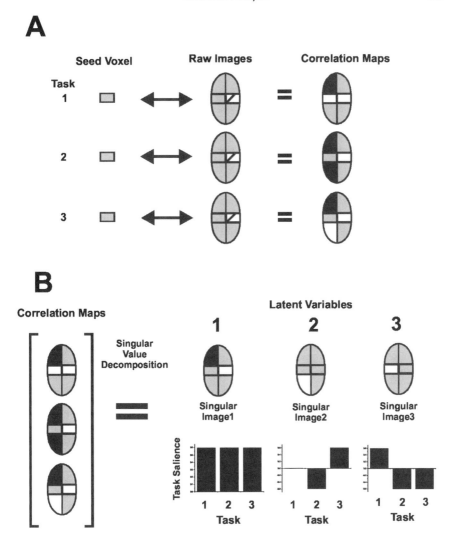

FIGURE 5.2. Graphic representation of the steps involved in a partial least squares analysis of seed voxel correlations. Panel A: A seed voxel is selected from the middle of the right side of the image (indicated by the black hash mark) within each of three tasks and correlated with the rest of the six-voxel image, resulting in one correlation map per task. Black represents a strong negative correlation, and white a strong positive. In panel B the three correlation maps are stacked into one large matrix and decomposed with singular value decomposition, resulting in three latent variable (LV) pairs. Each pair consists of the singular image, which is an image representation of the weights (saliences) for voxels, and the weights or saliences across tasks or the task profile (bottom of each LV). As with the correlations, black represents a strong negative salience, and white a strong positive. LV1 is a common pattern of seed voxel correlations, LV2 distinguishes the correlation maps from tasks 2 versus 3, and LV3 contrasts the map for task 1 with tasks 2 and 3.

mon correlation of the seed voxel with itself and the contralateral frontal regions. The singular image in LV2 has a negative salience at a posterior location, and the profile across the tasks contrasts tasks 2 and 3, so the LV depicts a posterior difference in seed–voxel correlation patterns. Finally, LV3 shows the salience at the contralateral homologue for the seed voxel, and the task profile contrasts task 1 with tasks 2 and 3. Although the results of the seed PLS analysis in Figure 5.2 could have easily been distilled from the examination of the within-task correlation maps, it is much more difficult when images contain several thousand voxels, as with positron emission tomography (PET) or functional magnetic imaging (fMRI) data (and real data are seldom as clean). The seed PLS analysis can also be extended to include more than one seed voxel, or a seed voxel and a behavior measure (McIntosh et al., 1997; Lenartowicz & McIntosh, 2005). The interpretation of the singular image and task profiles is the same as that for the single seed voxel analysis, but a given singular image may show different task profiles for each seed voxel/behavior measure (e.g., task commonalities for one seed voxel, task differences for another).

PLS has also been used for activation analysis to define distributed activity patterns that differentiate tasks or to determine whether task effects differ between different groups of subjects. The machinery for the "task PLS" analysis is identical to that for seed PLS, except that voxel-wise activity measures form the maps rather than correlations. In task PLS, these maps are usually mean centered such that activity is expressed as the deviation from the overall mean for the experiment. Mean centering improves the sensitivity of the analysis to task-dependent differences.

The more recent developments of PLS have made it possible to take advantage of time series information gained from electroencephalography (EEG) or functional MRI data (Lobaugh et al., 2001; McIntosh et al., 2004). Although the basic algorithm is identical to what is described above, the added temporal information enables the identification of similarities in the spatial patterns that relate to task or behavior, but show differences in the timing or duration of involvement (McIntosh & Lobaugh, 2004).

PLS can be used in any of the first three steps of network analysis. Task PLS identifies the dominant activity differences. Using the configuration for seed PLS, brain–behavior analysis can be done to identify similarities and differences in the spatial patterns that most closely relate to measured behavior. As mentioned above, the seed PLS is an analysis of functional connectivity, making it an ideal segue to estimation of effective connectivity (McIntosh et al., 1998).

Covariance Structural Equation Modeling

Covariance structural equation modeling (CSEM), or path analysis, is a multivariate analytic tool that is used to test hypotheses about the causal influences among measured or latent variables. One of the main purposes is to determine whether a hypothesized set of causal relationships is consistent with the observed data. The covariances between the variables are used to provide weights to proposed causal relationships in a manner similar to a multiple linear regression, which then indexes how well the proposed causal structure represents the observed covariance. CSEM is used extensively in psychology and other social sciences (Bollen, 1989). For example, structural equation modeling has been used to distinguish between inherited and environmentally determined influences on certain personality traits (Loehlin, 1987) and whether performances on several memory tasks are best accounted for by the influence of a unitary or bidimensional memory system (Nyberg, 1994). As applied to neuroimaging data, structural equation modeling combines interregional covariances and neuroanatomy. This is an important feature of the application of structural equation modeling to neuroimaging. The causal structure is determined from the anatomy, rather than hypothesized, and the major goal is to evaluate the experimentally induced changes in the effective connections between regions. Clarification of this point can be made with reference to Figure 5.1. The four regions (A, B, C, D) have their anatomical connections defined by the presence of paths u, v, w, x, y, z. This formally sets up a set of structural equations:

$$A = uB + e_A \tag{1}$$
$$B = e_B \tag{2}$$
$$C = vA + yB + e_C \tag{3}$$
$$D = wA + zD + e_D \tag{4}$$

where e indicates residual influences on the region of interest that are not captured by the other effects. Estimation of the values for each of the paths are the effective connections for the network and are derived by fitting the observed covariances among the four areas with a set of covariances that are calculated on the basis of the estimated effective connections. Specifically, if we rewrite the structural equations in a matrix format, such that **Y** is a vector containing the variances of regions A, B, C, D, and β is a square matrix of zeros except for cells containing the path coefficients:

$$\beta = \begin{bmatrix} 0 & u & 0 & 0 \\ 0 & 0 & 0 & 0 \\ v & y & 0 & x \\ w & z & 0 & 0 \end{bmatrix}$$

where the columns indicate the area sending the effect, and the rows the area receiving the effect. Finally, matrix E is a diagonal matrix containing the residual values for each region (e_A, e_B, e_C, e_D). The full matrix equation for the structural model would be

$$Y = \beta Y + E \tag{5}$$

To fit this equation, we can compute the observed covariances of the regions:

$$\sigma = Y^T Y \tag{6}$$

(where superscript T indicates transpose) and compare this to the implied covariance computed by

$$\Sigma = \mathrm{inv}(I - \beta)^{T} * (E^T E) * \mathrm{inv}(I - \beta) \tag{7}$$

where I is an identity matrix and inv indicates matrix inverse. The estimates for β and E are adjusted until differences between σ and Σ are as small as possible (in practice, this works until the change in difference between iterations reaches a minimum). Assuming that the anatomical network accurately captures the dominant connections that have been reported, it is likely that there would be other influences that contribute to the covariances of the system that are not included in the model. Thus, although the estimated path coefficients in β will be the optimal estimate of the effective connections model specified, the model per se may not explain all the variance and covariance in the data. However, it is perfectly legitimate to compare the estimated effective connections between two groups or tasks even when the overall model does not fit the data. This is because the estimated path coefficients are not greatly affected by the influences that are not included in the model (McIntosh & Gonzalez-Lima, 1994).

Figure 5.3 outlines the essential processes in the estimation of effective connectivity changes with CSEM. Once the nodes for the model are identified from prior analyses (Figure 5.3, top row), two decisions must be made. The first is the number of regions to model. For CSEM there is a mathematical limit to the total number of regions that can be analyzed, which is constrained by the number of observations per task/group. To maintain a full rank covariance matrix, the number of regions should be equal to or less than the number of observations. It is possible to exceed this limit, but only if constraints are placed on the final model to ensure that the estimated path coefficients are not unduly influenced by rank deficiency (linear dependency among regions). For example, we were able to model a network of 22 bilateral regions with a sample size of 12, by first modeling within-hemisphere effective connectivity, fixing those estimates, and then estimating interhemispheric effects (McIntosh et al., 1996b). The assumption of this model is that the interhemispheric effects are determined by intrahemispheric interactions.

The second consideration is the determination of the anatomical connections in the model (Figure 5.3, middle row). The anatomic connectivity between selected brain regions is derived from the neuroanatomy literature. This is not a trivial step, and it is at this stage that the theoretical persuasion

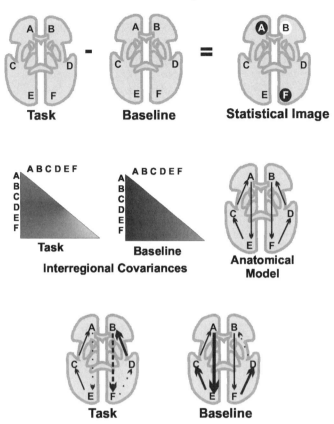

FIGURE 5.3. Graphic representation of essential steps in structural equation modeling for imaging data. In the top row, regions for the model are selected based partly on the statistical differences between task and baseline (regions A and F showing deactivation and B showing activation) and partly on theoretical considerations, such as anatomical completeness or a theoretical model (regions C, D, and E). In the middle row, the activity correlations between areas are computed within-task and the anatomical model is constructed based on published neuroanatomical work. Finally, in the bottom row, the correlations are used to derive path coefficients for each anatomical connection within task, yielding two functional models. Positive weights are solid lines, and negative dashed, with the thickness of the line indicating the size of the weight. The "deactivations" identified from the subtraction image in region A corresponds to a reduced involvement of region A, and the deactivation of F is because of strong negative feedback from region B. The activation in region B corresponds to its increased (suppressive) influence on F plus the stronger afferent influence from D.

of the investigator must guide the decision of which connections to include in a model. Any system of equations where there are unknowns to be solved will benefit from constraints to possible solutions. Using the anatomy of the system helps to constrain solutions. However, if all major and minor paths were to be included, most models would contain reciprocal loops between most areas, with some interconnections spanning regions, both feedforward and feedback. When all possible anatomical connections are included, it is likely that there would be either the same number of known and unknown elements or more unknown elements. In either case, an underdetermined system of equations would result and unique solutions would not be obtainable. In most cases, some compromise between anatomical accuracy and interpretability is needed. Any compromise would clearly be a simplification of what the reality of the interactions may be, and these compromises need to be made explicit for a complete understanding of the final model. There have been several published accounts in which the compromises in model building have been made explicit (McIntosh et al., 1994; Buchel & Friston, 1997; Kohler et al., 1998), although such specificity is often lacking in neurocognitive models that are loosely based on activation patterns. Any modeling effort, whether based on simulations, data fitting, or intuition, is necessarily a simplification of reality, and it is the degree of simplification that determines the utility of the model.

For most published accounts of CSEM in neuroimaging, the interregional covariances were computed within a condition and across participants. For fMRI and data from electrical or magnetic recordings (event-related potentials, ERP; or magnetoencephalography, MEG), covariances can be computed for an individual subject across tasks or across trials of the same task, because many more within-subject measures can be made (Buchel & Friston, 1997).

Path coefficients represent the proportion of the activity in one area that is determined by the activity of other areas that project to it. When the coefficients are based on functional activity measured across participants, they reflect what could be thought of as an average functional influence within a given task and index the reliability and sign of the influence. The final step includes the comparison of path coefficients across tasks to determine if the interactions within the functional network differ (Figure 5.3, bottom row). This is done by assuming that path coefficients are the same between tasks, and thereby the same implied covariance matrix (see Eq. 7 above), and by comparing this to the covariance matrix for each group. This overall measure of fit is compared to a model where the estimated path coefficients are allowed to vary between tasks, yielding a separate implied covariance matrix for each group. If the fit improves significantly when the coefficients are allowed to vary, this suggests that there is a significant difference in effective connections between tasks. Using this nested or stacked model approach, one may test for more specific differences involving individual paths (McIntosh et al., 1998).

Dorsal and Ventral Stream Processing
in Perceptual Matching

The first application of CSEM to human neuroimaging data examined the effective connections in the cortical–visual system (McIntosh et al., 1994). One well-established functional distinction in the brain is between object and spatial–visual pathways. The foundation for this dual organization can be traced at least as far back as Kleist in the 1930s (Kleist, 1935). One of its strongest expressions to date is in the dorsal and ventral cortical processing streams, described by Ungerleider and Mishkin (1982), which correspond to spatial and object processing pathways, respectively.

A similar duality was identified in humans with the aid of PET(Haxby et al., 1991). In this experiment, a match-to-sample task for faces was used to explore object vision. For spatial vision, a match-to-sample task for the location of a dot within a square was used. The results from right hemisphere analysis are presented in Figure 5.4 (left hemisphere interactions did not differ between tasks). Path coefficients along the ventral pathway from cortical area 19v extending into the frontal lobe were stronger in the face-matching model, and interactions along the dorsal pathway from area 19d to the frontal lobe were relatively stronger in the location-matching model. Among posterior areas, the differences in path coefficients were mainly in magnitude. Occipitotemporal interactions between area 19v and area 37 were stronger in the face-matching model, and the impact of area 17/18 to 19d and the occipitoparietal influences from area 19d to area 7 was stronger in the location-matching model.

The anatomical connections allowed for interactions between the dorsal and ventral pathways with connections from area 37 to area 7 and from area 7 to area 21. The interactions between these areas showed task-dependent differences in magnitude and sign. Thus, the strongest positive interactions in each model may have preferentially been in one pathway, but the parallel pathways were not functioning independently. Strong interactions between parallel pathways have been a consistent finding in all CSEM applications to imaging data. Therefore, although a certain pathway or area may be critical for a particular function, operations in the intact brain involve interactions between many regions. A second observation, and one that underscores the importance of network analysis, is that activation differences were restricted to posterior cortices, yet differences in interactions extended into prefrontal cortex. The overall magnitude of effective connections to prefrontal cortex was the same, but the signs of the effects differed between tasks (cf. Figure 5.1).

We extended this network analysis, comparing healthy older adults with young adults and patients with early Alzhiemer's dementia (DAT) with healthy elders in the face-matching version of the task (Horwitz et al., 1995). There were no group differences in accuracy on the task, though the healthy older adults and the patients with DAT were both somewhat slower than their respective comparison groups. When interactions along ventral stream areas

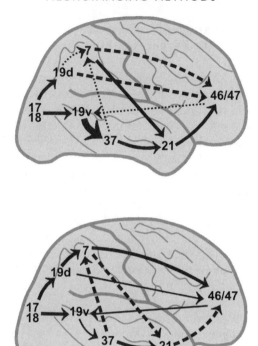

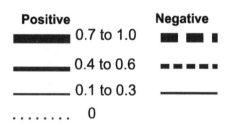

FIGURE 5.4. Effective connectivity between cortical areas in the right hemisphere for object and spatial vision operations. The numbers on the cortical surface refer to Brodmann areas (d, dorsal; v, ventral). The arrows represent the anatomical connections between areas, and the magnitude of the direct effect from one area to another is proportional to the arrow width for each path.

were assessed, two interesting results emerged (Figure 5.5). First, when compared with young adults, the older group had similar effective connections between posterior regions but showed additional feedback effects from prefrontal to occipitotemporal regions. Interestingly, when activation patterns were compared between young and old, prefrontal and occipitotemporal regions showed relatively greater activity in the older adults during the face-matching task. The results from the analysis of effective connectivity suggested this activity difference might be explained by increased interactions between these two areas in the older participants.

Activation patterns in the DAT group were similar to those in controls in the ventral stream areas, but members of the DAT group showed greater relative activation in dorsal prefrontal cortices as compared with controls. Using CSEM, the patients with DAT showed a pattern of interactions in the ventral stream network that was decidedly different from that of controls, with a disconnection of temporofrontal effects and a weak negative feedback effect from prefrontal to occipitotemporal cortex. Indeed, functional connections (correlations) between ventral stream areas were in general weaker in the DAT group. As a supplementary analysis, a functional connectivity analysis was done using a region in the prefrontal cortex where its correlations with the rest of the brain were examined. In the DAT group, a widespread pattern of functional connectivity was observed that was restricted to the prefrontal cortex, whereas controls showed stronger functional connections between prefrontal and occipital regions.

Functional Connectivity during Working Memory for Faces

As a continuation of the face-matching study described above, Haxby and colleagues (Haxby et al., 1995) explored the changes in activity patterns when a working memory component was added. They used a delayed match-to-sample task, with a parametric increase in delay between the sample and test faces. In young adults, there was a linear increase in activity of prefrontal, cingulate, and anterior temporal cortices, and a concomitant decrease in occipitotemporal cortices. Using a similar protocol, Grady and colleagues examined the changes in activity patterns in normal old adults and patients with DAT (Grady et al., 2001). Relative to young subjects, both groups showed slower reaction time in general, but all showed a linear increase in reaction time with increasing delay. Accuracy in the older adults was quite high across all delay levels (> 90%), whereas the DAT group showed a decrease in accuracy with increasing delay.

In terms of activity, many brain regions showed similar activity during these tasks in both young and older adults, including the left anterior prefrontal cortex, which had increased activity with delay, and the ventral extrastriate cortex, which showed decreased activity with delay. However, older adults had less activation overall and less modulation across delay in the right ventrolateral

Young Subjects

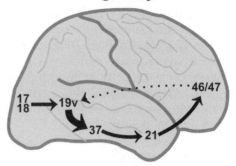

Healthy Old Subjects

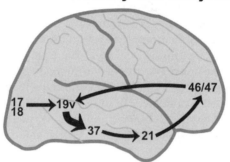

DAT Subjects

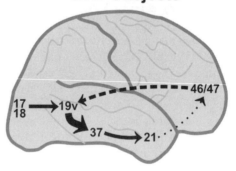

FIGURE 5.5. Effective connectivity between cortical areas in the right hemisphere for object vision operations (face matching) in young individuals, older individuals, and patients with mild Alzheimer's dementia (DAT). The numbers on the cortical surface refer to Brodmann's areas. The arrows represent the anatomical connections between areas, and the magnitude of the direct effect from one area to another is proportional to the arrow width for each path, as in Figure 5.4.

prefrontal cortex than did the young adults. Older adults also showed greater activation in the left dorsolateral–prefrontal cortex across all working memory (WM) delays and increased activity at short delays in the left occipitoparietal cortex, as compared with young adults. The DAT group had increased activity in the right prefrontal, anterior cingulate, and left amygdala. Increased activity in the right prefrontal cortex was associated with better memory performance in both older adults and the DAT group, and activity in the left amygdala was correlated with better performance in the patients with DAT. Based on these task and behavioral effects, functional connectivity of the right prefrontal cortex and left amygdala was examined in both groups by determining those areas whose activity was correlated with activity in these regions. In older adults, activity in the right prefrontal cortex was positively correlated with blood flow in the left prefrontal cortex, bilateral extrastriate and parietal areas, and the right hippocampus. In patients with DAT, activity in the right prefrontal cortex was correlated mainly with other prefrontal regions. Areas where activity was correlated with the left amygdala in patients with DAT included the bilateral posterior parahippocampal gyri, a number of left prefrontal regions, and the anterior and posterior cingulate, thalamus, and insula. Older adults had a relatively restricted set of regions where activity correlated with the left amygdala, mainly the temporal and occipital areas.

    The profound engagement of the amygdala in the DAT patient group may seem puzzling at first blush, but the fact that this region was not only more active in patients but also predicted relatively better memory performance warrants closer consideration. One potential explanation for the amygdala recruitment put forth by Grady and colleagues (Grady et al., 2001) was that the patients with DAT were focusing more on the emotional quality of the faces, which would thus enhance their memory. Although it was unlikely an overt strategy, this affective response would partially overcome the reduced capacity of the usual cognitive systems that would be engaged during encoding of the faces (e.g., medial temporal, anterior prefrontal). A second, and perhaps more contentious, possibility is that the differences in functional connectivity reflect a reorganization of the neural circuitry such that regions that are typically allied with one cognitive domain (i.e., affective processing) are recruited for somewhat different operations. Such reorganization would be enabled by existing anatomical relationships that may be unmasked when the dominant network is compromised. Such unmasking of connections has been observed in stroke (Bach y Rita, 1981; Chen et al., 2002; Lee & van Donkelaar, 1995), and may also occur in degenerative disorders.

Perceptual Memory and Corticolimbic Networks

Much of the research comparing different groups tends to focus on tasks in which there are possible differences in the cognitive strategies used to do a task. For example, in the case of learning a list of words, it is possible to design the experiment to ensure that the words are learned at an equivalent level across groups, but it is difficult to control for experiential differences that may affect performance in different groups (e.g., cohort effects). Moreover, there is a strong possibility that the fundamental difference in network operations may extend from basic sensory all the way to higher-order cognitive operations, despite the possibility that performance in sensory tasks may not differ between groups. On the basis of the work on perceptual matching of faces described above, we thought the potential for this possibility was strong, and we sought to investigate it using rudimentary visual stimuli made from single vertical sine wave gratings differing in spatial frequency (Della-Maggiore et al., 2000; McIntosh et al., 1999).

Young and older subjects' brain activity was measured using PET while they performed a short-term memory task (delayed visual discrimination) in which they determined which of two successively presented sine wave gratings had the highest spatial frequency. Memory load was manipulated by interposing a delay between the two gratings of either 500 ms or 4,000 ms. Memory performance was measured as the percent difference between the two gratings necessary to achieve 80% accuracy. This procedure, which is typical for psychophysical studies, enables adjustment for differences in contrast sensitivity across subjects and thus equates performance.

Memory performance was indeed equal between groups, and both showed a delay-related increase in threshold. The first question we asked was whether the similar performance across groups meant that the same neural systems were engaged. This was answered using behavior PLS, correlating memory performance within short and long delays and the corresponding data across subjects from each group.

Three stable patterns of brain–behavior correlations were extracted by the PLS analysis. The first pattern identified regions that were commonly correlated across both delays and age groups. In this pattern, lower thresholds (i.e., better performance) were associated with high activity in the occipital cortices and ventral posterior thalamus, and low activity in the left anterior prefrontal and bilateral inferior parietal cortices.

The second pattern identified by PLS was a delay effect that was common across groups. The dominant regions for the delay pattern are shown in Plate 5.1A, where the color assigned to a region indicates a negative or positive relation to behavior. Negative weights are seen in the medial occipital cortices, and positive weights bilaterally in the ventral striatum and inferior prefrontal cortex, and in the right inferior temporal cortex. This pattern was correlated inversely with the threshold across the two delays. At the short delay, higher activity in the medial occipital cortex and lower activity in the striatum, inferior prefrontal, and inferior temporal cortex was associated with better performance. At the long delay, the reverse was true. Interestingly, although the delay pattern was correlated with performance for both young and older adults, the strength of the correlations (functional connections) among regions within the delay pattern was higher in the young group. This age-related difference in interregional correlations suggests that the functional network underlying this form of short-term visual memory is degraded in older individuals.

If this is the case, how did older adults manage to perform as well as their younger counterparts on the task? One possible answer is that older subjects recruited new areas of the brain to help them compensate for the weakened state of the primary neural network. Support for this answer comes from the analysis of the third pattern identified by PLS, which differentiates the performance of older from young adults. The peak weights for this pattern are shown in Plate 5.1B. Negative weights were found in the left anterior and medial temporal cortices and more dorsally in the occipital cortex, and positive saliences were observed in the posterior thalamus and dorsomedial prefrontal cortices. As was found with the delay pattern, there was an age-related difference in the pattern of correlations between the brain regions showing this effect. However, in this case the interregional correlations were stronger in older adults than in the young. If the strong interregional correlations are an indication of a working functional network, then the PLS analysis suggests that a new network has emerged for older adults that is not present for young observers. One interpretation of this result is that old brains recruit new areas to perform a task to compensate for a lack of coherence among areas within the primary network used by young brains (the delay pattern).

These results, and their further elaboration (Della-Maggiore et al., 2000, 2002), demonstrate that there may be quite distinct patterns of network operations that support similar levels of behavioral output. The critical feature of this particular study was that this difference was observed in a rudimentary visual memory task, in which it is unlikely that the network differences reflect a difference in overt strategy.

Development of Network Theory: Neural Context

A concept that has come from the use of network analysis is that of a *neural context* (McIntosh, 1998, 2000b). Most brain regions receive inputs from many areas and then send projections to several others. At any instant, the interactions through anatomical connections may shift from one afferent/efferent source to another, resulting in a change in cognition or behavior. Across several different tasks, a brain area may show the same activity pattern but serve different functions because of the relation of that activity with other brain regions. The important factor is not that a particular event occurred at a particular site, but rather the *neural context* under which that event occurred—in other words, what was the rest of the brain doing? Neural context is closely related to the idea of "functional pluripotentialism," put forth by Filimonov (Luria, 1962), which states that no formation in the central nervous system is responsible solely for a single function and under certain conditions, a given formation may be involved in other functional systems and may participate in performance of other tasks.

A salient demonstration of neural context comes from a recent study examining functional connectivity of the medial temporal lobe (MTL) in relation to learning and awareness in healthy young adults (McIntosh et al., 2003). In a sensory learning paradigm, individuals were classified as *Aware* or *Unaware*, based on whether they noted that one of two tones predicted a visual event. Although only the Aware subjects acquired and reversed a differential response to the tones, both groups showed learned facilitation.

When we related brain activity (indexed by blood flow measured with PET) to behavior in each group, we observed that MTL activity related to facilitation in both groups. This was curious, given the suggestion that the MTL is critical for learning with awareness, but not when learning proceeds without awareness (Clark & Squire, 1998, 2000). Given the principle of neural context, it was possible that this common regional involvement in both the Aware and Unaware groups was an expression of contextual dependency. We then examined the functional connectivity of the MTL and observed completely different interactions of the MTL between groups (Figure 5.6). In the Aware group, dominant MTL interactions were observed for the prefrontal,

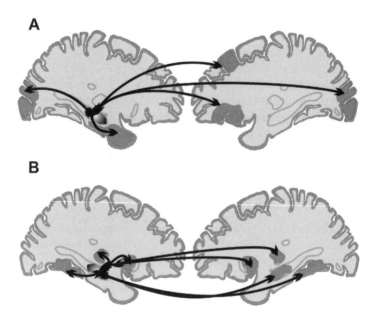

FIGURE 5.6. Summary of the dominant functional connections of the left medial temporal lobe (MTL) in learning with (A) and without (B) awareness. Panel A shows dominant interactions, indicated by bidirectional arrows, between MTL and occipital, temporal, and prefrontal cortices when learning proceeds with awareness. Panel B shows dominant interactions between MTL and thalamus, basal ganglia, and contralateral MTL when learning proceeds without awareness. The key feature is the common involvement of the MTL, but because the regions to which it is functionally connected differ, the MTL can be related to learning in both situations.

occipital, and temporal cortices, whereas in Unaware subjects, MTL interactions were more spatially restricted to inferotemporal, thalamus, and basal ganglia. The MTL was related to learning in both groups, but because the regions interacting with the MTL varied between groups, in only one case was learning accompanied by awareness. In other words, the difference in neural context serves as a possible explanation for the involvement of the MTL in both groups.

Catalysts and Critical Functions

A problem with the notion of a neural context is the observation that the expression of certain behaviors or cognitive states appears to rely critically on specific brain areas. The overt expression of declarative memory, for example, depends on the integrity of the MTL. Such dependencies have led many researchers to speculate that such regions form a part of the neurocognitive system whose constituents subserve that function, but this implies a rather static view of brain function.

An alternative perspective, and one consistent with the idea of neural context, is to consider neural dynamics as a critical feature to understanding functional dependencies such as the MTL and memory. Most often studied at the cellular level, such dynamics are thought to be vital in enabling neurons to code for rapid temporal shifts in the environment and to make rapid adjustments of effectors at time scales much smaller than any single cell can achieve (Milton & Mackey, 2000). It is quite likely that such dynamics are at play across many levels of organization in the brain, with a similar general outcome: that it allows for rapid integration of information and responding. These same dynamics are also likely to underlie contextual effects between interacting populations that will manifest as changes in similarly large-scale behaviors, such as attentional states, perceptions, memory types, and, quite likely, consciousness (Bressler & Kelso, 2001). We have speculated that shifting between behavioral states may require the integrity of certain key regions, which when damaged would result in a deficit in moving between states. Such a region may not necessarily participate in the processing within the particular state, but rather may enable the transition—it is a *behavioral catalyst* (McIntosh, 2004).

The likely feature of such catalysts is their anatomical relation to regions that are processing the primary information in the state in question. In the awareness study, the MTL was engaged in learning with and without awareness, interacting with regions that seemed to be related to learning in either attentive state. The MTL is anatomically connected with regions that were part of both patterns, providing the potential for the MTL to catalyze the transition between two different networks and thereby the movement from learning without awareness to learning with awareness. The critical point at which the MTL is needed is when learning moves to the conscious state.

Before this, the MTL can be engaged, by virtue of its anatomical links, without being critical for behavioral expression.

Considering regions that are critical for the expression of a function as potential catalysts emphasizes the dynamic nature of brain function. The temporal expansion of any behavior or cognitive function can be viewed as a series of transitions that require specific regions to be intact. In some cases, this dependence may reflect a network node that transmits information between regions (e.g., the lateral geniculate nucleus in the visual system). In other cases, key brain areas enable the change in dominant interactions from one set of regions to another. These are the catalysts.

When the idea of neural context and catalysts are extended to other patient groups, our understanding of the underlying disorder, and perhaps potential remediation, is significantly altered. For example, in the study discussed earlier about face working memory, it was observed that the amygdala was a more central part of the network supporting face memory in patients with DAT than in age-matched controls. Given that the brain networks respond to damage by reorganization of existing pathways (functional and structural), it is possible that the change in the role of the amygdala in patients with DAT reflects a change in its neural context. The new pattern of functional connections thus enables a similar emergent behavior from regions that were not as heavily recruited before. A similar scenario explains the outcome in the perceptual memory study, in which older subjects seem to recruit new networks to bolster reduced efficacy of other networks. The implication of these findings is that behavioral deficits, which are observed in the presence of deterioration or damage, may not simply be due to the loss of a particular brain region or connection, but rather due to a response of the system to that damage. Indeed, although reorganization may preserve function in some domains, it may come at the cost of behavior in other domains. By exploring brain networks and their relation to cognitive function and dysfunction, we are in a position to differentiate among these outcomes and perhaps make use of these measured network dynamics to evaluate recovery and the efficacy of therapeutic intervention.

Conclusion

Network analysis has been part of the neuroimaging tool kit for more than a decade. In that time, some consistent results have emerged that encourage the continued use and development of these methods. As we have demonstrated above, there is a potential for great insights into the operations of both "normal" and dysfunctional brains using network analytic approaches. We have been purposefully restrictive in our survey, but there is a substantial body of work that uses different aspects of network analysis in comparing patient groups with controls (Mentis et al., 2002; Carbon et al., 2003), as well as in case studies (Maguire et al., 2000, 2001). We firmly believe that a more routine examination of network operations in brain disorders will not only contribute to our basic understanding of these disorders, but will also suggest new routes of therapy that target network dynamics.

REFERENCES

Aertsen, A., Bonhoeffer, T., & Kruger, J. (1987). Coherent activity in neuronal populations: analysis and interpretation. In E. R. Caianiello (Ed.), *Physics of cognitive processes* (pp. 1–34). Singapore: World Scientific.

Bach y Rita, P. (1981). Central nervous system lesions: Sprouting and unmasking in rehabilitation. *Archives of Physical Medicine and Rehabilitation, 62*, 413–417.

Bollen, K. A. (1989). *Structural equations with latent variables.* New York: Wiley.

Bressler, S. L., & Kelso, J. A. S. (2001). Cortical coordination dynamics and cognition. *Trends in Cognitive Sciences, 5*, 26–36.

Buchel, C., & Friston, K. (1997). Modulation of connectivity in visual pathways by attention: Cortical interactions evaluated with structural equation modeling and fMRI. *Cerebral Cortex, 7*, 768–778.

Carbon, M., Ghilardi, M. F., Feigin, A., et al. (2003). Learning networks in health and Parkinson's disease: Reproducibility and treatment effects. *Human Brain Mapping, 19*, 197–211.

Chen, R., Cohen, L. G., & Hallett, M. (2002). Nervous system reorganization following injury. *Neuroscience, 111*, 761–773.

Clark, C. M., & Squire, L. R. (2000). Awareness and the conditioned eyeblink response. In D. S. Woodruff-Pak & J. E. Steinmetz (Eds.), *Eyeblink classical conditioning: Vol. I. Applications in humans* (pp. 229–253). Norwell, MA: Kluwer Academic.

Clark, R. E., & Squire, L. R. (1998). Classical conditioning and brain systems: The role of awareness. *Science, 280*, 77–81.

Della-Maggiore, V., Grady, C. L., & McIntosh, A. R. (2002). Dissecting the effect of aging on the neural substrates of memory: Deterioration, preservation or functional reorganization? *Reviews in the Neurosciences, 13*, 167–181.

Della-Maggiore, V., Sekuler, A. B., Grady, C. L., et al. (2000). Corticolimbic interactions associated with performance on a short-term memory task are modified by age. *Journal of Neuroscience, 20*, 8410–8416.

Friston, K. (1994). Functional and effective connectivity: A synthesis. *Human Brain Mapping, 2*, 56–78.

Friston, K. J., Frith, C., & Fracowiak, R. (1993). Time-dependent changes in effective connectivity measured with PET. *Human Brain Mapping, 1*, 69–79.

Friston, K. J., Buechel, C., Fink, G. R., et al. (1997). Psychophysiological and modulatory interactions in neuroimaging. *NeuroImage, 6*, 218–229.

Grady, C. L., Furey, M. L., Pietrini, P., et al. (2001). Altered brain functional connectivity and impaired short-term memory in Alzheimer's disease. *Brain, 124*, 739–756.

Haxby, J. V., Grady, C. L., & Horwitz, B. (1991). Two visual processing pathways in human extrastriate cortex mapped with positron emission tomography. In N. A. Lassen, D. H. Ingvar, M. E. Raichle, & L. Friberg (Eds.), *Brain work and mental activity* (Alfred Benzon Symposium 31) (pp. 324–333). Copenhagen: Munksgaard.

Haxby, J. V., Ungerleider, L. G., Horwitz, B., et al. (1995). Hemispheric differences in neural systems for face working memory: A PET-rCBF study. *Human Brain Mapping*, *3*, 68–82.

Horwitz, B., & Braun, A. R. (2004). Brain network interactions in auditory, visual and linguistic processing. *Brain and Language*, *89*, 377–384.

Horwitz, B., McIntosh, A. R., Haxby, J. V., et al. (1995). Network analysis of PET-mapped visual pathways in Alzheimer type dementia. *Neuroreport*, *6*, 2287–2292.

Jennings, J. M., McIntosh, A. R., Kapur, S., et al. (1998). Functional network differences in schizophrenia: A rCBF study of semantic processing. *Neuroreport*, *9*, 1697–1700.

Kleist, K. (1935). Über Form und Orstsblindheit bei Verletzungen des Hinterhautlappens. *Deutsch Z Nervenheilk*, *138*, 206–214.

Kohler, S., McIntosh, A. R., Moscovitch, M., et al. (1998). Functional interactions between the medial temporal lobes and posterior neocortex related to episodic memory retrieval. *Cerebral Cortex*, *8*, 451–461.

Lee, R. G., & van Donkelaar, P. (1995). Mechanisms underlying functional recovery following stroke. *Canadian Journal of Neurological Sciences*, *22*, 257–263.

Lenartowicz, A., & McIntosh, A. R. (2005). The role of anterior cingulate cortex in working memory is shaped by functional connectivity. *Journal of Cognitive Neuroscience*, *17*, 1026–1042.

Lobaugh, N. J., West, R., & McIntosh, A. R. (2001). Spatiotemporal analysis of experimental differences in event-related potential data with partial least squares. *Psychophysiology*, *38*, 517–530.

Loehlin, J. C. (1987). *Latent variable models: An introduction to factor, path, and structural analysis*. Hillsdale, NJ: Erlbaum.

Lukic, A. S., Wernick, M. N., & Strother, S. C. (2002). An evaluation of methods for detecting brain activations from functional neuroimages. *Artifical Intelligence in Medicine*, *25*, 69–88.

Luria, A. R. (1962). *Higher cortical functions in man*. New York: Basic Books.

Maguire, E. A., Mummery, C. J., & Buchel, C. (2000). Patterns of hippocampal–cortical interaction dissociate temporal lobe memory subsystems. *Hippocampus*, *10*, 475–482.

Maguire, E. A., Vargha-Khadem, F., & Mishkin, M. (2001). The effects of bilateral hippocampal damage on fMRI regional activations and interactions during memory retrieval. *Brain*, *124*, 1156–1170.

McIntosh, A. R. (2004). Contexts and catalysts: A resolution of the localization and integration of function in the brain. *Neuroinformatics*, *2*, 175–182.

McIntosh, A. R. (2000a). From location to integration: How neural interactions form the basis for human cognition. In E. Tulving (Ed.), *Memory, consciousness, and the brain: The Tallinn Conference* (pp. 346–363). Philadelphia: Psychology Press.

McIntosh, A. R. (2000b). Towards a network theory of cognition. *Neural Networks*, *13*, 861–876.

McIntosh, A. R. (1998). Understanding neural interactions in learning and memory using functional neuroimaging. *Annals of the New York Academy of Sciences*, *855*, 556–571.

McIntosh, A. R., Bookstein, F. L., Haxby, J. V., et al. (1996a). Spatial pattern analysis of functional brain images using partial least squares. *NeuroImage*, *3*, 143–157.

McIntosh, A. R., Cabeza, R. E., & Lobaugh, N. J. (1998). Analysis of neural interactions explains the activation of occipital cortex by an auditory stimulus. *Journal of Neurophysiology*, *80*, 2790–2796.

McIntosh, A. R., Chau, W. K., & Protzner, A. B. (2004). Spatiotemporal analysis of event-related fMRI data using partial least squares. *NeuroImage, 23,* 764–775.

McIntosh, A. R., & Gonzalez-Lima, F. (1998). Large-scale functional connectivity in associative learning: Interrelations of the rat auditory, visual and limbic systems. *Journal of Neurophysiology, 80,* 3148–3162.

McIntosh, A. R., & Gonzalez-Lima, F. (1994). Structural equation modeling and its application to network analysis in functional brain imaging. *Human Brain Mapping, 2,* 2–22.

McIntosh, A. R., & Gonzalez-Lima, F. (1991). Structural modeling of functional neural pathways mapped with 2-deoxyglucose: Effects of acoustic startle habituation on the auditory system. *Brain Research, 547,* 295–302.

McIntosh, A. R., Grady, C. L., Haxby, J. V., et al. (1996b). Changes in limbic and prefrontal functional interactions in a working memory task for faces. *Cerebral Cortex, 6,* 571–584.

McIntosh, A. R., Grady, C. L., Ungerleider, L. G., et al. (1994). Network analysis of cortical visual pathways mapped with PET. *Journal of Neuroscience, 14,* 655–666.

McIntosh, A. R., & Lobaugh, N. J. (2004). Partial least squares analysis of neuroimaging data: Applications and advances. *NeuroImage, 23*(Suppl. 1), S250–S263.

McIntosh, A. R., Nyberg, L., Bookstein, F. L., et al. (1997). Differential functional connectivity of prefrontal and medial temporal cortices during episodic memory retrieval. *Human Brain Mapping, 5,* 323–327.

McIntosh, A. R., Rajah, M. N., & Lobaugh, N. J. (2003). Functional connectivity of the medial temporal lobe relates to learning and awareness. *Journal of Neuroscience, 23,* 6520–6528.

McIntosh, A. R., Sekuler, A. B., Penpeci, C., et al. (1999). Recruitment of unique neural systems to support visual memory in normal aging. *Current Biology, 9,* 1275–1278.

Mentis, M. J., McIntosh, A. R., Perrine, K., et al. (2002). Relationships among the metabolic patterns that correlate with mnemonic, visuospatial, and mood symptoms in Parkinson's disease. *American Journal of Psychiatry, 159,* 746–754.

Milton, J. G., & Mackey, M. C. (2000). Neural ensemble coding and statistical periodicity: Speculations on the operation of the mind's eye. *Journal of Physiology—Paris, 94,* 489–503.

Nyberg, L. (1994). A structural equation modeling approach to the multiple memory systems question. *Journal of Experimental Psychology: Learning, Memory, and Cognition, 20,* 485–491.

Seminowicz, D. A., Mayberg, H. S., McIntosh, A. R., et al. (2004). Limbic-frontal circuitry in major depression: A path modeling metanalysis. *NeuroImage, 22,* 409–418.

Stephan, K. E. (2004). On the role of general system theory for functional neuroimaging. *Journal of Anatomy, 205,* 443–470.

Ungerleider, L. G., & Mishkin, M. (1982). Two cortical visual systems. In D. J. Ingle, M. A. Goodale, & R. J. W. Mansfield (Eds.), *Analysis of visual behavior* (pp. 549–586). Cambridge: MIT Press.

Welchew, D. E., Honey, G. D., Sharma, T., et al. (2002). Multidimensional scaling of integrated neurocognitive function and schizophrenia as a disconnexion disorder. *NeuroImage, 17,* 1227–1239.

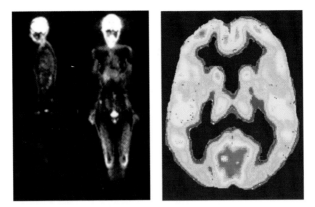

PLATE 1.1. Whole-body and brain images obtained with FDG in normal subjects. Note that in the whole-body images those organs are shown most intensely whose metabolism is the most intense (brain, heart, skeletal muscles) or wherein the excreted tracer accumulates (urinary bladder). In the brain image (average image obtained from seven young volunteers, horizontal slice) the cerebral cortex and the subcortical nuclei are metabolically active. Inside the cortex those parts are most active (primary visual cortex) whose cell and synaptic density is superior to the rest of the cortex.

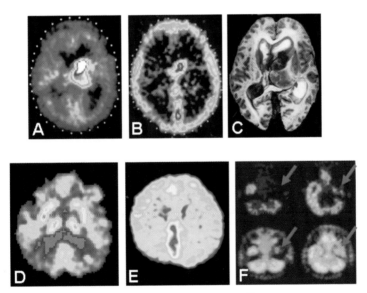

PLATE 1.2. Increased metabolic activity as a disease marker: (A) [^{11}C]methionine and (B) FDG scans of a metabolically active brain tumor (C). Note that in the FDG images the visual cortex shows normal metabolic uptake (cf. Plate 1.1). Decreased metabolic activity as a disease marker: FDG brain scans of (D) a patient with Alzheimer's disease, (E) a patient suffering from Creutzfeldt–Jakob disease, and a patient with epilepsy with a temporal lobe focus (F, lower panels). In the upper panels of (F), [^{11}C]flumazenil images are shown of the same patient with epilepsy. Red arrows indicate the regional metabolic decreased and receptor losses (GABA–benzodiazepine system) in the epileptic focus.

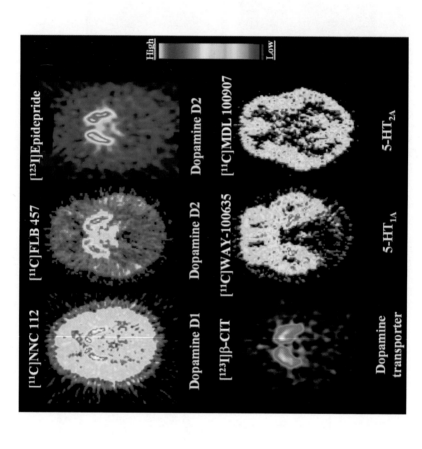

PLATE 1.3. [11]C radioligands used for the mapping of various central neuroreceptor and transporter systems.

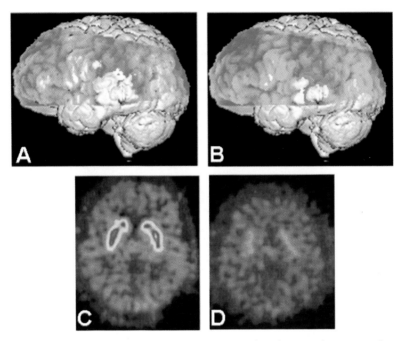

PLATE 1.4. The use of PET in therapy follow-up. Upper row: Three-dimensional reconstructed averaged blood flow images of 12 patients scanned before (pretreatment; A) and after (posttreatment; B) a 2-week-long treatment with vinpocetine in pharmacological doses. Only cortical regions with blood flow reaching the physiological levels are shown in color. The images indicate an improvement in cerebral blood flow as a result of drug treatment. Lower row: (C) Imaging the brain's dopamine-D2 receptor system with [11C]raclopride in a normal subject. (D) In a patient with schizophrenia, the successful chronic treatment with haloperidol significantly reduces the number of available dopamine receptors in the striatum, indicating that the drug binds to striatal dopamine D2/D3 receptors.

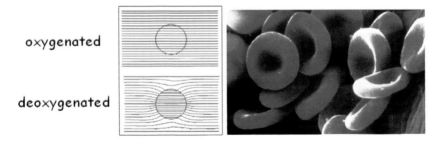

oxygenated

deoxygenated

PLATE 2.1. The photograph shows the irregular geometry of red blood cells. The diagrams show the effect that oxygenated red blood cells have on an applied magnetic field. Deoxygenated blood causes field distortions, which lead to spin-dephasing, decreasing the T2*-weighted MRI signal. Oxygenated blood has a reduced effect on the field, causing a reduction in field distortions, which leads to less dephasing, causing an increase in MRI signal.

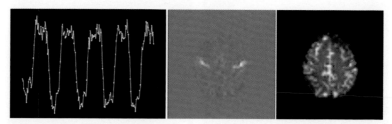

PLATE 2.2. An MRI time series obtained from the motor cortex during repeated finger tapping alternating with periods of rest. The middle image is a raw map of activation created by calculating the cross-correlation of the time series of each image voxel with a function that represents the expected neuronal response. The image on the right is a corresponding anatomical echo-planar image from the time series.

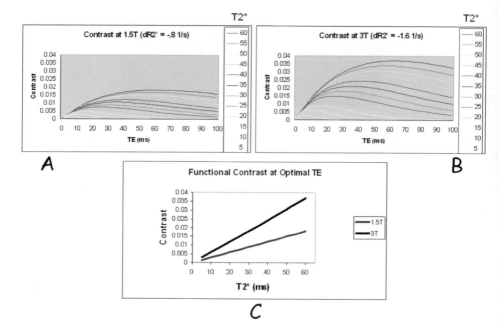

PLATE 2.3. Comparison of functional contrast between 1.5 Tesla and 3.0 Tesla field strengths as a function of echo time and baseline T2* (which varies over space with the quality of the shimming or, rather, the homogeneity of the macroscopic magnetic field). Because delta R2* is lower for 1.5T (A), the optimal functional contrast is not as high as with 3T (B). Nevertheless, baseline T2* generally decreases at high field strengths, so if baseline T2* is the same, the functional contrast increases approximately linearly with field strength, but since baseline T2* is decreased at higher field strengths, the echo time used is reduced slightly and the gains in functional contrast are less than linear (C).

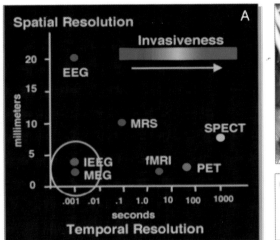
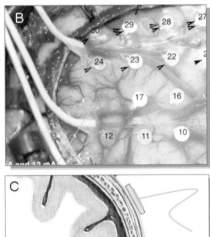

PLATE 3.1. Temporal and spatial resolution of various imaging and neurophysiological techniques. (A) Comparison of the modern imaging and neurophysiological techniques (IEEG, invasive electroencephalography; MEG, magnetoencephalography; MRS, magnetic resonance spectroscopy; fMRI, functional MRI; SPECT, single-photon emission cranial tomography; PET, positron emission tomography) with respect to their temporal (x-axis) and spatial (y-axis) resolution as well as invasiveness (colored scale in the right upper corner). Panel A minimally modified and published with generous permission from 4D-Neuroimaging.

(B) Position of the subdural electrodes placed directly on the cortical surface in the operating room. By design, these electrodes are embedded in the grid with a 10-mm distance between their centers. Thus, direct placement on the surface and short interelectrode distance account for superior spatial resolution of invasive EEG (iEEG) over scalp EEG and other imaging techniques.

(C) Relative position of the scalp electrode with regard to the brain cortex where presumed sources are contained. The distance from the surface of the cortex and scalp electrode is on the order of 6 10 mm. Intervening tissues have different electrical conductivities, leading to the attenuation, filtering, and distortion of the EEG signals. Along with longer interelectrode distance, this is a reason for significantly lower spatial resolution of scalp EEG, as shown in panel A.

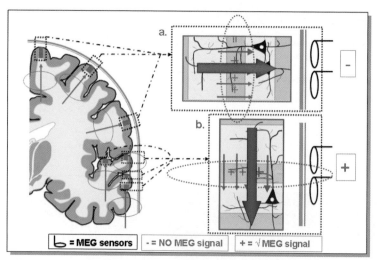

PLATE 3.2. Radial (a) versus tangential (b) sources as "seen" by MEG. Radial sources (red squares) are distributed along the crests of the gyri and tangential (blue squares) along the sulci. Parallel alignment of the apical dendrites (as shown in the enlargements of the respective sources [boxes a and b outlined by the broken black lines]) in the upper cortical layers is critical for spatial summation and their synchronous firing (represented by red and blue arrows, respectively) for temporal summation of neural activity. If the activity of a critical number of firing neurons (presumably > 105) is summated, it leads to a signal detectable by the MEG sensors (SQUIDS). Orientation of the source (thin and thick red and blue arrows) with respect to the skull (thick light brown line) is a critical geometric relationship governed by the right-hand rule of physics (see Figure 3.1, and pp. 76–77 for explanation). Because magnetic fields (represented by ellipses) are orthogonal to the corresponding intracellular currents (thin and thick arrows), those magnetic fields generated by the radial sources (enlarged, represented by the thick red arrow) will distribute parallel to the skull (represented by the thick red ellipse) and will not reach (indicated by "–") the MEG sensors indicated by the black icons. On the contrary, those magnetic fields (thick blue ellipse) corresponding to tangential sources (thick blue arrow) will distribute toward the skull and reach the sensors (indicated by "+"). Thus, MEG is "blind" to radial sources, but "sees" tangential sources. Nevertheless, owing to the different nature and principles governing electrical signals, as explained in the text (pp. 76–77), EEG will not only preferentially "see" radial sources, but will probably see strong tangential sources as well, depending on the signal-to-noise ratio. Parts of this image were kindly provided by Elekta Neuromag.

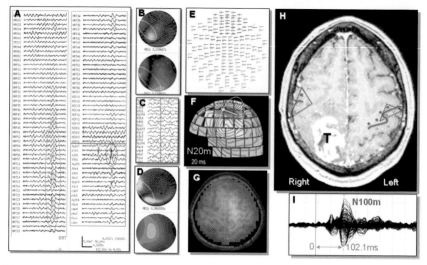

PLATE 3.3. Sample of typical MEG data and some representative clinical and research applications of MEG. (A) MEG acquires large amounts of data that require powerful computations and can be displayed and used in many different ways. It applies many methods that were initially established in the EEG field, including an intuitive first step of displaying raw data (recorded tracings in the intact form) for visual inspection. Even if we wrongly assume

an identical appearance of all waveforms on EEG and MEG, there is the problem of having enough screen space for displaying about 300 MEG channels (as opposed to about 20 traditional channels for scalp EEG) in legible form for meaningful visual review. In order to get around this, various types of columnar (blue boxes) or topographic (for instance, lobar: frontal, temporal, parietal, occipital) displays are used where several columns of MEG channels are displayed side by side at the expense of time interval displayed. Thus, instead of displaying 20 EEG channels over 10 s (traditional EEG display) on the screen, users display grouped columns of MEG channels over a shorter time interval (i.e., 1 s). Thus, while reviewing data one scrolls across a short time interval but is able to see a particular time instance in every channel displayed on a single or double screen. The segment shown is a part of a six-column display that originally included 275 MEG channels (blue boxes, only two out of six shown) and 18 EEG channels (red box). A left temporal spike is visible on EEG (red ellipse) and MEG (blue ellipse). It should be noted that only one-third of the MEG channels are shown for the purpose of illustration. This type of analysis is a good screening step for interesting features that should be analyzed further, depending on application.

(B) Along with identifying the waveforms of interest for further analysis, it is customary to review a field map of a particular peak or deflection in a waveform of interest (B). Different software packages have different display designs even when they display exactly the same waveform. It may be a round two-dimensional projection of the head with small circles representing sensors (B) where left is on the left and right on the right. Another common display design is a nine-projection (three left, three top, and three right—anterior, middle, and posterior projections, respectively) display of the sensor array (F), where sensors are represented as squares. The common feature is color designation of the magnetic field direction: A blue color represents incoming, and a red color outgoing, field with respect to the skull (see pp. 75–76 for the right-hand rule). Brightest color (B) or densest isocontour lines (F) represent respective maxima of the magnetic field as it comes in (blue) and exits (red) the cranium. A well-structured field map with clearly identifiable opposing maxima (within yellow ellipse) symmetrically positioned with respect to the zero line is an additional criterion used for accepting an ECD as a valid explanation of a particular deflection or peak. Thus, a spike identified on MEG and EEG tracings also has consistent field maps in both modalities (B). In contrast, a spike present on MEG (not shown), but not visible in EEG (C; a position of the corresponding MEG spike marked with red line), has only an appropriately structured MEG map (D, top, yellow ellipse) but not an EEG map (D, bottom).

If conducting a clinical study for epilepsy localization, one can apply an ECD model (see pp. 76–77) on identified spikes or sharps ("epileptiform discharges") and coregister calculated dipole solutions (panel H, yellow triangles) with the patient's MRI to generate magnetic source images (MSI). This provides three-dimensional views that can be used for surgical planning, as well as partial neuronavigational maps during image-guided surgery.

Head plot (E) is a practical display for showing regional distribution of the recorded signal; by showing the reflection of selected activity in each sensor, it allows visual inspection of its topographic features. Subsequently, one can decide what region is clinically or scientifically interesting for further analysis.

(H) Axial (horizontal) brain MRI section of a patient with a right parieto-occipital tumor (T) with coregistered sensory map generated by averaging brain MEG responses to the electrical stimulations applied to right and left hand and fingers. Green dots (left) or squares (right) represent equivalent current dipoles (ECD) corresponding with the major known physiological peaks of somatosensory evoked fields (SEF). This map outlines a sensory strip (postcentral gyrus) for the purpose of presurgical mapping of major anatomical and functional landmarks and can be derived for any body part if stimulated appropriately. Similarly, a motor strip containing motor functions within the precentral gyrus (red dots, left; red squares, right) can be identified by recording motor evoked fields associated with movements of the corresponding right and left muscles.

Identification of major sensory and/or motor landmarks helps to determine the exact location of the boundary between the sensory and motor cortex—the central sulcus (thick blue line, exactly overlaying the central sulcus for better visual clarity). Normal physiological relationship is preserved on the left side (circles), whereas the topography is completely changed by the growing tumor on the right side (squares). Note a triangle on the left that outlines the three physiological locations identified by MEG and their displaced counterparts on the right (also outlined with the triangle). This image would be an invaluable neuronavigational map for image-guided surgery.

The first and most stable peak on the median nerve SEF appears about 20 ms after a stimulus and is termed N20m (N = negative, m = magnetic) (F). A corresponding dipole is anteriorly directed (F, yellow arrow) and localized in the anterior rim of the postcentral gyrus or posterior bank of the central sulcus (H, on the left, dark green circle), unless displaced by a pathological process (H, on the right, dark green square).

Any spontaneous (A) or time-locked (I) signal can be averaged and conveniently displayed in the form of a butterfly plot for further review (for instance, fast identification of epileptic spikes) or analysis (averaging of time-locked signals). Having averaged signals displayed in this manner enables identification of major deflections or peaks and measurement of their latencies starting with time of stimulus (0 point marked with red cursor). Panel I shows averaged waveforms of auditory evoked fields recorded with MEG during auditory stimulations of a healthy volunteer with pure tones. A major deflection is N100m (N = negative, m = magnetic) that appears after 102.1 ms in this subject and would be localized in the superior temporal gyrus (data not shown). Among many increasingly popular research methods for assessing "global" or "regional" brain activity is synthetic aperture magnetometry (SAM) (Vrba & Robinson, 2001), a beam former technique (see pp. 80–81, this volume) that generates statistical maps of brain activity based on different predetermined parameters (frequency, peakedness, etc.) (G). In this example, it shows fast brain activity of predetermined frequency in association with a seizure focus localized in the right precentral gyrus. The brightest color represents statistically strongest activity. Recently, this approach has been used to research some aspects of "connectivity" as well as for language lateralization and/or localization.

Note. For better clarity and because of space limitations, some images have been resized, trimmed, and otherwise enhanced to convey key points.

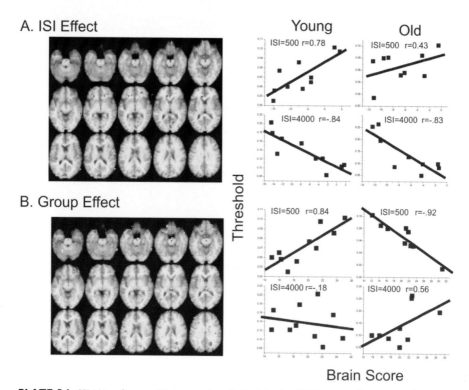

PLATE 5.1. ISI (A) and group (B) patterns from brain–behavior PLS image analysis. Scatterplots show the relation of individual participants' threshold with the brain scores derived from the singular image. Voxels most strongly related to the pattern in the scatterplots are shaded either red (positive weight) or blue (negative weight) on an axial structural MRI. The MRI is in standard stereotaxic atlas space with brain slices moving from ventral (extreme upper left of panels A and B) to dorsal (lower right corner of panels A and B).

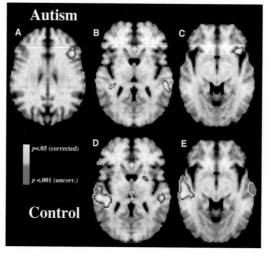

PLATE 6.1. Regional cerebral blood flow increases associated with passive verbal stimulation (listening to sentences, as compared with rest) in a group of five adults with autism (top row) and five matched normal controls (bottom row). Activation clusters are superimposed onto standard MRI in Talairach space. The autism group shows activation in right middle frontal (A), bilateral superior temporal (B), and right inferior frontal gyri (C), which contrasts with predominantly left-lateralizing temporal activation seen in the control group (D–E). Based on data from Müller et al. (1999a).

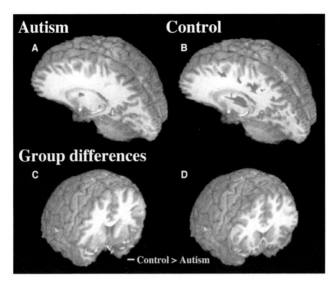

PLATE 6.2. Clusters of significant functional connectivity ($p < .05$; corrected) with area 17 (primary visual cortex) for autism (A) and normal control groups (B). Extensive connectivity in superior parietal, superior frontal, and thalamic regions seen for the control group (B) is reduced in the autism group (A). Direct group comparisons show significantly reduced functional connectivity in bilateral inferior and superior frontal gyri (C–D). Based on data from Villalobos et al. (2005).

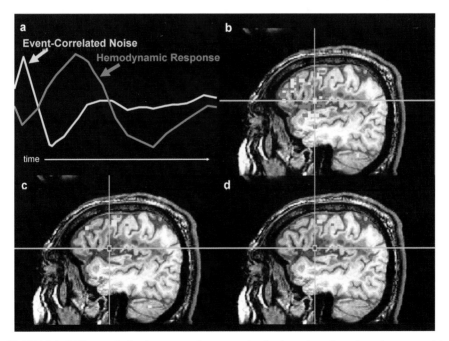

PLATE 8.1. Differences in the time course of event-correlated noise and true hemodynamic responses (a) allows for the separation of artifact from BOLD response. Artifacts from event-correlated noise (b) are reduced when the first two images are dropped from analyses (c) or when a selective detrending technique is used to mitigate artifacts (d).

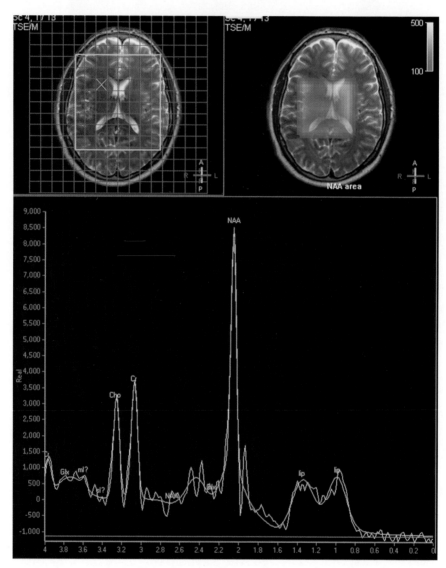

PLATE 9.1. Full-slice, chemical shift imaging of a healthy adult.

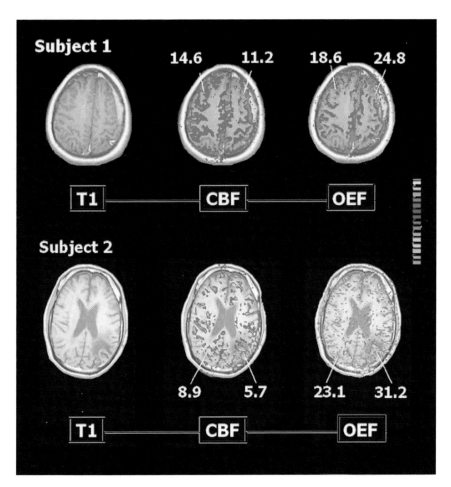

PLATE 9.2. The basic differences in CBF and OEF in two cases of TBI. For both cases, brain regions adjacent to lesion sites reveal diminished CBF and greater OEF as compared with homologous contralateral brain regions. Disruption of baseline cerebrovascular parameters following neurotrauma may have important implications for using blood flow-based measurements such as fMRI. Images here were obtained using ASL (QUIPPS) and a breath-holding task. The unit of measurement for CBF is ml/100gm/min and OEF is a ratio based on CBF and oxygen utilization. Data from Hillary and Biswal (2007).

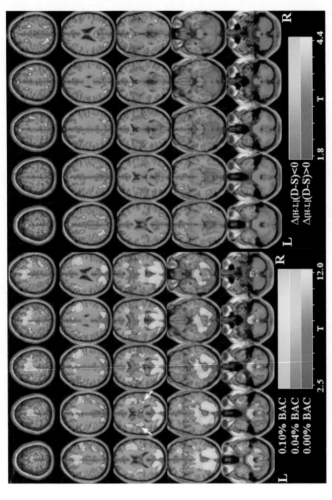

PLATE 11.1. Main effect group maps for (mean) sober, low-dose, and high-dose conditions and correlation with alcohol dose. Left: *T*-maps are displayed over the T₁-weighted template. Images were thresholded at $p < 0.05$ (corrected for multiple comparisons). All colored regions in the figure represent activations and are color-coded to discriminate the alcohol dosing level. The main effect SPM (statistical parametric mapping) group analysis for (1) (mean) sober (colored red/orange), (2) low dose (colored blue/cyan), and (3) high dose (colored green/yellow) are displayed on the same image for clarity. Alcohol dose results in a global decrease in contrast-to-noise and also some localized increases and decreases. Right: Comparison of the amplitude difference between the sober (S) and drug (D) conditions for the high (H) dose with the amplitude difference between the sober and intoxicated conditions for the low (L) dose, that is, ($\Delta_{H\pm L}$ [D – S]). *T*-maps are displayed over one of the normalized EPI (echo-planar imaging) images. Images were thresholded at $p < .05$ and a cluster size of 50 voxels. Dose-dependent decreases are depicted in blue/cyan, whereas dose-dependent increases are depicted in red/orange.

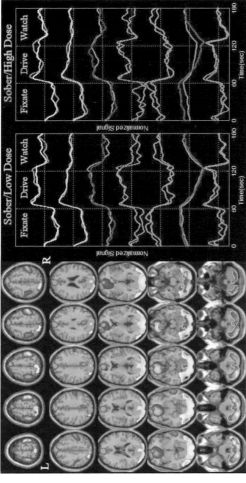

PLATE 11.2. Results from the fixed-average-spatial (FAS) analysis. Random effects group fMRI maps are thresholded at $p < .005$. A total of seven components are presented. A green component extends on both sides of the parieto-occipital sulcus including portions of the cuneus, precuneus, and the lingual gyrus. A yellow component contains mostly occipital areas. A white component contains bilateral visual association and parietal areas; and a component consisting of motor areas is depicted in red. Cerebellar areas are also depicted in red (but with a turquoise border). Orbitofrontal and anterior cingulate areas identified are depicted in blue. Finally, a component including medial frontal, parietal, and posterior cingulate regions is depicted in blue. Group-averaged time courses (right) for the fixate–drive–watch order are also depicted with similar colors for the sober versus low-dose and sober versus high-dose conditions (drug conditions are colored gray). The three repeated epochs are averaged and presented as fixation, drive, and watch.

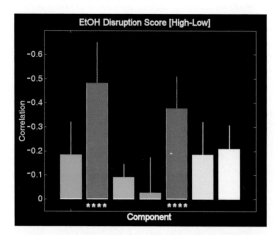

PLATE 11.3. Differences in disruption scores for the ICA (independent component analysis) time courses. Within-day correlations were computed between the sober condition and the drug condition on the same day as a measure of the amount of disruption induced by the alcohol. The differences in these correlations are presented for each component, with color corresponding to Plate 11.2. The high-dose condition was in all cases less correlated with its sober counterpart than was the low-dose condition (all values are negative). Significant ($p < .001$) differences were observed for the pink (orbitofrontal/anterior cingulate) and red (motor) components only.

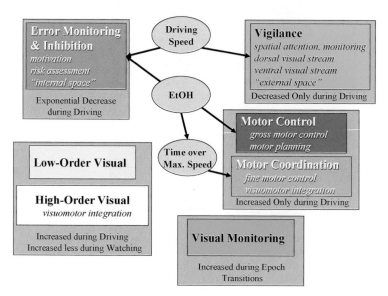

PLATE 11.4. Interpretation of imaging results. Extension of the results of our previous study examining speed-related changes (Calhoun et al., 2002). Colors correspond to those used in Plate 11.2. Components are grouped according to the averaged pattern demonstrated by their time courses. The speed-modulated components (previously found), as well as the EtOH component revealed in the present study, are indicated with arrows.

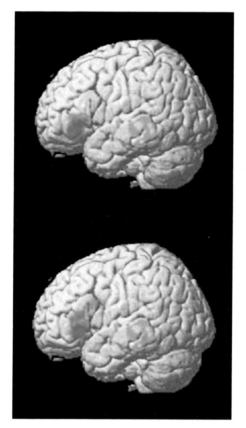

PLATE 12.1. Brain images showing left ventrolateral prefrontal activation during deep minus shallow encoding in 14 healthy controls (top) and 14 patients with schizophrenia. Results are surface-rendered in the sagittal plane on a smoothed brain image in SPM2. Colored areas indicate a difference in signal change exceeding a corrected *p*-value of .05.

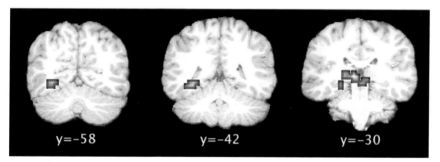

PLATE 12.2. Brain image showing greater patient versus control activation during deep minus shallow encoding in the left lingual gyrus, hippocampus, and thalamus. Results are rendered on a coronal brain slice in SPM2. Colored areas indicate a difference in signal change exceeding a corrected *p*-value of .05.

A

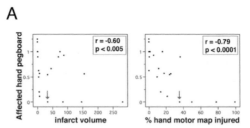

B

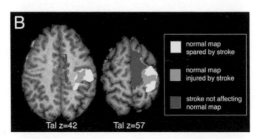

PLATE 14.1. (A) Infarct volume (top left) and fraction of hand motor map injured by stroke (top right) each show a significant inverse relationship with pegboard performance by the affected hand (normalized to pegboard results for the unaffected hand). However, the correlation is stronger and more significant in the latter case. Note that injury to >37% of the hand motor map was associated with total loss of hand motor function. The arrow indicates the patient whose images are displayed below. (B) Images from a patient whose stroke was mild–moderate in size (33 cm³), but injured 35% of the hand motor area and was associated with total loss of hand motor function. From Crafton et al. (2003). Copyright 2003 by Oxford University Press. Reprinted by permission.

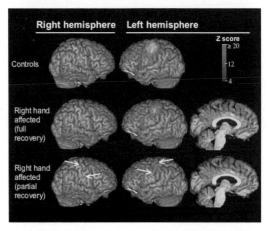

PLATE 14.2. Group maps from healthy controls, from patients with stroke affecting the right arm (left brain) and complete recovery, and from patients with stroke affecting the right arm and good but incomplete recovery, show a difference in activation site and size. Among patients, differences varied with level of recovery. All subjects tapped left index finger. The Talairach coordinates for center of activation for the activation cluster in the left primary sensorimotor cortex in those with complete recovery was (31, –21, 50), which was ventral as compared with those with partial recovery, among whom the center of activation was located at (30, –19, 54). In addition, patients with full recovery, versus partial recovery, showed 2.7-fold larger contralateral sensorimotor activation, with negligible differences in the supplementary motor area, despite no differences in finger-tapping force or in surface electromyogram (EMG) recordings. From Zemke et al. (2003). Copyright 2003 by Lippincott Williams & Wilkins. Reprinted by permission.

PART III

CLINICAL APPLICATIONS

CHAPTER 6

Functional Neuroimaging of Developmental Disorders

LESSONS FROM AUTISM RESEARCH

Ralph-Axel Müller

Any attempt to cover neuroimaging contributions to the large number of disorders that can be considered neurodevelopmental within a single chapter would be overly ambitious. Disturbances or defects can affect the developing nervous system in countless different sites and ways, and the resulting spectrum of impairments is vast. In a first approach, neurodevelopmental disorders can be grouped into three distinct classes: (1) disorders that result from some kind of disturbance (e.g., neuromigrational) or lesion (e.g., stroke) during intrauterine or early postnatal phases; (2) those caused by defects of a single gene or a well-defined chromosomal locus; and (3) those known to be predominantly genetic in nature, but involve multiple different genetic (and epigenetic) risk factors.

Among the disorders of type (1), there are subtypes that demonstrate the astounding potential of the developing brain for compensatory reorganization. The most positive examples of developmental plasticity come from cases of perinatal or early postnatal stroke, or from neurodegenerative diseases such as Sturge–Weber syndrome or Rasmussen's encephalitis, which usually affect only one cerebral hemisphere, leaving the other intact. For instance, behavioral studies have documented the often surprisingly good language outcome in patients with early left-hemisphere lesions (Nass & Stiles, 1996; Vicari et al., 2000), although etiology (Curtiss et al., 2001; Pulsifer et al., 2004) and the presence or absence of seizures are important predictive variables (Isaacs et al., 1996; Muter et al., 1997). Similar positive outcomes have been reported for patients who underwent hemispherectomy following early-onset left hemisphere disease (Curtiss & de Bode, 1999; Jonas et al., 2004; Vargha-Khadem et al., 1997; Vargha-Khadem & Mishkin, 1997). Functional neuroimaging studies in groups of patients with early lesions (Müller et al., 1999b; Staudt et al., 2002) and in a single patient with hemispherotomy (Hertz-Pannier et al., 2002) generally suggest that compensatory plasticity and good language outcome may be supported by neurofunctional reorganization, in particular atypical involvement of right hemisphere regions homotopic to the classical left perisylvian language areas (Broca's and Wernicke's). Although, as mentioned, the integrity of the right hemisphere is an important prognostic factor, it currently remains uncertain what other clinical variables drive or prevent interhemispheric reorganization for language (Liegeois et al., 2004).

There is additional evidence showing that not all neurodevelopmental disorders of type (1) will have relatively beneficial outcomes. On the contrary, very early neurodevelopmental disturbances derailing basic organizational stages of brain development may result in severe brain malformations with negative prognosis. This has been shown through controlled lesion experiments in animals. For instance, Kolb and colleagues (1996) observed reduced functional sparing when bilateral frontal or parietal resections were performed at postnatal day 1, as compared with day 10, in rats. These time points approximately correspond to human gestational month 5 and postnatal month 6, respectively. In cats, Villablanca and colleagues (1993a, 1993b) showed good recovery after left frontal cortical ablation at postnatal days 8–14, whereas similar ablation during the third gestational trimester resulted in severe sensorimotor impairments. According to Kolb and Gibb (2001), animal lesion models overall suggest that "damage [at the] time of neural migration and the initiation of synaptic formation . . . is associated with dismal outcome" (p. 179). In humans, neuromigrational disturbances, as seen in cortical dysplasia and heterotopia, are typically associated with epilepsy and cognitive impairment (Palmini et al., 1995; Raymond et al., 1995). Neurotoxins, such as ethanol, that are known to affect neuronal survival (Farber & Olney, 2003) and migration have profound and lifelong effects on the central nervous system (CNS). Fetal exposure to alcohol is often associated with microcephaly, neuronal apoptosis (Farber & Olney, 2003), white matter reduction (especially in parietal lobes; Archibald et al., 2001), reduced size of the caudate nuclei (Chen et al., 2003; Mattson, 2000), and, in severe cases, widespread cerebral dysgenesis and malformation (Coulter et al., 1993).

The catalog of neurodevelopmental disorders of type (2) has become longer in the past decade because for some disorders that had been previously described in clinical–behavioral terms, relatively simple genetic causes have been identified. One such example is Williams syndrome, a disorder initially characterized on the basis of a diverse set of features, such as atypical "elfin" faces, supravalvular aortic stenosis, deficient bodily growth, hypercalcemia, and severe visuospatial deficits in the context of often apparently good verbal abilities (Donnai & Karmiloff-Smith, 2000). In the early 1990s the genetic cause of the disorder was identified as a microdeletion of the elastin gene and adjacent genes on chromosome 7 (Ewart et al., 1993; Morris, 2004). Another example is Rett syndrome, initially defined in clinical terms on the basis of regressive loss of praxic and communicative abilities in young girls, with an outcome of severe retardation. In the late 1990s it was discovered that up to 90% of subjects with sporadic (nonfamilial) Rett syndrome presented with a mutation in the *MECP2* gene, a transcriptional repressor on the X chromosome (Shahbazian & Zoghbi, 2002).

The investigation of neurodevelopmental disorders of type (2) is attractive because knowledge of affected genetic loci promises to open windows to links between genes of phenotypes. However, even in single-gene disorders these links appear to be highly complex. Williams syndrome, for instance, affects numerous bodily and neural systems. Even when phenotypic traits are largely limited to the brain, these traits affect diverse functional systems. An even more telling example comes from the recently described heritable disorder associated with language impairment that was identified in multiple members of family KE. This disorder was first described from a linguistic perspective as a selective impairment within the grammatical (more precisely, morphosyntactic) domain (Gopnik & Crago, 1991). In 1998 it was linked to a locus on chromosome 7 (7q31), and the gene was suggestively labeled "*SPCH1*" (Fisher et al., 1998). The finding was greeted with enthusiasm by some in the linguistic community whose research had been based—following the groundbreaking work by Chomsky (1965)—on the theory of a genetically anchored language ability ("universal grammar") distinguishing humans from nonhuman primates. For instance, the most eloquent current spokesman for the Chomskian view, Steve Pinker (2001), saw the identified gene as playing "a causal role in the development of the normal brain circuitry that underlies language and speech" (p. 465).

Upon careful consideration, however, the disorder in family KE tells a very different story. First, more comprehensive clinical and neuropsychological evaluation of affected members was inconsistent with a selective morphosyntactic deficit, demonstrating a broad picture of impairments including reduced nonverbal IQ, orofacial apraxia, and reduced phonological working memory (Vargha-Khadem et al., 1995; Watkins et al., 2002). Second, the gene initially called *SPCH1* was more accurately classified as a gene encoding forkhead transcription factors, therefore more aptly called *FOXP2* (Lai et al., 2001). Forkhead proteins are transcription factors that are involved in diverse, very basic developmental events, such as cell differentiation and proliferation (Marcus & Fisher, 2003). Disappointingly for those who expect to have identified a "language gene," *FOXP2* is expressed during embryonic development, not only in the brain, but also in other organs such as the lungs and the heart. Recent findings of a cosegregation of one coding change of *FOXP2* with verbal apraxia could reflect a more specific link, but it remains clear that defects of the *FOXP2* gene will account for only a very small fraction of developmental language impairments (MacDermot et al., 2005). In conclusion, what appeared the most promising discovery in the study of the genetic origins of language turned out to be a tale of caution (for discussion, see Fisher, 2005; Müller, 2004, 2005).

This chapter is dedicated to neuroimaging of developmental disorders of type (3), which can be justly considered the most challenging type. One of the most puzzling of these disorders is autism, which is the focus of the rest of this chapter. Contrary to the disorders described above, autism is known to be strongly genetic, but probably involves many different genetic (in addition to epigenetic) risk factors located on several chromosomes. This developmental complexity raises special issues in the use of functional neuroimaging.

Autism

Autism is a neurodevelopmental disorder with a high prevalence of 2–4 in 1,000 children (Baird et al., 2006; Fombonne et al., 2006). The disorder affects multiple domains of cognitive, perceptuomotor, and sociobehavioral functions (Rapin, 1997; Tager-Flusberg et al., 2001). The rate of mental retardation in the autistic population is about 75%, and the vast majority of affected individuals require lifelong institutional or therapeutic support (Rapin & Katzman, 1998).

By today's consensus, autism requires explanation in neurological terms. However, comprehensive models of neuropathological development in autism are not currently established. Diagnosis of autism is typically made relatively late (at about age 3 years), whereas crucial etiological events may occur much earlier in postnatal or prenatal development. In addition, since many different etiological pathways (Trottier et al., 1999) may result in cognitive-behavioral phenotypes that fulfill diagnostic criteria for autism (American Psychiatric Association, 2000), the probability of identifying *consistent* abnormalities in brain imaging or event-related potential (ERP) studies is reduced (see below).

From twin studies it is known that genetic factors are heavily involved in autism (Bailey et al., 1995). Linkage studies have further identified numerous potential genetic loci, but the current consensus on specific sites of susceptibility for autism remains limited (Folstein & Mankoski, 2000; Korvatska et al., 2002; Muhle et al., 2004). Furthermore, some studies suggest that nongenetic etiological mechanisms, such as viral infection (Lotspeich & Ciaranello, 1993; Tanoue et al., 1988) or neurotoxic exposure in utero (Edelson & Cantor, 1998; Rodier et al., 1997; Stromland et al., 1994) may increase the risk of autism. Finally, autism spectrum disorders are often associated with other medical disorders (Gillberg & Coleman, 1996; Miller et al., 2005)—such as tuberous sclerosis (Gillberg et al., 1994)—even though it is unclear whether such associations relate to mental retardation rather than autism per se (Barton & Volkmar, 1998).

A unique genetic or epigenetic cause of autism is therefore unlikely. Consequently, we have to expect that there are multiple etiological pathways and patterns of neurodevelopmental disturbances that ultimately result in a cognitive-behavioral phenotype fulfilling the diagnostic criteria for autism. From this perspective, it is not surprising that numerous brain regions have been reported as affected in diverse neuroanatomical studies, sometimes without replication (reviewed in Akshoomoff et al., 2002; Brambilla et al., 2003). Findings of abnormality have been reported for the frontal (Carper & Courchesne, 2005; Herbert et al., 2004), parietal (Courchesne et al., 1993), and lateral temporal lobes (Rojas et al., 2005; Zilbovicius et al., 2000), the cingulate region (Abell et al., 1999; Haznedar et al., 1997), the corpus callosum (Egaas et al., 1995; Piven et al., 1997; Waiter et al., 2005), the hippocampal formation and amygdala (Bauman & Kemper, 1994; Otsuka et al., 1999; Raymond et al., 1996; Saitoh et al., 2001; Schumann et al., 2004), as well as the basal ganglia (Hollander et al., 2005; Sears et al., 1999), the thalamus (Tsatsanis et al., 2003), and the brainstem (Hashimoto et al., 1995a; Rodier, 2002). Besides these, the brain region that has received most attention is the cerebellum. Cerebellar abnormalities have been identified in a number of studies (Courchesne et al., 1988, 1994a; Gaffney et al., 1987; Hashimoto et al., 1995b; Murakami et al., 1989; Otsuka et al., 1999), some of which indicated specifically a reduced size of the posterior vermis (lobules VI–VII; Courchesne et al., 1988, 2001; Murakami et al., 1989). In postmortem studies the most consistent finding has been reduced numbers or size of cerebellar Purkinje neurons (Bailey et al., 1998; Palmen et al., 2004). However, cerebellar findings have not been replicated in an equally large number of magnetic resonance (MR) volumetric studies (reviewed in Brambilla et al., 2003). The degree to which cerebellar findings are specific to autism has thus not been definitively established.

Functional Neuroimaging in Autism

Starting in the mid-1980s, functional imaging techniques, such as positron emission tomography (PET) and single-photon emission computed tomography (SPECT), began to be applied to the study of autism. These studies were usually limited to single conditions, with subjects being scanned at rest, with eyes closed (Horwitz et al., 1988; Rumsey et al., 1985) or open (George et al., 1992; McKelvey et al., 1995; Mountz et al., 1995; Schifter et al., 1994; Sherman et al., 1984), or during sedation (Chiron et al., 1995; De Volder et al., 1987; Ohnishi et al., 2000; Zilbovicius et al., 2000). Only in a few studies, cognitive conditions were controlled through experimental conditions, such as verbal learning (Haznedar et al., 1997) and continuous performance tasks (Buchsbaum et al., 1992; Heh et al., 1989; Siegel et al., 1992). Some of these early studies yielded intriguing results. For instance, Horwitz and colleagues (1988) found reduced correlation in regional glucose metabolism between frontal, parietal, thalamic, and neostriatal regions in young men with autism, suggesting disruptions of functional networks. As I describe below, this study anticipates some of the promising approaches in current functional neuroimaging research on autism. All in all, however, it is hard to draw conclusions from the single-condition PET and SPECT studies noted above because of the diversity and even inconsistency of many findings. For one example, in the very first such study, Rumsey and colleagues (1985) observed widespread hypermetabolism in young autistic men. Contrary to this, Herold and colleagues (1988) reported normal rates of glucose metabolism and regional cerebral blood flow in a small sample of young men with autism. De Volder et al. (1987) also found normal rates of glucose metabolism in autistic children and adolescents (including females).

The literature on single-condition functional imaging studies is reviewed in detail by Chugani (2000). Inconsistencies in this literature can be attributed to several factors: differences in mental condition (task performance, rest, sedation); differences in inclusionary criteria (age, gender) as well as in diagnostic criteria for autism; and differences in the selection of comparison groups (e.g., healthy controls, siblings, individuals with mental retardation). Some of the shortcomings in early studies have been overcome in more recent functional neuroimaging work of a different type—that is, task-induced activation studies. Further progress has been driven by the need in the autism field in general to tighten diagnostic criteria. Thus, it has become standard to include only subjects who fulfill criteria on the retrospective Autism Diagnostic Interview (ADI-R; Rutter et al., 1995) and the Autism Diagnostic Observation Schedule (ADOS; Lord et al., 2001), in addition to those in the text revision of the *Diagnostic and Statistical Manual of Mental Disorders* (4th ed.) (DSM-IV-TR; American Psychiatric Association, 2000). Whether this truly eliminates sample heterogeneity is in doubt, as discussed above, but diagnostic progress in the past decade or two has certainly added to the replicability of findings.

Task-induced activation studies differ from the earlier PET and SPECT studies described above in that they do not assess absolute levels of activity in a single state (e.g., regional glucose metabolic rate at rest), but *compare* relative levels of activity between two or more different cognitive states. Task-induced studies are therefore, at least in theory, more controlled, avoiding such ill-defined conditions as so-called rest. There is good reason to assume that for a healthy adult the "resting state" is one of potentially intense mental activity (Binder et al., 1999; Raichle et al., 2001). There is also little confidence that every healthy adult will respond in identical ways to an unfamiliar setting in a scanner, which in functional MRI is also restraining and noisy. In other words, the resting state invites uncontrolled mental function as well as individual variability of such function. It is reasonable to expect that such variability is even greater in clinical populations, as for instance in people with autism. Keeping subjects on-task continuously while monitoring behavior (using button-press responses, for example) is probably the best available method to control effects of the experimental setting.

Cognitive specificity in task-induced studies has enabled autism researchers to target functional domains of interest in much more direct ways than was previously possible. For example, a structural imaging study may target the amygdala because this structure is known for its involvement in socio-emotional functions that are impaired in autism (Schumann et al., 2004); or a single-state PET study may target the superior temporal lobe, based on hypotheses of auditory dysfunction in autism (Zilbovicius et al., 2000). In these cases, functional specificity is indirectly attained through selection of an anatomical region of interest, based on the assumed function of this region in the healthy brain. In task-induced studies, on the other hand, specificity is directly attained by selection of a cognitive or sensorimotor task paradigm tapping into domains of known or expected impairments in autism. The rationale for this approach is very straightforward. For instance, in the very first task-induced study of autism by Happé and colleagues (1996), comprehension of narratives requiring "theory of mind" or mentalizing—known to be impaired in autism (Baron-Cohen et al., 1985; Happé & Frith, 1996)—was compared with comprehension of physical stories (assumed unaffected in autism) during PET scanning, which showed differentially localized activity in medial frontal cortex in participants with autism spectrum disorders, as compared with control subjects.

Imaging Studies of Social Cognition

Given the salience of sociocommunicative deficits among the diagnostic criteria for autism (American Psychiatric Association, 2000), it will come as no surprise that the bulk of currently available task-induced neuroimaging studies have focused on functions related to social cognition. Among these, the largest set has been dedicated to face processing. For instance, a study by Schultz and colleagues (2000) suggested that face perception in autism was associated with activity patterns in lateral portions of the inferior temporal lobe typically found for non-face object perception in healthy controls. A study by Pierce et al. (2001) supported reduced activity in the "fusiform face area" (FFA) in autism during face perception, but not the complementary activity in the lateral inferior temporal gyrus. Hubl and colleagues (2003) also observed reduced FFA activity in 10 participants with autism during face processing, but found enhanced activation in the medial occipital lobe in their autism group, as compared with controls.

More recently it has become clear that the results from these earlier studies cannot be simply construed as the reflection of a defective FFA in autism. Hadjikhani and colleagues (2004) partially replicated the design of the study by Schultz et al. (2000), but had subjects passively view faces, objects, and scrambled faces. In their study, activity in the fusiform face area was clearly present in autistic subjects during face viewing. It is therefore possible that the nature of the task and the response modality (passive viewing versus sameness judgments by button press of two simultaneously shown stimuli in the study by Schultz et al.) may affect the presence or absence of FFA activation in autism. A recent follow-up study by Pierce and colleagues (2004) supports the conclusion that the FFA is not simply defective in autism, but modulated in atypical ways in certain task settings. In this study, participants with autism performed gender judgments while viewing familiar faces (family and friends) and strange faces. Contrary to their earlier study (Pierce et al., 2001), which also involved gender discrimination, FFA activity was present in autistic subjects for faces of strangers and even more robustly for familiar faces.

At least two general lessons can be drawn from face perception studies in autism. First, they show that results from a single-task paradigm may erroneously suggest some localized neurofunctional defect, whereas reduced activity may be more reasonably explained by an unusual response to a particular type of task and by atypical ways in which functional systems in the autistic brain cooperate. For instance, absence or presence of FFA activity in the studies reviewed above may be linked to orthogonal tasks (sameness judgments), which may have reduced attentional upregulation of FFA activity in subjects with autism, but not in control subjects. If so, the true underlying abnormality would be related to attentional functions (see below).

To appreciate the second more general lesson derived from the face perception studies, let us assume (counterfactually) that absence of FFA activity in response to faces in autism had been definitively replicated in a number of studies. What would such a finding actually explain? Avoidance of eye contact is one of the core diagnostic criteria for autism (American Psychiatric Association, 2000; Baird et al., 2000). This implies that subjects with autism look at faces much less frequently than typically developing children (Klin et al., 2002). In other words, domain-specific stimulation is strongly reduced in autism. It is further well known that experience and activity are important factors that shape the neurofunctional organization of cerebral cortex during development. Animal studies, for example, show that a prospective "auditory cortex" in the superior temporal lobe will assume visual function if afferent information from the retina is rerouted via the thalamic medial geniculate nucleus (Sur & Leamey, 2001). Human studies show that congenitally blind subjects, who process tactile information much more intensely than seeing subjects (e.g., in Braille reading), "use" their occipital cortices for tactile functions (Sadato et al., 2002). Professional musicians, who have engaged in intense sensorimotor practice on their instruments over many years, show respective expansions of perirolandic sensorimotor maps (Elbert et al., 1995). Against this background, even if neuroimaging could demonstrate reduced FFA involvement during face perception in autism, it would be reasonable to explain such reduction as a reflection of normal experience-based neurofunctional plasticity. This underscores the need for caution when it comes to interpreting unusual regional activation patterns in autism as reflections of brain defects. At the same time, if it is true that atypical response in FFA to faces is a result of atypical experience with faces in autism, a deeper question still remains: What elementary early-onset neurofunctional abnormalities may explain reduced face perception experience in autism? The need for answering such elementary questions first in autism research is discussed in more detail below.

A few functional imaging studies have examined responses in the autistic brain specifically to emotional expressions of faces. Critchley and colleagues (2000) presented subjects with happy or angry faces (versus neutral faces in a control condition) in an implicit passive viewing task and an explicit judgment task. Overall, participants with autism showed lower than normal activity in the right FFA. A site close to the left amygdala was active during the implicit condition in controls, but activated only during the explicit task in subjects with autism. This specific finding could suggest that passive viewing of faces may not be as automatically engaging for autistic individuals as it is for healthy control subjects. Such an interpretation would contrast in interesting ways with the results of the nonemotional face processing studies discussed above, which suggested that an explicit task that is unrelated or orthogonal to face processing per se may reduce FFA activity in autism. Taken together, the findings may imply that FFA will activate in autism in the context of explicit processing of facial emotion, but not when an additional task (e.g., gender discrimination) is given. A study by Piggot et al. (2004) further implies that FFA activity in high-functioning autism may be normal for verbal labeling of emotional face expressions, but slightly reduced for nonverbal matching of such expressions.

In a more recent study, Hall and coworkers (2003) tested autistic men on emotional matching of facial expressions with voices, comparing this to a gender-matching condition. Even though this task design was thus very different from the one used by Critchley and colleagues (2000), Hall et al. also observed diminished activity in the right FFA in their autism group. Baron-Cohen and colleagues (1999) presented only parts of facial stimuli, containing eyes and brows, to young adults with autism. The task was to select the emotional state of a pair of eyes from two words (e.g., "unconcerned" vs. "concerned") presented at the bottom of a screen. This task was considered to tap into theory of mind because it required empathizing. In the control condition, subjects had to make gender decisions in an analogous design. Controls showed highly distributed activation in bilateral frontal, temporal, and parietal lobes, whereas much less significant activation was seen in participants with autism, mostly in the right hemisphere. Although an expected group difference was found in the left amygdala, where subjects with autism showed less activation than did controls, a number of significant group effects in perisylvian cortices could probably be attributed to differential response to verbal components of the task. Welchew and colleagues (2005) recently examined functional connectivity during viewing of facial expressions and found that medial temporal structures, such as amygdala and parahippocampal gyrus, were affected by "disconnectivity" in men with autism or Asperger syndrome.

One further neuroimaging study examined theory of mind in autism. In this PET study, Castelli and colleagues (2002) showed subjects triangles moving around on a screen. In one condition, the movement was random, whereas in a theory-of-mind condition, triangles appeared to mentalize, that is, to anticipate or manipulate the other triangle's mental state. A group of autistic adults showed normal levels of activation for the theory-of-mind (compared to the random) condition in extrastriate visual cortex, but significantly less activation than normal controls in three other regions of the right hemisphere: a basal temporal region close to the amygdala, the superior temporal sulcus, and medial prefrontal area 9.

These results are important because they highlight the more consistent findings (among a wealth of nonreplicated results) in studies of social cognition and face processing in autism. First, atypical activity in the amygdala or its vicinity is a relatively consistent finding (but see Piggot et al., 2004, for a counterexample). It is also supported by evidence from other experimental techniques, such as postmortem cellular examination and structural imaging (Baron-Cohen et al., 2000; Sweeten et al., 2002). However, it clearly does not imply total absence of function in the autistic amygdala (Pierce et al., 2004). Second, the superior temporal sulcus is known for its involvement in the perception of biological motion (Puce & Perrett, 2003). Lack of activity in this area may reflect a reduced ability in autism to perceive visual stimuli as biological motion—even when such a perception is factually an illusion (as in the triangle study by Castelli and colleagues). One other functional neuroimaging study on voice processing (as compared with nonbiological tones) supports the finding of reduced activity in the superior temporal sulcus in autism (Gervais et al., 2004). Third, beginning with early imaging studies (Baron-Cohen et al., 1994; Happé et al., 1996), the role of the medial prefrontal cortex in social cognition has been documented (Ramnani & Miall, 2004). Both the studies by Happé et al. (1996) and Castelli et al. (2002) did indeed report atypical activation in this region for participants with autism. However, the specific findings were quite different. Happé and colleagues found that normal activity for a theory-of-mind task located in Brodmann's area 8 was displaced and located more inferior and anterior in area 9 in a group of five subjects with Asperger syndrome. Contrary to this, Castelli and colleagues saw an absence of normal activation in area 9 in autistic adults for their version of a theory-of-mind task. Strictly speaking, these results are contradictory, but it remains likely that social cognition impairments in autism involve atypical medial prefrontal function, in addition to abnormalities in the amygdala and the superior temporal sulcus.

Imaging Studies of Language

Bearing in mind that language acquisition is commonly delayed in autism and that many lower-functioning individuals with autism never acquire phrase speech (Lord et al., 2004), the number of functional imaging studies of language in autism is surprisingly small. In an early small-sample PET study (Müller et al., 1999a), adults with autism—when listening to short sentences—showed blood flow increases in perisylvian cortex that lacked the leftward asymmetry seen in a normal control group (Plate 6.1). However, when autistic subjects had to generate their own sentences, prompted by sentences and cue words (e.g., "He was listening to the radio—*television*"), normal perisylvian leftward asymmetry was found and left inferior frontal activation appeared normal. A number of results from techniques other than task-related neuroimaging have suggested atypical hemispheric asymmetries in language-related areas (Chiron et al., 1995; Gendry Meresse et al., 2005; Herbert et al., 2002; Rojas et al., 2005). The results of our PET study (Müller et al., 1999a) may indicate that atypical language-related asymmetries are task dependent in high-functioning individuals with autism, that is, affect only subcomponents of the language system (e.g., receptive functions). A follow-up analysis (Müller et al., 1998) limited to four autistic males, however, did suggest reduced left dorsolateral prefrontal activity, as well as atypical rightward asymmetry of thalamic activation during sentence generation. A more recent PET study by Boddaert et al. (2003), again in a small sample of five adults with autism, yielded evidence consistent with atypical receptive asymmetries. This study used synthetic speech-like stimuli for passive listening (as compared with rest). Leftward asymmetry of activation in the superior temporal cortex, as observed in healthy controls, was reversed in the autism group.

In a functional magnetic resonance imaging (fMRI) study, Just and colleagues (2004a) applied a sentence comprehension paradigm in a comparatively large sample of 17 high-functioning individuals with autism. In comparison with a low-level baseline task (visual fixation), both autism and control groups showed extensive activation in occipitoparietal, lateral temporal, premotor, and inferior frontal areas. Direct statistical group comparisons for identifying activation differences were not reported. However, the study also included functional connectivity analyses, suggesting generally reduced interregional cooperation during language processing in the autism group (for discussion, see below). More recently, Gaffrey and coworkers (2007) studied semantic category decisions in 10 adolescents and young adults with autism spectrum disorder, also using fMRI. A matched control group showed extensive left inferior frontal activation, which was also seen—though less robustly—in the autism group. The main finding on direct group comparisons was much stronger activation in extrastriate cortex in the participants with autism, suggesting that semantic organization in autism may rely heavily on visual imagery. This is consistent with a study by Kana and colleagues (2006), who found greater than normal activity in visual cortex in autistic adolescents and adults for sentence comprehension, especially for low-imagery sentences. Enhanced extrastriate activation in adults with autism has also been reported by Koshino et al. (2005) for an *n*-back verbal working memory task, which again would indicate an unusual visual strategy for processing linguistic stimuli (here: letters).

Imaging Studies of Attention and Sensorimotor Functions

Although not included among the diagnostic criteria, attentional impairments have for a long time been considered an elementary disturbance in autism, potentially accounting for higher cognitive deficits. In early electrophysiological studies, reduced amplitude of endogenous event-related potentials (N_c and auditory P3b) was considered evidence for attentional dysfunction (Courchesne, 1987; Courchesne et al., 1989). More recent behavioral data indicate selective deficits in the ability to shift attention in autism. In one study, participants with autism had problems in quickly shifting attention from the visual to the auditory domain and vice versa, whereas they performed normally when required to focus attention within the auditory or visual domain, or when given more time (> 2.5 s) for attention shifts between sensory modalities (Courchesne et al., 1994b). These deficits could be related to cerebellar pathology in autism, given that patients with acquired cerebellar lesions show attentional deficits similar to those found in subjects with autism (Akshoomoff & Courchesne, 1992; Courchesne et al., 1994b) and that functional MRI studies in healthy adults have demonstrated cerebellar involvement in nonmotor attentional processes (Allen et al., 1997; Le et al., 1998). Another neuroanatomical site of interest with regard to attentional impairments is the parietal lobe. Volume loss in the parietal lobes has been found in a subset of subjects with autism (Courchesne et al., 1993). Like patients with acquired parietal lesions (Posner et al., 1984), autistic subjects with parietal volume loss (but not those without) show deficits in redirecting attention in visual space, manifesting an abnormally narrow "spotlight" of attention (Townsend & Courchesne, 1994; Townsend et al., 1996).

More recently, the indirect evidence for links between cerebellar and parietal anatomical involvement and attentional deficits in autism has been complemented by functional neuroimaging results. In a study by Belmonte and Yurgelun-Todd (2003), six subjects with autism spectrum disorders performed a visuospatial covert attention-shifting task, in which detection of an oddball target in one location shifted covert attention to the opposite location. The autism group showed unusual ventral occipital activity, whereas activation in superior parietal lobes that was prominent in healthy controls was absent. Haist and coworkers (2005) found reduced inferior parietal activity in autistic adolescents and adults during spatial attention shifting when intervals between cues and response were short (100 ms). Allen and Courchesne (2003) focused on the cerebellum in a study of visual attention in eight autistic individuals. Subjects selectively attended and responded to either a shape or a color in any given task block. A parametric design allowed the investigators to examine the effects of task difficulty, with stimuli presented at three different interstimulus intervals. Activation in several regions of the posterior cerebellum tended to be reduced in the autism group (as compared with matched controls) even when subjects were matched for performance. The study by Allen and Courchesne had a limited field of view, with only four coronal slices through the cerebellum. Although parietal effects were not statistically examined, attention-related parietal activity appeared bilaterally reduced in the autism group, compared with controls.

A few studies have investigated basic sensorimotor functions in autism. Gomot and colleagues (2006) observed reduced activity in the left anterior cingulate cortex in a group of autistic children during detection of novel and deviant tones in an auditory oddball paradigm. Allen and colleagues (2003, 2004) contrasted their attentional findings in the cerebellum with those for simple thumb movement. The results suggested that the cerebellum showed specific activational reduction associated with attention, whereas activity related to movement was actually greater than normal. In particular, motor-related activation in participants with autism extended into posterior cerebellar regions that were involved in attentional functions in healthy controls. Allen et al. (2004) also observed that reduced anatomical size of the anterior cerebellum and the posterior lobule VII correlated with enhanced activation extent (volume of activation) during thumb movement. As mentioned above, reduced cerebellar volume has been hypothesized to be developmentally related to autistic pathology (Courchesne, 1997; Courchesne et al., 1988). The finding of correlated overactivation for simple motor functions in cerebellar regions of volume loss may indicate neurofunctional sequelae of cerebellar pathology in autism.

A further study (Müller et al., 2001), also on simple finger movement (visually prompted button pressing with the index finger of the preferred hand), yielded information on cerebral activation patterns consistent with those of the aforementioned studies by Allen and colleagues. Even though groupwise activation analyses for a sample of eight autistic men showed only a slight reduction of normal activation in motor, premotor, and supplementary motor cortices, inspection of the data for individual subjects revealed that these differences were due to unusual scattering of motor-related activation into parietal and prefrontal brain areas in a number of individuals with autism—a pattern not seen in a single control subject (Figure 6.1). This observation, together with the results from Allen et al. (2004), could reflect elementary disturbances in neurofunctional organization in autism, potentially related to the finding of abnormal brain growth curves in early autistic development (Carper et al., 2002; Courchesne et al., 2001). According to a very simple hypothesis, early-developing functions (e.g., simple motor control) require greater than normal processing territory in cerebral cortex (presumably due to reduced processing efficiency of autistic cortex; Casanova et al., 2002) at the expense of later-developing higher cognitive functional systems. A further fMRI study examining slightly more complex visuomotor coordination, in which subjects had to perform button press sequences prompted by visual cues, yielded results consistent with this model, that is, a spread of acti-

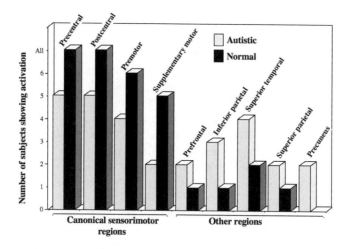

FIGURE 6.1. Number of subjects per group (autism versus normal control) showing activation ($p < .05$; corr.) in regions of interest during unilateral finger tapping. Bars on the left ("canonical sensorimotor regions") indicate activations in contralateral regions expected to activate in a simple motor task; bars on the right show activation in other regions of the hemisphere contralateral to the movement. The prefrontal region includes all portions of the superior, middle, and inferior frontal gyri not included in the sensorimotor regions. Whereas fewer autistic than control subjects show activations in canonical sensorimotor regions, the inverse is seen for other regions in the frontal, parietal, and temporal lobes. Based on data from Müller et al. (2001).

vation in autistic subjects beyond normal premotor and superior parietal sites into the prefrontal and inferior parietal cortex (Müller et al., 2003).

Task-induced neuroimaging studies of learning in autism are currently not available, except for one study on procedural digit sequence learning (Müller et al., 2004). This experiment used the visuomotor design of a previous study mentioned above (Müller et al., 2003), but examined changes over time associated with learning. Both an autism group (consisting of eight men) and a matched control group relied heavily on premotor and superior parietal activity during early stages of performing a repeating eight-digit sequence. Reduced reaction times in the later phases of the experiment indicated learning effects, which were associated with overall decreased premotor activity in controls, but increased premotor involvement in the autism group. Although this was not predicted based on the hypothesis of early-developing functions "invading" what is normally polymodal association cortex, it may be considered a complementary finding, adding up to a more general hypothesis of neurofunctional organization in autism. This hypothesis implies that (1) early-emerging sensorimotor functions require too much cortical processing territory and therefore spread into adjacent cortices that are normally involved in complex polymodal processing and (2) high-functioning autistic individuals develop strategies for solving more complex tasks that rely heavily on sensorimotor components. This latter hypothesis is supported by abnormal premotor cortex involvement in learning, but also by the finding of atypical activation in extrastriate visual cortex during semantic decision and verbal working memory, as described above.

Limits and Promises of Functional Neuroimaging in Autism

Functional neuroimaging has experienced an astounding growth in the past two decades. When fMRI was established in the early 1990s as an alternative to PET in its ability to map out regional brain activation (Belliveau et al., 1991), this growth became exponential because widely available clinical MRI scanners could be easily upgraded for echo-planar imaging and fMRI use. Today, several thousand fMRI studies are published every year, and even for the study of developmental disorders, such as attention deficit disorder or autism, which pose extreme problems of subject cooperation regarding head motion and task compliance, fMRI has become an important source of evidence. However, enthusiasm about functional neuroimaging techniques needs to be viewed in context, with its historical baggage and future promises.

Past: The Brain as a Map

Many basic assumptions of modern functional neuroimaging have a long history in the prescientific study of the brain and in early neurology, which was dominated by the idea of brain organization as a functional landscape or "map" (Clarke & Dewhurst, 1972). Interestingly, today's most important professional organization representing functional neuroimaging research still abides by this metaphor, calling itself the Organization for Human Brain Mapping (*www.humanbrainmapping.org*). An exhaustive discussion of the roots and limitations of this metaphor in neurology and cognitive neuroscience is beyond the scope of this chapter (see, e.g., Müller, 1992; Sternberg, 1990). Suffice it to state here that there is a growing awareness in cognitive and clinical neuroscience that localization of function (or dysfunction) per se may not be explanatory (e.g., Mesulam, 1998). Some conceptual elements of this awareness have a long history. For instance, the notion of functional systems being organized, not as serially lined up "centers" (Lichtheim, 1885), but as distributed networks can be traced back at least to the work of Pierre Flourens in the early 19th century (cf. Clarke & Dewhurst, 1972). Directly relevant to the study of clinical disorders, neurologists of the late 19th and early 20th centuries, such as Hughlings-Jackson (1878) and Head (1926), explained behavioral changes in lesion patients as resulting from brain systems that remain *intact* following brain damage—contrary to the conventional focus on links between lesion site and behavioral impairment, which is still dominant in today's cognitive neuropsychology. Animal work by Lashley

(1950) following this "holistic" tradition in neurology had a groundbreaking impact on emerging modern concepts of distributed neuronal representations and the developmental plasticity of multipotential cortex (cf. O'Leary & Nakagawa, 2002).

Present: The Limits of Deficit "Blobology"

The traditional metaphor of the brain as a functional map, which today continues to dominate cognitive neuroscience, has direct repercussions for neuroimaging studies of developmental disorders. Adopting the terminology of Thomas Kuhn (1962), the dominant "paradigm" of imaging research in healthy adults has been to localize cognitive components of function to one or a few brain regions, typically presented as colorful blobs on standardized brain anatomy that reflect clusters of voxels (image volume elements) that survive corrected significance thresholds for an activation statistic. The obvious adaptation of this paradigm to the clinical realm and to developmental disorders is to localize components of impairment to specific brain regions in similar ways. As discussed above, the literature on face processing in autism initially took this approach. However, this view is questionable because it is unlikely that brain regions, such as the fusiform gyrus, work independently to fulfill a specific function such as face perception. To anyone familiar with the relative homogeneity of cortical architecture across different regions and the density of connections between cortical regions and between subcortex, cerebellum, and cerebral cortex, this modular idea of the autonomous and "encapsulated" function of a brain region will appear highly unlikely. The idea was formulated in its purest form by Fodor (1983), who postulated that perceptual systems were modular—that is, domain specific, informationally encapsulated (without access to processing in other modules), innate, and associated with a fixed neural architecture. Given that Fodor's book was primarily meant as a provocation (a "potboiler," as pointed out by Fodor, 1985, p. 33) and that from a neuroscientific view his ideas appear mostly unfounded (Müller, 1996), the impact of his book on the cognitive sciences has been surprisingly deep. For an example relevant to the clinical discussion in this chapter, Baron-Cohen (1992) and, more recently, Scholl and Leslie (2001) have argued for a modular status of "theory of mind," referring to Fodor's abovementioned criteria. The claim implies that autism may be explained in terms of a "broken module." The more general assumption for developmental disorders is that certain modules may be selectively affected in certain disorders, presumably due to specific genetic defects, whereas for the remainder of the developing neurocognitive systems "residual normality" can be assumed (for a critique, see Thomas & Karmiloff-Smith, 2002).

The issue of "residual normality" has been debated in neurology for centuries. It is not limited to the developmental setting, but it arises in analogous ways in the study of adult patients with brain damage, as mentioned in the previous section. Following in the footsteps of Hughlings-Jackson (1878) and

Head (1926), modern clinical neuroscience has begun to understand that an acquired brain damage, even when it appears focal on a computed tomography (CT) or MRI scan, can be fully understood only if reorganizational changes in the rest of the brain are taken into account. The brain outside the lesion may appear structurally intact, but may not be functionally "normal," in either a positive or a negative sense. For example, studies in adults with left perisylvian stroke have shown that right-hemisphere brain regions homotopic to the classical language areas become more involved in language processing than they are in the "normal" adult brain (Leff et al., 2002; Ohyama et al., 1996; Thulborn et al., 1999). Recent animal stroke models also demonstrate enhanced neurogenesis in the hippocampal dentate gyrus following middle cerebral artery ischemia, which may support postlesional compensatory changes (Tureyen et al., 2004). From these perspectives, the residual brain could be considered *supernormal* because it compensates for the loss of tissue in a variety of ways. In other respects, postlesional changes in the residual brain may imply *subnormality*—that is, additional loss of function. A good example is the reduced function of the contralateral cerebellum in patients with unilateral cerebral stroke, a phenomenon called crossed cerebellar diaschisis (Gold & Lauritzen, 2002; Pantano et al., 1986).

"Residual normality" is thus clearly not present in adult patients with acquired focal lesion. Much less so can we expect it in developmental disorders, for at least two reasons. First, developmental brain impairments are usually not focal. Among the types of neurodevelopmental disorders discussed at the beginning of this chapter, cases of type (1) in which a brain lesion is truly focal are probably quite rare. Among types (2) and (3) (i.e., disorders that are predominantly caused by genetic risk), focal brain impairment is highly improbable, as discussed above. Second, damage to a functional region or system is likely to have different consequences depending on developmental stage. A striking illustration of this was discussed at the beginning of this chapter. Children with early-onset damage to the left hemisphere usually show much better language outcome than adults with comparable left-hemisphere damage. This can be attributed to the greater plasticity of the developing brain, and it is likely that greater synaptic density in the child's brain is one of the parameters related to this plasticity.

Another more specific example of the differential roles of functional systems across development relates to the neurotransmitter serotonin (5-HT) and autism. There is some evidence from neuroimaging research (Chugani, 2002; Chugani et al., 1999), as well as from blood plasma and pharmacological studies (Buitelaar & Willemsen-Swinkels, 2000) for serotonergic abnormalities in autism. Although the precise roles of serotonin transporter and serotonin receptor genes in autism have not been fully elucidated, their involvement in this disorder appears probable (Veenstra-VanderWeele & Cook, 2004). Interestingly, the role of serotonin changes dramatically during development. In the mature brain, serotonin functions as a neurotransmitter active in widely distributed projections from the raphe nuclei in the brainstem and is considered important for attentional regulation (Schwartz, 2000), as well as sensory gating, inhibition, and a variety of affective and endocrine functions (Anderson & Lombroso, 2002). During development, however, serotonin plays neurotrophic roles with an impact on neuronal differentiation, myelination, synaptogenesis, and dendritic development (Whitaker-Azmitia, 2001). Abnormal serotonin metabolism at critical developmental stages may affect thalamocortical afferents (Chugani, 2004) as well as laminar and columnar cortical organization (Janusonis et al., 2004). Therefore, even if autism could be explained solely on the basis of serotonergic abnormalities, these would still imply a variety of effects, some of which resulting from disturbances of early cortical organization, others involving functional systems, such as attention, sensory gating, or inhibition, for which serotonin plays an important role in the mature nervous system.

The preceding example underscores that "residual normality" cannot be expected in developmental disorders (for detailed argument and peer discussion, see Thomas & Karmiloff-Smith, 2002). This conclusion has repercussions for functional neuroimaging in these disorders. Although the metaphor of "functional mapping" may be a useful paradigm in adult neuroimaging (though it will certainly come to be considered crude and misleading in the future), it is to be treated with utmost caution in developmental disorders. From all that we know today, it is unrealistic to expect that the phenotype of a developmental disorder—even if it is caused by a single-gene defect—could be explained by a focal brain regional abnormality (Fisher, 2005; Müller, 2005). This implies that the conventional lesion approach of adult cognitive neuropsychology, according to which damage to a brain area with resulting specific impairment indicates that the impaired function was localized to the damaged site premorbidly (and is analogously localized in the healthy brain), is questionable in developmental disorders. An example regarding abnormal activity patterns in the fusiform gyrus during face perception in autism was discussed above. Similar considerations concern the possibility of atypical perisylvian asymmetries for language in autism.

Recent MR volumetric work by Herbert and colleagues (2002) showed that leftward volumetric asymmetries commonly seen in typically developing children were reversed in children with autism when large brain regions were measured, whereas examination of small subregions (Herbert et al., 2005) revealed complex patterns of partially exaggerated leftward asymmetry (as in the planum temporale) and partially reversed asymmetry (as in the frontal operculum). As mentioned above, there are only few functional neuroimaging studies of language in autism. Some of these are consistent with the hypothesis of atypical asymmetries in autism (Boddaert et al., 2003; Müller et al., 1998, 1999a), whereas others have yielded evidence for apparently typical leftward asymmetry in the inferior frontal cortex (Broca's area) in autism during sentence comprehension (Just et al., 2004b) and semantic category decision (Gaffrey et al., 2007). The question of atypical asymmetries in autism may have to be raised in much more specific ways. For example, it may depend on the nature of the task (e.g., passive stimulation with verbal material versus active production or judgment), and there may be greater individual variability within the autism population with the possibility of atypical language asymmetries being related to atypical hand preferences (Escalante-Mead et al., 2003; Soper et al., 1986). A deeper issue is our limited understanding of the developmental causes for functional brain asymmetries; that is, it is not fully understood why typically developing young children begin to prefer one hand over the other, why they typically use predominantly the left hemisphere for language-related functions, and how these two developmental processes relate to each other. I do not discuss the evidence relevant to these questions in this chapter because it would stray too far from the topic of functional neuroimaging. However, the issue highlights the importance of a developmental perspective. Such a perspective should be the obvious choice in the study of developmental disorders. However, since subjects can usually be included in functional neuroimaging studies only as adults or adolescents, given the high demands on cooperation, the evidence provided by most such studies is not developmental per se, but requires developmental interpretation.

A straightforward, but potentially nondevelopmental interpretation of imaging findings in autism would be to say, for example, "Autistic individuals have problems with face perception because the fusiform face area does not function normally" (as debunked above), or, "Children with autism have language delays because language asymmetries (structural or functional) are abnormal." Such interpretations are as tempting as they are misleading. As argued earlier, it is very likely that effects of experience and activity (interaction with the environment) continuously alter neurofunctional organization in autism throughout childhood. Therefore, abnormalities observed in older children or adults are at least in part a reflection of atypical experience rather than an indication of a *cause* of impairment. This raises the issue of belated study in neuroimaging, that is, the study of a disorder long after the onset of pathogenesis.

Future: Development and Integration

Technical Advances

There are two possible technical solutions to the problem of belated study. The first one is to adapt neuroimaging techniques such as fMRI that are typically used in older children and adults to the study of infants and young children. Some pioneering work suggests that this is indeed possible. Dehaene-Lambertz and colleagues (2002) studied 20 nonsedated infants, ages 2–3 months, during speech stimulation and found evidence for leftward asymmetry of temporal lobe activation. Interestingly, this group of researchers could even obtain usable data from 5 infants who remained awake throughout the procedure. Temporal activation associated with speech stimuli was found in sleeping as well as in awake subjects. A similar study using nonverbal auditory stimuli found effects in the superior temporal cortex in neonates (Anderson et al., 2001), including preterm babies as young as 25 weeks of gestation. Notably, blood-oxygen-level-dependent (BOLD) effects were positive in some, but negative in the majority of the neonates, with no obvious correlation between gestational or postnatal age and BOLD polarity.

This highlights the unresolved issue of maturational changes in the physiology underlying the BOLD response in fMRI studies of young children. In one study, an abrupt shift at about 8 weeks of age from positive to negative BOLD response associated with visual stimulation was reported (Yamada et al., 2000). Born and colleagues (1998, 2002a) reported BOLD inversion even in older children up to the age of 71 months. However, these results may have been affected by the use of sedatives, given that Dehaene-Lambertz and colleagues (2002) found consistently positive BOLD responses in the study of unsedated 2- to 3-month-olds. Alternatively or additionally, polarity of BOLD response may interact with the functional system examined. Most reports of BOLD negativity come from visual studies (Born et al., 1998, 2002b; Meek et al., 1998; Muramoto et al., 2002; Yamada et al., 2000), whereas auditory studies of infants and neonates (Anderson et al., 2001; Dehaene-Lambertz et al., 2002) and even of the fetus *in utero* (Moore et al., 2001) have shown mostly positive BOLD responses. Based on the limited available evidence, factors such as age, physiological state (awake, natural sleep, sedated), and functional system may interact in determining polarity of the BOLD response. This complicates the prospect of neuroimaging studies in developmental disorders at ages that promise minimal effects of postnatal plasticity and reorganization and therefore a clearer picture of the primary pathological effects on functional brain organization.

A second solution to the problem of belated study is the use of techniques that can be better adapted to the study of young children. Positron emission tomography (PET) has the advantage of a quiet experimental setting, as compared with noisy fMRI data acquisition, but is considered unethical in children except for those with severe neurological conditions (Morton et al., 1996). Event-related potential (ERP) and magnetoencephalographic (MEG) studies are also performed in relatively nondistracting environments, although they are sensitive to head motion, which is hard to prevent in young children. Besides a number of ERP studies in children with autism below age 8 years (Bruneau et al., 1999; Dawson et al., 1986, 1995; Martineau et al., 1992; Ogawa et al., 1982; Roux et al., 1997), there have been some recent promising applications of MEG in the study of the auditory system in children with autism ages 8 years and older (Gage et al., 2003a, 2003b). Although temporal resolution of ERP and MEG is greatly superior to that of fMRI and PET, spatial resolution is inferior. Near-infrared spectroscopy (NIRS) is a technique that relies on effects of blood oxygenation on tissue absorption of near-infrared light. This completely noninvasive technique has been used extensively for clinical purposes in neonates (Nicklin et al., 2003). A few studies have applied this technique in neurologically healthy neonates and infants and were able to show expected oxygenation effects over occipital and temporal sites during visual (Meek et al., 1998) and auditory stimulation (Zaramella et al., 2001), respectively. However, the spatial resolution of NIRS is low and its application has been mostly limited to gross examination of basic sensorimotor functions, despite a few attempts to study more complex affective (Hoshi & Chen, 2002) and executive functions (Hoshi, 2003; Schroeter et al., 2004).

A Developmental Understanding of Cognitive Outcome

Technical progress may certainly contribute to solving the problem of belated study in the coming years, but the more fundamental challenge for the study of developmental disorders is a change in perspective—away from the common adultocentrist view of children as little adults on their way to completion and toward a constructivist understanding of development, that is, one that views the cognitive system at any stage as erected on the building blocks of previous stages. This perspective, of course, belongs to Swiss psychologist Jean Piaget and his school (Piaget, 1979), which in the context of the "cognitive revolution" of the 1960s (Gardner, 1987) came to be considered quasi-empiricist and incompatible with the radical antibehaviorism of Chomsky and his followers (Piattelli-Palmarini, 1980). Piaget's biggest "sin" in this historical context was to deny language the innate and autonomous status on which Chomskian generative grammar and its offshoots in psycholinguistics were founded. As discussed above, the repercussions of this Chomskian view can still be felt in the study of developmental disorders, in particular when it comes to defining language impairments in disorders such as specific language impairment, Williams syndrome, or autism.

However, alternative views of language acquisition, which take into account developmental precursors, are gaining more ground (Bates et al., 2003; Carpenter et al., 1998). These have important implications for developmental disorders. For example, the question of whether language capacity is compromised in autism can be reformulated: Are any of the precursor or ingredient functions of language acquisition impaired, and may this be the cause of delays in language acquisition? "Ingredients" of language can be defined as neurocognitive functions that emerge before the onset or during the course of language acquisition and that are prerequisites for normal language development (Müller, 2005). As already discussed, interactive mechanisms of language acquisition are likely to be compromised in autism (Baltaxe & Simmons, 1975). For a specific example, there is overall consensus that imitation is delayed in autism (Williams et al., 2004). This may reflect more general delays in sensorimotor integration. Imitation deficits have been shown to correlate with impaired social cooperation in young children with autism (Rogers et al., 2003). Furthermore, joint attention, which is intimately related with and probably a predictor for language acquisition (Bates et al., 2003; Markus et al., 2000), is impaired in autism (Bruinsma et al., 2004; Charman, 2003).

Baron-Cohen et al. (1997) observed that children with autism, when presented with a novel object in combination with a novel word, followed a speaker's direction of gaze much less often than typically developing and nonautistic mentally retarded children. Joint attention deficits in autism have been found to correlate with delays in language acquisition (Bono et al., 2004; Mundy et al., 1990), which suggests that reduced joint attention undermines normal strategies for lexical learning. What appears as a language disorder may thus be developmentally explained on the basis of more elementary impairments.

Support for the model of language ingredients comes from neuroimaging evidence, which has demonstrated participation of the left inferior frontal cortex (Broca's area) in many seemingly nonlinguistic functions. Among these are imitation (Buccino et al., 2004; Iacoboni et al., 1999), motor preparation (Krams et al., 1998) and complex motor planning (Fincham et al., 2002), sequence learning (Haslinger et al., 2002), action imagery (Binkofski et al., 2000) and observation (Buccino et al., 2001), rule shifting (Konishi et al., 1998), response selection (Thompson-Schill et al., 1997), response inhibition (Kemmotsu et al., 2005; Rubia et al., 2001), and working memory (Chen & Desmond, 2005). Adult cognitive neuroscience tends to be agnostic with regard to the unexpected apparent overlap of functional specializations in Broca's area. A developmental perspective, however, offers clues. Rather than asking why in adults all those nonlinguistic functions *also* populate a relatively small piece of cortical tissue in the inferior frontal gyrus, a developmental perspective considers many of those nonlinguistic functions as language ingredients. From this perspective, Broca's area is pivotal for language learning because a number of functional pathways providing crucial components for language learning converge in this brain area by the second year of life (Müller & Basho, 2004). This argument has been partially made previously in regard to the mirror neuron system (Rizzolatti & Arbib, 1998), but it should also be noted that convergence of the dorsal visual stream (grossly related to the mirror neuron system) with afferents from the ventral visual stream (Di Virgilio & Clarke, 1997; Petrides & Pandya, 2002) providing information about objects in the world is equally important for an understanding of the role of Broca's area.

Network Impairments

A model of language development emerging from language ingredient functions is important for the study of developmental disorders such as autism or specific language impairment because it acknowledges that atypical language organization may be a secondary outcome of impaired development of ingredient functions, such as imitation, joint attention, or complex motor planning. On the neurofunctional level, an understanding of cognitive impairment as emerging from more elementary sensorimotor impairments translates into a focus on distributed networks, as opposed to localized modules. Staying with the example of language impairment, a developmental neurofunctional approach has to consider all systems that may function as language precursors or ingredients. Disturbances in any of these systems may result in secondary language deficits. Therefore, developmental cognitive neuroscience needs to examine the integrity of the neural systems involved in potential ingredient functions. It becomes clear that an exclusive focus on what are considered left perisylvian "language areas" in the adult brain is insufficient. Instead, extensive regions outside the left perisylvian cortex are likely to cooperate in enabling the young child to begin acquiring words and grammar. The developmental and constructivist perspective therefore highlights the distributed organization of emerging cognitive systems. This in turn means that impairments in a given domain, such as language, can be explained as either a result of damage to one or several regions in a distributed system or an abnormality in the way multiple regions cooperate. In other words, issues of brain connectivity and the integrity of white matter come to the forefront.

One promising bottom-up approach relates to the role of the dorsal visual stream and the mirror neuron system—a system first described in monkeys that includes neurons with increased firing during action planning *and* action observation (Fadiga et al., 2000; Rizzolatti et al., 2002). It has been argued that this system plays a pivotal role in the phylogenetic emergence of language and in child language acquisition (Rizzolatti & Arbib, 1998), and that defects in the mirror neuron system may explain joint attention deficits and language delays in autism (Williams et al., 2001). fMRI studies of visuomotor functions (Müller et al., 2001, 2003, 2004) have documented atypical patterns of parietal and frontal activity, which suggest that the dorsal stream in autism is atypically organized. This view of the dorsal stream follows recent evidence of this pathway's being a system of "vision for action" (rather than solely a system supporting visuospatial functions), which incorporates portions of the prefrontal cortex (Goodale & Westwood, 2004).

The study of functional networks and pathways, such as the mirror neuron system, requires imaging techniques that go beyond the detection of local activation and toward the measurement of interregional cooperation. Recent structural MRI studies have documented abnormal growth patterns of white matter in autistic children, with atypical overgrowth in the first years of life followed by lack of normal growth (Carper & Courchesne, 2005; Carper et al., 2002; Courchesne et al., 2001). Herbert and colleagues (2004) showed that white matter increases in autism are region specific, with prominent involvement of the frontal lobes, and strongly affect late-myelinating radiate components of white matter. A technique that directly assesses white matter integrity is diffusion-tensor MRI (DTI). Very little DTI evidence is currently available for autism. One study (Barnea-Goraly et al., 2004) found reduced diffusion anisotropy, which is considered a measure of white matter integrity, in a large number of regions across all four forebrain lobes in boys with autism.

An alternative approach to the study of neural network organization is functional connectivity MRI (fcMRI), which is based on interregional low-frequency correlations of the BOLD signal in fMRI. Although their precise underlying physiology remains to be fully elucidated (cf Obrig et al., 2000), such BOLD cross-correlations have been shown to reflect functional connectivity in numerous previous studies (Allen et al., 2005; Biswal et al., 1995; Cordes et al., 2000; Greicius et al., 2003; Hampson et al., 2004; Jiang et al., 2004; Koch et al., 2002; Koechlin et al., 2003; Lowe et al., 2000; Stamatakis et al., 2005; Stein et al., 2000; Xiong et al., 1999). In a clinical study, Quigley and colleagues (2003) found that the robust fcMRI effects between homotopic sensorimotor regions seen in healthy subjects were absent in patients with callosal agenesis. Although fcMRI approaches probably do not exclusively reflect monosynaptic axonal connections, they are likely to relate (at least indirectly) to anatomical connectivity and white matter integrity.

In one recent study (Villalobos et al., 2005), functional connectivity along the dorsal stream was examined in autistic individuals and matched control subjects during visuomotor coordination. The main result was that functional connectivity between primary visual cortex and bilateral inferior frontal area 44 was significantly reduced in autism (Plate 6.2)—a result that is consistent with the hypothesis of mirror neuron defects (see above). Just and colleagues (2004a), examining interregional BOLD covariance associated with language processing, reported across-the-board reductions of functional connectivity within cerebral cortex and hypothesized that the autistic brain is generally characterized by underconnectivity. Additional studies by the same group of researchers on sentence comprehension (Kana et al., 2006) and an executive (Tower of London) task (Just et al., 2007) largely support generalized underconnectivity. However, the findings by Villalobos and colleagues (2005)—showing partly intact occipitoparietal functional connectivity—as well as recent results suggesting partial *overconnectivity* between subcortex (thalamus, caudate nuclei) and some cerebral cortical regions (Mizuno et al., 2006; Turner et al., 2006) imply that regionally specific models of connectivity in autism may be more promising than one of overall underconnectivity (see also Koshino et al., 2005).

Conclusion

The wide availability of noninvasive functional neuroimaging techniques, in particular fMRI, has in the past few years greatly boosted the role of neuroimaging and activation mapping in the study of developmental disorders. Task-induced neuroimaging affords twofold specificity because it permits the investigator to examine specific *anatomical* loci under well-controlled *functional* conditions. When using fMRI in the study of developmental disorders, such as autism, it is tempting to focus on functional domains of impaired outcome. However, since functional neuroimaging techniques are today largely limited to application in older children and adults, it is hard to distinguish apparent abnormalities of activation patterns that are direct reflections of the disorder itself from effects of abnormal experience or compensatory plasticity. One must therefore be wary of interpreting atypical activation patterns (e.g., absence of activation in the fusiform face area) as *explanations* of functional deficits (e.g., impaired face perception). The need for developmental disorders to be studied from a developmental perspective—self-explanatory as it may sound—is not always evident in the neuroimaging literature. From a developmental perspective, it is highly unlikely that neurodevelopmental disorders can be accounted for in terms of modular and localized defects, with one functional system being impaired and the remaining functional systems unaffected. Instead, a developmental perspective requires an understanding of how elementary functional systems interact in the emergence of more complex functional systems. For neuroimaging, this implies that we have to go beyond simply mapping out differences and toward models of network cooperation. In this context, recent technical advances in diffusion-tensor imaging and functional connectivity MRI are promising.

ACKNOWLEDGMENTS

Preparation of this chapter was supported by the National Institutes of Health (Grant Nos. R01-DC006155, and R01-NS43999).

REFERENCES

Abell, F., Krams, M., Ashburner, J., et al. (1999). The neuroanatomy of autism: A voxel-based whole brain analysis of structural scans. *NeuroReport, 10*(8), 1647–1651.

Akshoomoff, N., Pierce, K., & Courchesne, E. (2002). The neurobiological basis of autism from a developmental perspective. *Development and Psychopathology, 14*(3), 613–634.

Akshoomoff, N. A., & Courchesne, E. (1992). A new role for the cerebellum in cognitive operations. *Behavioral Neuroscience, 106*(5), 731–738.

Allen, G., Buxton, R. B., Wong, E. C., et al. (1997). Attentional activation of the cerebellum independent of motor involvement. *Science, 275*, 1940–1943.

Allen, G., & Courchesne, E. (2003). Differential effects of developmental cerebellar abnormality on cognitive and motor functions in the cerebellum: An fMRI study of autism. *American Journal of Psychiatry, 160*(2), 262–273.

Allen, G., McColl, R., Barnard, H., et al. (2005). Magnetic resonance imaging of cerebellar–prefrontal and cerebellar–parietal functional connectivity. *NeuroImage, 28*(1), 39–48.

Allen, G., Müller, R.-A., & Courchesne, E. (2004). Cerebellar function in autism: fMRI activation during a simple motor task. *Biological Psychiatry, 56*, 269–278.

American Psychiatric Association. (2000). *Diagnostic and statistical manual of mental disorders* (4th ed., text rev.). Washington, DC: Author.

Anderson, A. W., Marois, R., Colson, E. R., et al. (2001). Neonatal auditory activation detected by functional magnetic resonance imaging. *Magnetic Resonance Imaging, 19*(1), 1–5.

Anderson, G. M., & Lombroso, P. J. (2002). Genetics of childhood disorders: XLV. Autism, Part 4: Serotonin in autism. *Journal of the American Academy of Child and Adolescent, 41*(12), 1513–1516.

Archibald, S. L., Fennema-Notestine, C., Gamst, A., et al. (2001). Brain dysmorphology in individuals with severe prenatal alcohol exposure. *Developmental Medicine and Child Neurology, 43*(3), 148–154.

Bailey, A., Le Couteur, A., Gottesman, I., et al. (1995). Autism as a strongly genetic disorder: Evidence from a British twin study. *Psychological Medicine, 25*(1), 63–77.

Bailey, A., Luthert, P., Dean, A., et al. (1998). A clinicopathological study of autism. *Brain, 121*, 889–905.

Baird, G., Charman, T., Baron-Cohen, S., et al. (2000). A screening instrument for autism at 18 months of age: A 6-year follow-up study. *Journal of the American Academy of Child and Adolescent Psychiatry, 39*(6), 694–702.

Baird, G., Simonoff, E., Pickles, A., et al. (2006). Prevalence of disorders of the autism spectrum in a population cohort of children in South Thames: The Special Needs and Autism Project (SNAP). *Lancet, 368*(9531), 210–215.

Baltaxe, C. A., & Simmons, J. Q. D. (1975). Language in childhood psychosis: A review. *Journal of Speech and Hearing Disorders, 40*(4), 439–458.

Barnea-Goraly, N., Kwon, H., Menon, V., et al. (2004). White matter structure in autism: Preliminary evidence from diffusion tensor imaging. *Biological Psychiatry, 55*(3), 323–326.

Baron-Cohen, S. (1992). Debate and argument: On modularity and development in autism: A reply to Burack. *Journal of Child Psychology and Psychiatry and Allied Disciplines, 33*(3), 623–629.

Baron-Cohen, S., Baldwin, D. A., & Crowson, M. (1997). Do children with autism use the speaker's direction of gaze strategy to crack the code of language? *Child Development, 68*(1), 48–57.

Baron-Cohen, S., Leslie, A. M., & Frith, U. (1985). Does the autistic child have a "theory of mind"? *Cognition, 21*, 37–46.

Baron-Cohen, S., Ring, H., Moriarty, J., et al. (1994). Recognition of mental state terms: Clinical findings in children with autism and a functional neuroimaging study of normal adults. *British Journal of Psychiatry, 165*(5), 640–649.

Baron-Cohen, S., Ring, H. A., Bullmore, E. T., et al. (2000). The amygdala theory of autism. *Neuroscience and Biobehavioral Reviews, 24*(3), 355–364.

Baron-Cohen, S., Ring, H. A., Wheelwright, S., et al. (1999). Social intelligence in the normal and autistic brain: An fMRI study. *European Journal of Neuroscience, 11*(6), 1891–1898.

Barton, M., & Volkmar, F. (1998). How commonly are known medical conditions associated with autism? *Journal of Autism and Developmental Disorders, 28*(4), 273–278.

Bates, E., Thal, D., Finlay, B., et al. (2003). Early language development and its neural correlates. In I. Rapin & S. Segalowitz (Eds.), *Handbook of neuropsychology: Vol. 8. Child neurology* (2nd ed., pp. 525–592). Amsterdam: Elsevier.

Bauman, M. L., & Kemper, T. L. (1994). Neuroanatomic observations of the brain in autism. In M. L. Bauman & T. L. Kemper (Eds.), *The neurobiology of autism* (pp. 119–145). Baltimore: Johns Hopkins University Press.

Belliveau, J. W., Kennedy, D. N., Jr., McKinstry, R. C., et al. (1991). Functional mapping of the human visual cortex by magnetic resonance imaging. *Science, 254*(5032), 716–719.

Belmonte, M. K., & Yurgelun-Todd, D. A. (2003). Functional anatomy of impaired selective attention and compensatory processing in autism. *Cognitive Brain Research, 17*(3), 651–664.

Binder, J. R., Frost, J. A., Hammeke, T. A., et al. (1999). Conceptual processing during the conscious resting state. A functional MRI study. *Journal of Cognitive Neuroscience, 11*(1), 80–95.

Binkofski, F., Amunts, K., Stephan, K. M., et al. (2000). Broca's region subserves imagery of motion: A combined cytoarchitectonic and fMRI study. *Human Brain Mapping, 11*(4), 273–285.

Biswal, B., Yetkin, F. Z., Haughton, V. M., et al. (1995). Functional connectivity in the motor cortex of resting human brain using echo-planar MRI. *Magnetic Resonance in Medicine, 34*(4), 537–541.

Boddaert, N., Belin, P., Chabane, N., et al. (2003). Perception of complex sounds: Abnormal pattern of cortical activation in autism. *American Journal of Psychiatry, 160*(11), 2057–2060.

Bono, M. A., Daley, T., & Sigman, M. (2004). Relations among joint attention, amount of intervention and language gain in autism. *Journal of Autism and Developmental Disorders, 34*(5), 495–505.

Born, A. P., Law, I., Lund, T. E., et al. (2002a). Cortical deactivation induced by visual stimulation in human slow-wave sleep. *NeuroImage, 17*(3), 1325–1335.

Born, A. P., Rostrup, E., Miranda, M. J., et al. (2002b). Visual cortex reactivity in sedated children examined with perfusion MRI (FAIR). *Magnetic Resonance Imaging, 20*(2), 199–205.

Born, P., Leth, H., Miranda, M. J., et al. (1998). Visual activation in infants and young children studied by functional magnetic resonance imaging. *Pediatric Research, 44*(4), 578–583.

Brambilla, P., Hardan, A., di Nemi, S. U., et al. (2003). Brain anatomy and development in autism: Review of structural MRI studies. *Brain Research Bulletin, 61*(6), 557–569.

Bruinsma, Y., Koegel, R. L., & Koegel, L. K. (2004). Joint attention and children with autism: A review of the literature. *Mental Retardation and Developmental Disabilities Research Reviews, 10*(3), 169–175.

Bruneau, N., Roux, S., Adrien, J. L., et al. (1999). Auditory associative cortex dysfunction in children with autism: Evidence from late auditory evoked potentials (N1 wave-T complex). *Clinical Neurophysiology, 110*(11), 1927–1934.

Buccino, G., Binkofski, F., Fink, G. R., et al. (2001). Action observation activates premotor and parietal areas in a somatotopic manner: An fMRI study. *European Journal of Neuroscience, 13*(2), 400–404.

Buccino, G., Binkofski, F., & Riggio, L. (2004). The mirror neuron system and action recognition. *Brain and Language, 89*(2), 370–376.

Buchsbaum, M. S., Siegel, B. V., Wu, J. C., et al. (1992). Brief report: Attention performance in autism and regional brain metabolic rate assessed by positron emission tomography. *Journal of Autism and Developmental Disorders, 22*, 115–125.

Buitelaar, J. K., & Willemsen-Swinkels, S. H. (2000). Medication treatment in subjects with autistic spectrum disorders. *European Child and Adolescent Psychiatry, 9*(Suppl. 1), I85–I97.

Carpenter, M., Nagell, K., & Tomasello, M. (1998). Social cognition, joint attention, and communicative competence from 9 to 15 months of age. *Monographs of the Society for Research in Child Development, 63*(4), i–vi, 1–143.

Carper, R. A., & Courchesne, E. (2005). Localized enlargement of the frontal cortex in early autism. *Biological Psychiatry, 57*(2), 126–133.

Carper, R. A., Moses, P., Tigue, Z. D., et al. (2002). Cerebral lobes in autism: Early hyperplasia and abnormal age effects. *NeuroImage, 16*(4), 1038–1051.

Casanova, M. F., Buxhoeveden, D. P., Switala, A. E., et al. (2002). Minicolumnar pathology in autism. *Neurology, 58*(3), 428–432.

Castelli, F., Frith, C., Happe, F., et al. (2002). Autism, Asperger syndrome and brain mechanisms for the attribution of mental states to animated shapes. *Brain, 125*(Pt. 8), 1839–1849.

Charman, T. (2003). Why is joint attention a pivotal skill in autism? *Philosophical Transactions of the Royal Society of London. Series B: Biological Sciences, 358*(1430), 315–324.

Chen, S. H., & Desmond, J. E. (2005). Cerebrocerebellar networks during articulatory rehearsal and verbal working memory tasks. *NeuroImage, 24*(2), 332–338.

Chen, W. J., Maier, S. E., Parnell, S. E., et al. (2003). Alcohol and the developing brain: Neuroanatomical studies. *Alcohol Research and Health, 27*(2), 174–180.

Chiron, C., Leboyer, M., Leon, F., et al. (1995). SPECT of the brain in childhood autism: Evidence for a lack of normal hemispheric asymmetry. *Developmental Medicine and Child Neurology, 37*, 849–860.

Chomsky, N. (1965). *Aspects of the theory of syntax.* Cambridge, MA: MIT Press.

Chugani, D. (2000). Autism. In M. Ernst & J. Rumsey (Eds.), *The foundation and future of functional neuroimaging in child psychiatry* (pp. 171–188). New York: Cambridge University Press.

Chugani, D. C. (2004). Serotonin in autism and pediatric epilepsies. *Mental Retardation and Developmental Disabilities Research Reviews, 10*(2), 112–116.

Chugani, D. C. (2002). Role of altered brain serotonin mechanisms in autism. *Molecular Psychiatry, 7*(Suppl. 2), S16–S17.

Chugani, D. C., Muzik, O., Behen, M., et al. (1999). Developmental changes in brain serotonin synthesis capacity in autistic and nonautistic children. *Annals of Neurology, 45*(3), 287–295.

Clarke, E., & Dewhurst, K. (1972). *An illustrated history of brain function.* Oxford, UK: Sanford.

Cordes, D., Haughton, V. M., Arfanakis, K., et al. (2000). Mapping functionally related regions of brain with functional connectivity MR imaging. *American Journal of Neuroradiology, 21*(9), 1636–1644.

Coulter, C. L., Leech, R. W., Schaefer, G. B., et al. (1993). Midline cerebral dysgenesis, dysfunction of the hypothalamic-pituitary axis, and fetal alcohol effects. *Archives of Neurology, 50*(7), 771–775.

Courchesne, E. (1987). A neurophysiological view of autism. In E. Schopler & G. B. Mesibov (Eds.), *Neurobiological issues in autism* (pp. 285–324). New York: Plenum Press.

Courchesne, E. (1997). Brainstem, cerebellar and limbic neuroanatomical abnormalities in autism. *Current Opinion in Neurobiology, 7*, 269–278.

Courchesne, E., Karns, C. M., Davis, H. R., et al. (2001). Unusual brain growth patterns in early life in patients with autistic disorder: An MRI study. *Neurology, 57*(2), 245–254.

Courchesne, E., Lincoln, A. J., Yeung-Courchesne, R., et al. (1989). Pathophysiologic findings in nonretarded autism and receptive developmental language disorder. *Journal of Autism and Developmental Disorders, 19*(1), 1–7.

Courchesne, E., Press, G. A., & Yeung-Courchesne, R. (1993). Parietal lobe abnormalities detected with MR in patients with infantile autism. *American Journal of Roentgenology, 160*(2), 387–393.

Courchesne, E., Saitoh, O., Yeung-Courchesne, R., et al. (1994a). Abnormality of cerebellar vermian lobules VI and VII in patients with infantile autism: Identification of hypoplastic and hyperplastic subgroups by MR imaging. *American Journal of Roentgenology, 162*, 123–130.

Courchesne, E., Townsend, J., Akshoomoff, N. A., et al. (1994b). Impairment in shifting attention in autistic and cerebellar patients. *Behavioral Neuroscience, 108*(5), 848–865.

Courchesne, E., Yeung-Courchesne, R., Press, G. A., et al. (1988). Hypoplasia of cerebellar vermal lobules VI and VII in autism. *New England Journal of Medicine, 318*(21), 1349–1354.

Critchley, H. D., Daly, E. M., Bullmore, E. T., et al. (2000). The functional neuroanatomy of social behavior: Changes in cerebral blood flow when people with autistic disorder process facial expressions. *Brain, 123*, 2203–2212.

Curtiss, S., & de Bode, S. (1999). Age and etiology as predictors of language outcome following hemispherectomy. *Developmental Neuroscience, 21*(3–5), 174–181.

Curtiss, S., de Bode, S., & Mathern, G. W. (2001). Spoken language outcomes after hemispherectomy: Factoring in etiology. *Brain and Language, 79*(3), 379–396.

Dawson, G., Finley, C., Phillips, S., et al. (1986). Hemispheric specialization and the language abilities of autistic children. *Child Development, 57*, 1440–1453.

Dawson, G., Klinger, L., Panagiotides, H., et al. (1995). Subgroups of autistic children based on social behavior display distinct patterns of brain activity. *Journal of Abnormal Child Psychology, 23*, 569–583.

Dehaene-Lambertz, G., Dehaene, S., & Hertz-Pannier, L. (2002). Functional neuroimaging of speech perception in infants. *Science, 298*(5600), 2013–2015.

De Volder, A. G., Bol, A., Michel, C., et al. (1987). Brain glucose metabolism in children with the autistic syndrome: Positron emission analysis. *Brain and Development, 9*, 581–587.

Di Virgilio, G., & Clarke, S. (1997). Direct interhemispheric visual input to human speech areas. *Human Brain Mapping, 5*, 347–354.

Donnai, D., & Karmiloff-Smith, A. (2000). Williams syndrome: From genotype through to the cognitive phenotype. *American Journal of Medical Genetics, 97*(2), 164–171.

Edelson, S. B., & Cantor, D. S. (1998). Autism: Xenobiotic influences. *Toxicology and Industrial Health, 14*(4), 553–563.

Egaas, B., Courchesne, E., & Saitoh, O. (1995). Reduced size of corpus callosum in autism. *Archives of Neurology, 52*(8), 794–801.

Elbert, T., Pantev, C., Wienbruch, C., et al. (1995). Increased cortical representation of the fingers of the left hand in string players. *Science, 270*, 305–307.

Escalante-Mead, P. R., Minshew, N. J., & Sweeney, J. A. (2003). Abnormal brain lateralization in high-functioning autism. *Journal of Autism and Developmental Disorders, 33*(5), 539–543.

Ewart, A. K., Morris, C. A., Ensing, G. J., et al. (1993). A human vascular disorder, supravalvular aortic stenosis, maps to chromosome 7. *Proceedings of the*

National Academy of Sciences of the United States of America, 90(8), 3226–3230.

Fadiga, L., Fogassi, L., Gallese, V., et al. (2000). Visuomotor neurons: Ambiguity of the discharge or "motor" perception? *International Journal of Psychophysiology, 35*(2–3), 165–177.

Farber, N. B., & Olney, J. W. (2003). Drugs of abuse that cause developing neurons to commit suicide. *Brain Research: Developmental Brain Research, 147*(1–2), 37–45.

Fincham, J. M., Carter, C. S., van Veen, V., et al. (2002). Neural mechanisms of planning: A computational analysis using event-related fMRI. *Proceedings of the National Academy of Sciences of the United States of America, 99*(5), 3346–3351.

Fisher, S. E. (2005). Dissection of molecular mechanisms underlying speech and language disorders. *Applied Psycholinguistics, 26*, 111–128.

Fisher, S. E., Vargha-Khadem, F., Watkins, K. E., et al. (1998). Localisation of a gene implicated in a severe speech and language disorder. *Nature Genetics, 18*(2), 168–170.

Fodor, J. A. (1985). Précis of "The Modularity of Mind." *Behavioral and Brain Sciences, 8*, 1–42.

Fodor, J. A. (1983). *The modularity of mind*. Cambridge, MA: MIT Press.

Folstein, S. E., & Mankoski, R. E. (2000). Chromosome 7q: Where autism meets language disorder? *American Journal of Human Genetics, 67*(2), 278–281.

Fombonne, E., Zakarian, R., Bennett, A., et al. (2006). Pervasive developmental disorders in Montreal, Quebec, Canada: Prevalence and links with immunizations. *Pediatrics, 118*(1), e139–e150.

Gaffney, G. R., Tsai, L. Y., Kuperman, S., et al. (1987). Cerebellar structure in autism. *American Journal of Diseases of Children, 141*, 1330–1332.

Gaffrey, M. S., Kleinhans, N. M., Haist, F., et al. (2007). Atypical brain organization for lexical semantic decision in autism spectrum disorders: fMRI evidence of increased visual imagery. *Neuropsychologia, 45*, 1672–1684.

Gage, N. M., Siegel, B., Callen, M., et al. (2003a). Cortical sound processing in children with autism disorder: An MEG investigation. *NeuroReport, 14*(16), 2047–2051.

Gage, N. M., Siegel, B., & Roberts, T. P. (2003b). Cortical auditory system maturational abnormalities in children with autism disorder: An MEG investigation. *Brain Research: Developmental Brain Research, 144*(2), 201–209.

Gardner, H. (1987). *The mind's new science* (2nd ed.). New York: Basic Books.

Gendry Meresse, I., Zilbovicius, M., Boddaert, N., et al. (2005). Autism severity and temporal lobe functional abnormalities. *Annals of Neurology, 58*(3), 466–469.

George, M. S., Costa, D. C., Kouris, K., et al. (1992). Cerebral blood flow abnormalities in adults with infantile autism. *Journal of Nervous and Mental Disease, 180*, 413–417.

Gervais, H., Belin, P., Boddaert, N., et al. (2004). Abnormal cortical voice processing in autism. *Nature Neuroscience, 7*(8), 801–802.

Gillberg, C., & Coleman, M. (1996). Autism and medical disorders: A review of the literature. *Developmental Medicine and Child Neurology, 38*(3), 191–202.

Gillberg, I. C., Gillberg, C., & Ahlsen, G. (1994). Autistic behaviour and attention deficits in tuberous sclerosis: A population-based study. *Developmental Medicine and Child Neurology, 36*(1), 50–56.

Gold, L., & Lauritzen, M. (2002). Neuronal deactivation explains decreased cerebellar blood flow in response to focal cerebral ischemia or suppressed neocortical function. *Proceedings of the National Academy of Sciences of the United States of America, 99*(11), 7699–7704.

Gomot, M., Bernard, F. A., Davis, M. H., et al. (2006). Change detection in children with autism: An auditory event-related fMRI study. *NeuroImage, 29*(2), 475–484.

Goodale, M. A., & Westwood, D. A. (2004). An evolving view of duplex vision: Separate but interacting cortical pathways for perception and action. *Current Opinion in Neurobiology, 14*(2), 203–211.

Gopnik, M., & Crago, M. B. (1991). Familial aggregation of a developmental language disorder. *Cognition, 39*(1), 1–50.

Greicius, M. D., Krasnow, B., Reiss, A. L., et al. (2003). Functional connectivity in the resting brain: A network analysis of the default mode hypothesis. *Proceedings of the National Academy of Sciences of the United States of America, 100*(1), 253–258.

Hadjikhani, N., Joseph, R. M., Snyder, J., et al. (2004). Activation of the fusiform gyrus when individuals with autism spectrum disorder view faces. *NeuroImage, 22*(3), 1141–1150.

Haist, F., Adamo, M., Westerfield, M., et al. (2005). The functional neuroanatomy of spatial attention in autism spectrum disorder. *Developmental Neuropsychology, 27*(3), 425–458.

Hall, G. B., Szechtman, H., & Nahmias, C. (2003). Enhanced salience and emotion recognition in autism: A PET study. *American Journal of Psychiatry, 160*(8), 1439–1441.

Hampson, M., Olson, I. R., Leung, H. C., et al. (2004). Changes in functional connectivity of human MT/V5 with visual motion input. *NeuroReport, 15*(8), 1315–1319.

Happé, F., Ehlers, S., Fletcher, P. C., et al. (1996). "Theory of mind" in the brain: Evidence from a PET scan study of Asperger syndrome. *NeuroReport, 8,* 197–201.

Happé, F., & Frith, U. (1996). The neuropsychology of autism. *Brain, 119*(4), 1377–1400.

Hashimoto, T., Tayama, M., Miyazaki, M., et al. (1995a). Developmental brain changes investigated with proton magnetic resonance spectroscopy. *Developmental Medicine and Child Neurology, 37*(5), 398–405.

Hashimoto, T., Tayama, M., Murakawa, K., et al. (1995b). Development of the brainstem and cerebellum in autistic patients. *Journal of Autism and Developmental Disorders, 25*(1), 1–18.

Haslinger, B., Erhard, P., Weilke, F., et al. (2002). The role of lateral premotor–cerebellar–parietal circuits in motor sequence control: A parametric fMRI study. *Cognitive Brain Research, 13*(2), 159–168.

Haznedar, M. M., Buchsbaum, M. S., Metzger, M., et al. (1997). Anterior cingulate gyrus volume and glucose metabolism in autistic disorder. *American Journal of Psychiatry, 154,* 1047–1050.

Head, H. (1926). *Aphasia and kindred disorders of speech.* Cambridge, UK: Cambridge University Press.

Heh, C. W. C., Smith, R., Wu, J., et al. (1989). Positron emission tomography of the cerebellum in autism. *American Journal of Psychiatry, 146,* 242–245.

Herbert, M. R., Harris, G. J., Adrien, K. T., et al. (2002). Abnormal asymmetry in language association cortex in autism. *Annals of Neurology*, *52*(5), 588–596.

Herbert, M. R., Ziegler, D. A., Deutsch, C. K., et al. (2005). Brain asymmetries in autism and developmental language disorder: A nested whole-brain analysis. *Brain*, *128*(Pt. 1), 213–226.

Herbert, M. R., Ziegler, D. A., Makris, N., et al. (2004). Localization of white matter volume increase in autism and developmental language disorder. *Annals of Neurology*, *55*(4), 530–540.

Herold, S., Frackowiak, R. S. J., Le Couteur, A., et al. (1988). Cerebral blood flow and metabolism of oxygen and glucose in young autistic adults. *Psychological Medecine*, *18*, 823–831.

Hertz-Pannier, L., Chiron, C., Jambaque, I., et al. (2002). Late plasticity for language in a child's non-dominant hemisphere: A pre- and post-surgery fMRI study. *Brain*, *125*(Pt. 2), 361–372.

Hollander, E., Anagnostou, E., Chaplin, W., et al. (2005). Striatal volume on magnetic resonance imaging and repetitive behaviors in autism. *Biological Psychiatry*, *58*(3), 226–232.

Horwitz, B., Rumsey, J. M., Grady, C. L., et al. (1988). The cerebral metabolic landscape in autism: Intercorrelations of regional glucose utilization. *Archives of Neurology*, *45*, 749–755.

Hoshi, Y. (2003). Functional near-infrared optical imaging: Utility and limitations in human brain mapping. *Psychophysiology*, *40*(4), 511–520.

Hoshi, Y., & Chen, S.-J. (2002). Regional cerebral blood flow changes associated with emotions in children. *Pediatric Neurology*, *27*, 275–281.

Hubl, D., Bolte, S., Feineis-Matthews, S., et al. (2003). Functional imbalance of visual pathways indicates alternative face processing strategies in autism. *Neurology*, *61*(9), 1232–1237.

Hughlings-Jackson, J. (1878). On affections of speech from disease of the brain. *Brain*, *1*, 304–330.

Iacoboni, M., Woods, R. P., Brass, M., et al. (1999). Cortical mechanisms of human imitation. *Science*, *286*(5449), 2526–2528.

Isaacs, E., Christie, D., Vargha-Khadem, F., et al. (1996). Effects of hemispheric side of injury, age at injury, and presence of seizure disorder on functional ear and hand asymmetries in hemiplegic children. *Neuropsychologia*, *34*, 127–137.

Janusonis, S., Gluncic, V., & Rakic, P. (2004). Early serotonergic projections to Cajal-Retzius cells: Relevance for cortical development. *Journal of Neuroscience*, *24*(7), 1652–1659.

Jiang, T., He, Y., Zang, Y., et al. (2004). Modulation of functional connectivity during the resting state and the motor task. *Human Brain Mapping*, *22*(1), 63–71.

Jonas, R., Nguyen, S., Hu, B., et al. (2004). Cerebral hemispherectomy: Hospital course, seizure, developmental, language, and motor outcomes. *Neurology*, *62*(10), 1712–1721.

Just, M. A., Cherkassky, V. L., Keller, T. A., et al. (2007). Functional and anatomical cortical underconnectivity in autism: Evidence from an fMRI study of an executive function task and corpus callosum morphometry. *Cerebral Cortex*, *17*, 951–961.

Just, M. A., Cherkassky, V. L., Keller, T. A., et al. (2004a). Cortical activation and synchronization during sentence comprehension in high-functioning autism: Evidence of underconnectivity. *Brain*, *127*(Pt. 8), 1811–1821.

Just, M. A., Newman, S. D., Keller, T. A., et al. (2004b). Imagery in sentence comprehension: An fMRI study. *NeuroImage, 21*(1), 112–124.

Kana, R. K., Keller, T. A., Cherkassky, V. L., et al. (2006). Sentence comprehension in autism: Thinking in pictures with decreased functional connectivity. *Brain, 129,* 2484–2493.

Kemmotsu, N., Villalobos, M. E., Gaffrey, M. S., et al. (2005). Activity and functional connectivity of inferior frontal cortex associated with response conflict. *Cognitive Brain Research, 24,* 335–342.

Klin, A., Jones, W., Schultz, R., et al. (2002). Visual fixation patterns during viewing of naturalistic social situations as predictors of social competence in individuals with autism. *Archives of General Psychiatry, 59*(9), 809–816.

Koch, M. A., Norris, D. G., & Hund-Georgiadis, M. (2002). An investigation of functional and anatomical connectivity using magnetic resonance imaging. *NeuroImage, 16*(1), 241–250.

Koechlin, E., Ody, C., & Kouneiher, F. (2003). The architecture of cognitive control in the human prefrontal cortex. *Science, 302*(5648), 1181–1185.

Kolb, B., & Gibb, R. (2001). Early brain injury, plasticity, and behavior. In C. A. Nelson & M. Luciana (Eds.), *Handbook of developmental cognitive neuroscience* (pp. 175–190). Cambridge, MA: MIT Press.

Kolb, B., Petrie, B., & Cioe, J. (1996). Recovery from early cortical damage in rats: VII. Comparison of the behavioural and anatomical effects of medial prefrontal lesions at different ages of neural maturation. *Behavioural Brain Research, 79*(1–2), 1–13.

Konishi, S., Nakajima, K., Uchida, I., et al. (1998). Transient activation of inferior prefrontal cortex during cognitive set shifting. *Nature Neuroscience, 1*(1), 80–84.

Korvatska, E., Van de Water, J., Anders, T. F., et al. (2002). Genetic and immunologic considerations in autism. *Neurobiology of Disease, 9*(2), 107–125.

Koshino, H., Carpenter, P. A., Minshew, N. J., et al. (2005). Functional connectivity in an fMRI working memory task in high-functioning autism. *NeuroImage, 24*(3), 810–821.

Krams, M., Rushworth, M. F., Deiber, M. P., et al. (1998). The preparation, execution and suppression of copied movements in the human brain. *Experimental Brain Research, 120*(3), 386–398.

Kuhn, T. (1962). *The structure of scientific revolutions.* Chicago: University of Chicago Press.

Lai, C. S., Fisher, S. E., Hurst, J. A., et al. (2001). A forkhead-domain gene is mutated in a severe speech and language disorder. *Nature, 413*(6855), 519–523.

Lashley, K. S. (1950). In search of the engram. In Symposia of the Society for Experimental Biology, *Physiological mechanisms in animal behavior* (Vol. IV, pp. 454–482). Cambridge, UK: Cambridge University Press.

Le, H. T., Pardo, J. V., & Hu, X. (1998). 4T-fMRI study of nonspatial shifting of selective attention: Cerebellar and parietal contributions. *Journal of Neurophysiology, 79,* 1535–1548.

Leff, A., Crinion, J., Scott, S., et al. (2002). A physiological change in the homotopic cortex following left posterior temporal lobe infarction. *Annals of Neurology, 51*(5), 553–558.

Lichtheim, L. (1885). On aphasia. *Brain, 7,* 433–484.

Liegeois, F., Connelly, A., Cross, J. H., et al. (2004). Language reorganization in children with early-onset lesions of the left hemisphere: An fMRI study. *Brain, 127*(Pt. 6), 1229–1236.

Lord, C., Risi, S., & Pickels, A. (2004). Trajectory of language development in autistic spectrum disorders. In M. Rice & S. Warren (Eds.), *Developmental language disorders: From phenotypes to etiologies* (pp. 7–29). Mahwah, NJ: Erlbaum.

Lord, C., Rutter, M., DiLavore, P., et al. (2001). *Autism Diagnostic Observation Schedule*. Los Angeles: Western Psychological Services.

Lotspeich, L. J., & Ciaranello, R. D. (1993). The neurobiology and genetics of infantile autism. *International Review of Neurobiology, 35*, 87–129.

Lowe, M. J., Dzemidzic, M., Lurito, J. T., et al. (2000). Correlations in low-frequency BOLD fluctuations reflect corticocortical connections. *NeuroImage, 12*(5), 582–587.

MacDermot, K. D., Bonora, E., Sykes, N., et al. (2005). Identification of *FOXP2* truncation as a novel cause of developmental speech and language deficits. *American Journal of Human Genetics, 76*(6), 1074–1080.

Marcus, G. F., & Fisher, S. E. (2003). *FOXP2* in focus: What can genes tell us about speech and language? *Trends in Cognitive Science, 7*(6), 257–262.

Markus, J., Mundy, P., Morales, M., et al. (2000). Individual differences in infant skills as predictors of child–caregiver joint attention and language. *Social Development, 9*(3), 302–315.

Martineau, J., Roux, S., Adrien, J. L., et al. (1992). Electrophysiological evidence of different abilities to form cross-modal associations in children with autistic behavior. *Electroencephalography and Clinical Neurophysiology, 82*, 60–66.

Mattson, S. N. (2000). *Prenatal alcohol exposure: Effects on brain structure and function* (10th Special Report to the U.S. Congress, pp. 285–299). Bethesda, MD: National Institute on Alcohol Abuse and Alcoholism.

McKelvey, J. R., Lambert, R., Mottron, L., et al. (1995). Right-hemisphere dysfunction in Asperger's syndrome. *Journal of Child Neurology, 10*, 310–314.

Meek, J. H., Firbank, M., Elwell, C. E., et al. (1998). Regional hemodynamic responses to visual stimulation in awake infants. *Pediatric Research, 43*(6), 840–843.

Mesulam, M.-M. (1998). From sensation to cognition. *Brain, 121*, 1013–1052.

Miller, M. T., Stromland, K., Ventura, L., et al. (2005). Autism associated with conditions characterized by developmental errors in early embryogenesis: A mini review. *International Journal of Developmental Neuroscience, 23*(2–3), 201–219.

Mizuno, A., Villalobos, M. E., Davies, M. M., et al. (2006). Partially enhanced thalamo-cortical functional connectivity in autism. *Brain Research, 1104*(1), 160–174.

Moore, R. J., Vadeyar, S., Fulford, J., et al. (2001). Antenatal determination of fetal brain activity in response to an acoustic stimulus using functional magnetic resonance imaging. *Human Brain Mapping, 12*(2), 94–99.

Morris, C. A. (2004). Genotype–phenotype correlations: Lessons from Williams syndrome research. In M. Rice & S. Warren (Eds.), *Developmental language disorders: From phenotypes to etiologies* (pp. 355–369). Mahwah, NJ: Erlbaum.

Morton, C. T., Casey, B., Cohen, J., et al. (1996). Is research in normal and ill children involving radiation exposure ethical? [letter and replies]. *Archives of General Psychiatry, 53*(11), 1059–1061.

Mountz, J. M., Tolbert, L. C., Lill, D. W., et al. (1995). Functional deficits in autistic disorder: Characterization by technetium-99m-HMPAO and SPECT. *Journal of Nuclear Medicine, 36*(7), 1156–1162.

Muhle, R., Trentacoste, S. V., & Rapin, I. (2004). The genetics of autism. *Pediatrics, 113*(5), e472–e486.

Müller, R.-A. (2005). Neurocognitive studies of language impairment: The "bottom-up" approach. *Applied Psycholinguistics*, 26, 65–78.

Müller, R.-A. (2004). Genes, language disorders, and developmental archaeology: What role can neuroimaging play? In M. Rice & S. Warren (Eds.), *Developmental language disorders: From phenotypes to etiologies* (pp. 291–328). Mahwah, NJ: Erlbaum.

Müller, R.-A. (1996). Innateness, autonomy, universality? Neurobiological approaches to language. *Behavioral and Brain Sciences*, 19(4), 611–631.

Müller, R.-A. (1992). Modularity, holism, connectionism: Old conflicts and new perspectives in aphasiology and neuropsychology. *Aphasiology*, 6, 443–475.

Müller, R.-A., & Basho, S. (2004). Are nonlinguistic functions in "Broca's area" prerequisites for language acquisition? fMRI findings from an ontogenetic viewpoint. *Brain and Language*, 89, 329–336.

Müller, R.-A., Behen, M. E., Rothermel, R. D., et al. (1999a). Brain mapping of language and auditory perception in high-functioning autistic adults: A PET study. *Journal of Autism and Developmental Disorders*, 29, 19–31.

Müller, R.-A., Cauich, C., Rubio, M. A., et al. (2004). Abnormal patterns of frontal activity during digit sequence learning in high-functioning autistic patients. *Biological Psychiatry*, 56(5), 323–332.

Müller, R.-A., Chugani, D. C., Behen, M. E., et al. (1998). Impairment of dentato–thalamo–cortical pathway in autistic men: Language activation data from positron emission tomography. *Neuroscience Letters*, 245, 1–4.

Müller, R.-A., Kleinhans, N., Kemmotsu, N., et al. (2003). Abnormal variability and distribution of functional maps in autism: An fMRI study of visuomotor learning. *American Journal of Psychiatry*, 160, 1847–1862.

Müller, R.-A., Pierce, K., Ambrose, J. B., et al. (2001). Atypical patterns of cerebral motor activation in autism: A functional magnetic resonance study. *Biological Psychiatry*, 49, 665–676.

Müller, R.-A., Rothermel, R. D., Behen, M. E., et al. (1999b). Language organization in patients with early and late left hemisphere lesion: A PET study. *Neuropsychologia*, 37, 545–557.

Mundy, P., Sigman, M., & Kasari, C. (1990). A longitudinal study of joint attention and language development in autistic children. *Journal of Autism and Developmental Disorders*, 20(1), 115–128.

Murakami, J. W., Courchesne, E., Press, G. A., et al. (1989). Reduced cerebellar hemisphere size and its relationship to vermal hypoplasia in autism. *Archives of Neurology*, 46(6), 689–694.

Muramoto, S., Yamada, H., Sadato, N., et al. (2002). Age-dependent change in metabolic response to photic stimulation of the primary visual cortex in infants: Functional magnetic resonance imaging study. *Journal of Computer Assisted Tomography*, 26(6), 894–901.

Muter, V., Taylor, S., & Vargha-Khadem, F. (1997). A longitudinal study of early intellectual development in hemiplegic children. *Neuropsychologia*, 35, 289–298.

Nass, R., & Stiles, J. (1996). Neurobehavioral consequences of congenital focal lesions. In Y. Frank (Ed.), *Pediatric behavioral neurology* (pp. 149–178). Boca Raton, FL: CRC Press.

Nicklin, S. E., Hassan, I. A., Wickramasinghe, Y. A., et al. (2003). The light still shines, but not that brightly? The current status of perinatal near infrared spectroscopy. *Archives of Disease in Childhood: Fetal and Neonatal Edition*, 88(4), F263–F268.

Obrig, H., Neufang, M., Wenzel, R., et al. (2000). Spontaneous low frequency oscillations of cerebral hemodynamics and metabolism in human adults. *NeuroImage*, *12*(6), 623–639.

Ogawa, T., Sugiyama, A., Ishiwa, S., et al. (1982). Ontogenic development of EEG-asymmetry in early infantile autism. *Brain and Development*, *4*(6), 439–449.

Ohnishi, T., Matsuda, H., Hashimoto, T., et al. (2000). Abnormal regional cerebral blood flow in childhood autism. *Brain*, *123*(Pt. 9), 1838–1844.

Ohyama, M., Senda, M., Kitamura, S., et al. (1996). Role of the nondominant hemisphere and undamaged area during word repetition in poststroke aphasics: A PET activation study. *Stroke*, *27*(5), 897–903.

O'Leary, D. D., & Nakagawa, Y. (2002). Patterning centers, regulatory genes and extrinsic mechanisms controlling arealization of the neocortex. *Current Opinion in Neurobiology*, *12*(1), 14–25.

Otsuka, H., Harada, M., Mori, K., et al. (1999). Brain metabolites in the hippocampus–amygdala region and cerebellum in autism: An 1H-MR spectroscopy study. *Neuroradiology*, *41*(7), 517–519.

Palmen, S. J., Van Engeland, H., Hof, P. R., et al. (2004). Neuropathological findings in autism. *Brain*, *127*(12), 2572–2583.

Palmini, A., Gambardella, A., Andermann, F., et al. (1995). Intrinsic epileptogenicity of human dysplastic cortex as suggested by corticography and surgical results. *Annals of Neurology*, *37*(4), 476–487.

Pantano, P., Baron, J. C., Samson, Y., et al. (1986). Crossed cerebellar diaschisis. *Brain*, *109*, 677–694.

Petrides, M., & Pandya, D. N. (2002). Comparative cytoarchitectonic analysis of the human and the macaque ventrolateral prefrontal cortex and corticocortical connection patterns in the monkey. *European Journal of Neuroscience*, *16*(2), 291–310.

Piaget, J. (1979). *L'Épistémologie génétique* (3rd ed.). Paris: Presses Universitaires De France.

Piattelli-Palmarini, M. (Ed.). (1980). *Language and learning*. Cambridge, MA: Harvard University Press.

Pierce, K., Haist, F., Sedaghat, F., et al. (2004). The brain response to personally familiar faces in autism: Findings of fusiform activity and beyond. *Brain*, *127*(Pt. 12), 2703–2716.

Pierce, K., Müller, R.-A., Ambrose, J. B., et al. (2001). Face processing occurs outside the "fusiform face area" in autism: Evidence from functional MRI. *Brain*, *124*, 2059–2073.

Piggot, J., Kwon, H., Mobbs, D., et al. (2004). Emotional attribution in high-functioning individuals with autistic spectrum disorder: A functional imaging study. *Journal of the American Academy of Child and Adolescent Psychiatry*, *43*(4), 473–480.

Pinker, S. (2001). Talk of genetics and vice versa. *Nature*, *413*(6855), 465–466.

Piven, J., Bailey, J., Ranson, B. J., et al. (1997). An MRI study of the corpus callosum in autism. *American Journal of Psychiatry*, *154*(8), 1051–1055.

Posner, M. I., Walker, J. A., Friedrich, F. J., et al. (1984). Effects of parietal injury on covert orienting of attention. *Journal of Neuroscience*, *4*(7), 1863–1874.

Puce, A., & Perrett, D. (2003). Electrophysiology and brain imaging of biological motion. *Philosophical Transactions of the Royal Society of London. Series B: Biological Sciences*, *358*(1431), 435–445.

Pulsifer, M. B., Brandt, J., Salorio, C. F., et al. (2004). The cognitive outcome of hemispherectomy in 71 children. *Epilepsia*, *45*(3), 243–254.

Quigley, M., Cordes, D., Turski, P., et al. (2003). Role of the corpus callosum in functional connectivity. *American Journal of Neuroradiology*, *24*(2), 208–212.

Raichle, M. E., MacLeod, A. M., Snyder, A. Z., et al. (2001). A default mode of brain function. *Proceedings of the National Academy of Sciences of the United States of America*, *98*(2), 676–682.

Ramnani, N., & Miall, R. C. (2004). A system in the human brain for predicting the actions of others. *Nature Neuroscience*, *7*(1), 85–90.

Rapin, I. (1997). Autism. *New England Journal of Medicine*, *337*, 97–104.

Rapin, I., & Katzman, R. (1998). Neurobiology of autism. *Annals of Neurology*, *43*(1), 7–14.

Raymond, A. A., Fish, D. R., Sisodiya, S. M., et al. (1995). Abnormalities of gyration, heterotopias, tuberous sclerosis, focal cortical dysplasia, microdysgenesis, dysembryoplastic neuroepithelial tumour and dysgenesis of the archicortex in epilepsy: Clinical, EEG and neuroimaging features in 100 adult patients. *Brain*, *118*(Pt. 3), 629–660.

Raymond, G. V., Bauman, M. L., & Kemper, T. L. (1996). Hippocampus in autism: A Golgi analysis. *Acta Neuropathologica*, *91*(1), 117–119.

Rizzolatti, G., & Arbib, M. A. (1998). Language within our grasp [see comments]. *Trends in Neurosciences*, *21*(5), 188–194.

Rizzolatti, G., Fogassi, L., & Gallese, V. (2002). Motor and cognitive functions of the ventral premotor cortex. *Current Opinion in Neurobiology*, *12*(2), 149–154.

Rodier, P. M. (2002). Converging evidence for brain stem injury in autism. *Development and Psychopathology*, *14*(3), 537–557.

Rodier, P. M., Ingram, J. L., Tisdale, B., et al. (1997). Linking etiologies in humans and animal models: Studies of autism. *Reproductive Toxicology*, *11*(2–3), 417–422.

Rogers, S. J., Hepburn, S. L., Stackhouse, T., et al. (2003). Imitation performance in toddlers with autism and those with other developmental disorders. *Journal of Child Psychology and Psychiatry*, *44*(5), 763–781.

Rojas, D. C., Camou, S. L., Reite, M. L., et al. (2005). Planum temporale volume in children and adolescents with autism. *Journal of Autism and Developmental Disorders*, *35*(4), 479–486.

Roux, S., Bruneau, N., Garreau, B., et al. (1997). Bioclinical profiles of autism and other developmental disorders using a multivariate statistical approach. *Biological Psychiatry*, *42*(12), 1148–1156.

Rubia, K., Russell, T., Overmeyer, S., et al. (2001). Mapping motor inhibition: Conjunctive brain activations across different versions of go/no-go and stop tasks. *NeuroImage*, *13*(2), 250–261.

Rumsey, J. M., Duara, R., Grady, C., et al. (1985). Brain metabolism in autism: Resting cerebral glucose utilization rates as measured with positron emission tomography. *Archives of General Psychiatry*, *42*, 448–455.

Rutter, M., Lord, C., & LeCouteur, A. (1995). *Autism Diagnostic Interview—Revised* (3rd ed.). Chicago: University of Chicago Press.

Sadato, N., Okada, T., Honda, M., et al. (2002). Critical period for cross-modal plasticity in blind humans: A functional MRI study. *NeuroImage*, *16*(2), 389–400.

Saitoh, O., Karns, C. M., & Courchesne, E. (2001). Development of the hippocampal formation from 2 to 42 years: MRI evidence of smaller area dentata in autism. *Brain, 124*(Pt. 7), 1317–1324.

Schifter, T., Hoffman, J. M., Hatten, H. P., et al. (1994). Neuroimaging in infantile autism. *Journal of Child Neurology, 9*, 155–161.

Scholl, B. J., & Leslie, A. M. (2001). Minds, modules, and meta-analysis. *Child Development, 72*(3), 696–701.

Schroeter, M. L., Zysset, S., Wahl, M., et al. (2004). Prefrontal activation due to Stroop interference increases during development: An event-related fNIRS study. *NeuroImage, 23*(4), 1317–1325.

Schultz, R. T., Gauthier, I., Klin, A., et al. (2000). Abnormal ventral temporal cortical activity during face discrimination among individuals with autism and Asperger syndrome [see comments]. *Archives of General Psychiatry, 57*(4), 331–340.

Schumann, C. M., Hamstra, J., Goodlin-Jones, B. L., et al. (2004). The amygdala is enlarged in children but not adolescents with autism; the hippocampus is enlarged at all ages. *Journal of Neuroscience, 24*(28), 6392–6401.

Schwartz, J. H. (2000). Neurotransmitters. In E. R. Kandel, J. H. Schwartz, & T. M. Jessell (Eds.), *Principles of neural science* (4th ed., pp. 280–297). New York: Elsevier.

Sears, L. L., Vest, C., Mohamed, S., et al. (1999). An MRI study of the basal ganglia in autism. *Progress in Neuro-Psychopharmacology and Biological Psychiatry, 23*(4), 613–624.

Shahbazian, M. D., & Zoghbi, H. Y. (2002). Rett syndrome and MeCP2: Linking epigenetics and neuronal function. *American Journal of Human Genetics, 71*(6), 1259–1272.

Sherman, M., Nass, R., & Shapiro, T. (1984). Brief report: Regional cerebral blood flow in autism. *Journal of Autism and Developmental Disorders, 14*, 439–446.

Siegel, B. V., Jr., Asarnow, R., Tanguay, P., et al. (1992). Regional cerebral glucose metabolism and attention in adults with a history of childhood autism. *Journal of Neuropsychiatry and Clinical Neurosciences, 4*(4), 406–414.

Soper, H. V., Satz, P., Orsini, D. L., et al. (1986). Handedness patterns in autism suggest subtypes. *Journal of Autism and Developmental Disorders, 16*(2), 155–167.

Stamatakis, E. A., Marslen-Wilson, W. D., Tyler, L. K., et al. (2005). Cingulate control of fronto-temporal integration reflects linguistic demands: A three-way interaction in functional connectivity. *NeuroImage, 28*(1), 115–121.

Staudt, M., Lidzba, K., Grodd, W., et al. (2002). Right-hemispheric organization of language following early left-sided brain lesions: Functional MRI topography. *NeuroImage, 16*(4), 954–967.

Stein, T., Moritz, C., Quigley, M., et al. (2000). Functional connectivity in the thalamus and hippocampus studied with functional MR imaging. *American Journal of Neuroradiology, 21*(8), 1397–1401.

Sternberg, R. J. (1990). *Metaphors of mind: Conceptions of the nature of intelligence.* Cambridge, UK: Cambridge University Press.

Stromland, K., Nordin, V., Miller, M., et al. (1994). Autism in thalidomide embryopathy: A population study. *Developmental Medicine and Child Neurology, 36*(4), 351–356.

Sur, M., & Leamey, C. A. (2001). Development and plasticity of cortical areas and networks. *Nature Reviews Neuroscience, 2*(4), 251–262.

Sweeten, T. L., Posey, D. J., Shekhar, A., et al. (2002). The amygdala and related structures in the pathophysiology of autism. *Pharmacology, Biochemistry and Behavior, 71*(3), 449–455.

Tager-Flusberg, H., Joseph, R., & Folstein, S. (2001). Current directions in research on autism. *Mental Retardation and Developmental Disabilities Research Reviews, 7*(1), 21–29.

Tanoue, Y., Oda, S., Asano, F., et al. (1988). Epidemiology of infantile autism in southern Ibaraki, Japan: Differences in prevalence in birth cohorts. *Journal of Autism and Developmental Disorders, 18*(2), 155–166.

Thomas, M., & Karmiloff-Smith, A. (2002). Are developmental disorders like cases of adult brain damage? Implications from connectionist modeling. *Behavioral and Brain Sciences, 25*(6), 727–750.

Thompson-Schill, S. L., D'Esposito, M., Aguirre, G. K., et al. (1997). Role of left inferior prefrontal cortex in retrieval of semantic knowledge: A reevaluation. *Proceedings of the National Academy of Sciences of the United States of America, 94*(26), 14792–14797.

Thulborn, K. R., Carpenter, P. A., & Just, M. A. (1999). Plasticity of language-related brain function during recovery from stroke. *Stroke, 30*(4), 749–754.

Townsend, J., & Courchesne, E. (1994). Parietal damage and narrow "spotlight" spatial attention. *Journal of Cognitive Neuroscience, 6*, 220–232.

Townsend, J., Courchesne, E., & Egaas, B. (1996). Slowed orienting of covert visual–spatial attention in autism: Specific deficits associated with cerebellar and parietal abnormality. *Development and Psychopathology, 8*, 563–584.

Trottier, G., Srivastava, L., & Walker, C. D. (1999). Etiology of infantile autism: A review of recent advances in genetic and neurobiological research [see comments]. *Journal of Psychiatry and Neuroscience, 24*(2), 103–115.

Tsatsanis, K. D., Rourke, B. P., Klin, A., et al. (2003). Reduced thalamic volume in high-functioning individuals with autism. *Biological Psychiatry, 53*(2), 121–129.

Tureyen, K., Vemuganti, R., Sailor, K. A., et al. (2004). Transient focal cerebral ischemia-induced neurogenesis in the dentate gyrus of the adult mouse. *Journal of Neurosurgery, 101*(5), 799–805.

Turner, K. C., Frost, L., Linsenbardt, D., et al. (2006). Atypically diffuse functional connectivity between caudate nuclei and cerebral cortex in autism. *Behavioral and Brain Functions, 2*, 34–45.

Vargha-Khadem, F., Carr, L. C., Isaacs, E., et al. (1997). Onset of speech after left hemispherectomy in a nine-year-old boy. *Brain, 120*, 159–182.

Vargha-Khadem, F., & Mishkin, M. (1997). Speech and language outcome after hemispherectomy in childhood. In I. Tuxhorn, H. Holthausen, & H. E. Boenigk (Eds.), *Paediatric epilepsy syndromes and their surgical treatment* (pp. 774–784): John Libbey.

Vargha-Khadem, F., Watkins, K. E., Alcock, K., et al. (1995). Praxic and nonverbal cognitive deficits in a large family with a genetically transmitted speech and language disorder. *Procedures of the National Academy of Sciences of the United States of America, 92*, 930–933.

Veenstra-VanderWeele, J., & Cook, E. H. (2004). Molecular genetics of autism spectrum disorder. *Molecular Psychiatry, 9*(9), 819–832.

Vicari, S., Albertoni, A., Chilosi, A. M., et al. (2000). Plasticity and reorganization during language development in children with early brain injury. *Cortex, 36*(1), 31–46.

Villablanca, J. R., Hovda, D. A., Jackson, G. F., et al. (1993a). Neurological and behavioral effects of a unilateral frontal cortical lesion in fetal kittens: I. Brain morphology, movement, posture, and sensorimotor tests. *Behavioural Brain Research*, 57(1), 63–77.

Villablanca, J. R., Hovda, D. A., Jackson, G. F., et al. (1993b). Neurological and behavioral effects of a unilateral frontal cortical lesion in fetal kittens: II. Visual system tests, and proposing an "optimal developmental period" for lesion effects. *Behavioural Brain Research*, 57(1), 79–92.

Villalobos, M. E., Mizuno, A., Dahl, B. C., et al. (2005). Reduced functional connectivity between V1 and inferior frontal cortex associated with visuomotor performance in autism. *NeuroImage*, 25, 916–925.

Waiter, G. D., Williams, J. H., Murray, A. D., et al. (2005). Structural white matter deficits in high-functioning individuals with autistic spectrum disorder: A voxel-based investigation. *NeuroImage*, 24(2), 455–461.

Watkins, K. E., Dronkers, N. F., & Vargha-Khadem, F. (2002). Behavioural analysis of an inherited speech and language disorder: Comparison with acquired aphasia. *Brain*, 125(Pt. 3), 452–464.

Welchew, D. E., Ashwin, C., Berkouk, K., et al. (2005). Functional disconnectivity of the medial temporal lobe in Asperger's syndrome. *Biological Psychiatry*, 57(9), 991–998.

Whitaker-Azmitia, P. M. (2001). Serotonin and brain development: Role in human developmental diseases. *Brain Research Bulletin*, 56(5), 479–485.

Williams, J. H., Whiten, A., & Singh, T. (2004). A systematic review of action imitation in autistic spectrum disorders. *Journal of Autism and Developmental Disorders*, 34(3), 285–299.

Williams, J. H., Whiten, A., Suddendorf, T., et al. (2001). Imitation, mirror neurons and autism. *Neuroscience Biobehavioral Review*, 25(4), 287–295.

Xiong, J., Parsons, L. M., Gao, J. H., et al. (1999). Interregional connectivity to primary motor cortex revealed using MRI resting state images. *Human Brain Mapping*, 8(2–3), 151–156.

Yamada, H., Sadato, N., Konishi, Y., et al. (2000). A milestone for normal development of the infantile brain detected by functional MRI. *Neurology*, 55(2), 218–223.

Zaramella, P., Freato, F., Amigoni, A., et al. (2001). Brain auditory activation measured by near-infrared spectroscopy (NIRS) in neonates. *Pediatric Research*, 49(2), 213–219.

Zilbovicius, M., Boddaert, N., Belin, P., et al. (2000). Temporal lobe dysfunction in childhood autism. *American Journal of Psychiatry*, 157, 1988–1993.

CHAPTER 7

Functional Magnetic Resonance Imaging in Neurosurgical Planning for Temporal Lobe Epilepsy

LANGUAGE, MEMORY, AND SEIZURE OUTCOME

Brenna C. McDonald
Andrew J. Saykin

Epilepsy is among the neurological disorders for which there has been a rapid realization of the potential direct clinical applications of functional magnetic resonance imaging (fMRI) for improving patient care. To date, much of the literature has focused on the utility of fMRI in common surgical epilepsy populations, particularly temporal lobe epilepsy (TLE). For patients under consideration for surgical resection to treat TLE, fMRI has shown the potential to replace invasive and potentially risky presurgical evaluation techniques and is already being used for such purposes under some circumstances. This chapter reviews recent applications of fMRI to the understanding of language and memory functioning in TLE, including presurgical lateralization and localization of brain regions critical to these cognitive processes and use of fMRI activation patterns to predict postsurgical outcome. It should be noted that although a comprehensive review of these areas is beyond the scope of this chapter, additional lines of research have also examined the utility of integration of other diagnostic tools with fMRI to improve localization of the epileptogenic zone (e.g., using electroencephalogram (EEG)-triggered fMRI; for review, see Hamandi et al., 2004; Lemieux, 2004), and have utilized fMRI in extratemporal epilepsy subtypes. In this chapter, however, we focus on current findings regarding language and memory processing in TLE, given the potential importance of these findings for postsurgical outcome, as well as for the future elimination of current invasive methods of evaluation. We also include examples of fMRI language mapping as conducted in our epilepsy center, demonstrating the clinical utility of these techniques for adults and children with epilepsy.

Characteristics of TLE

Epilepsy is among the most common neurological disorders, with an overall incidence, excluding febrile convulsions and single seizures, estimated at 40–70 cases per 100,000 persons per year (Sander & Shorvon, 1996), and a prevalence of 5–10 cases per 1,000 persons (Bell & Sander, 2001; Hauser, 1998). The incidence is high in childhood, decreases in young adulthood, and rises again in elderly populations (Sander et al., 1990). Partial seizures, including those with secondary generalization, are the most common seizure subtype, accounting for 40% in one population-based study (Sander et al., 1990), with 11% of those with newly diagnosed seizures having complex partial seizures. By definition, complex partial seizures are a focal-onset form of epilepsy, most commonly involving the temporal lobe (Babb & Brown, 1987; Williamson et al., 1987).

TLE demonstrates a strong tendency to be medically refractory; therefore, patients may be considered for surgical resection to treat their epilepsy. Such resection may include either a standard anterior temporal lobectomy (ATL) or a selective amygdalohippocampectomy. The selective procedure is most typically used in patients with localized medial temporal lobe (MTL) seizure onset, as the sparing of nonepileptogenic regions of the temporal lobe has been hypothesized to have the potential to minimize negative cognitive outcomes postsurgically, while leading to seizure control comparable to that gained from the larger ATL resection (Paglioli et al., 2006). Research has been equivocal regarding the benefits of the selective versus the standard surgical procedure in terms of prevention of cognitive decline postsurgically, with some studies demonstrating significant memory changes even in patients undergoing a selective resection, particularly in patients with an epileptic focus in the dominant temporal lobe, though such declines may be less severe than those noted for patients undergoing a standard procedure (Gleissner et al., 2002; Goldstein & Polkey, 1993; Helmstaedter et al., 1996, 1997). In a randomized trial, however, surgical resection for TLE was shown to be superior to drug treatment (Wiebe et al., 2001) in terms of seizure control.

Although the potential for significant improvement in seizure frequency, including possible cure of epilepsy, is a significant factor in favor of surgery, appropriate surgical candidates must be selected on the basis of careful presurgical assessment. In addition to inpatient video/EEG monitoring, routine presurgical evaluation includes high-resolution structural MRI scans utilizing scan sequences and parameters tailored to detect structural abnormalities that may indicate a seizure focus. Practice standards in presurgical assessment of patients with TLE also include detailed neuropsychological assessment and intracarotid amobarbital testing (the IAT, or "Wada" test) (American Academy of Neurology, 1996; National Institutes of Health, 1990; Rausch, 1992; Tatum et al., 2000). Neuropsychological testing establishes a presurgical baseline for cognitive functioning, as in addition to medical contraindications to temporal lobe resection, cognitive factors can preclude surgical treatment. In particular, the integrity of language and memory abilities come under close scrutiny in TLE, given the critical role temporal lobe structures play in these functions and the potential risk for postsurgical language and memory deficits. A major focus of fMRI research in epilepsy populations has therefore been on characterizing language and memory functions in TLE.

fMRI Language Studies in TLE

Lateralization and Localization of Language Functions

Initial fMRI studies of TLE focused on the lateralization and localization of language functions. One such line of research has investigated correspondence between hemispheric dominance for language as determined by the IAT with that demonstrated by examining fMRI laterality asymmetries, commonly referred to as asymmetry indices (AIs) or laterality indices (LIs; this abbreviation is used here across studies for consistency, though the terminology used in source citations varies). "Typical" language dominance is conventionally defined as clear left-hemisphere dominance for language activation, and "atypical" dominance includes right-hemisphere dominance or bilateral representation of language activation during fMRI language probes. To date, most studies comparing IAT and fMRI language dominance have found very high concordance between fMRI and IAT conclusions. Differences have typically reflected a nondiagnostic study in one modality, or bilateral representation of language in one modality but not the other (Adcock et al., 2003; Baciu et al., 2001; Benson et al., 1999; Gaillard et al., 2002; Lehéricy et al., 2000), rather than frank disagreement between fMRI and IAT results, though such discrepancy has been noted in a very few studies (e.g., Rutten et al., 2002; Worthington et al., 1997). Most studies have demonstrated concordance between IAT and fMRI language lateralization in upwards of 80% of subjects (Adcock et al, 2003; Benson et al., 1999; Rutten et al., 2002; Carpentier et al., 2001; Woermann et al., 2003), with several groups reporting complete agreement between modalities (Baciu et al., 2001; Bahn et al., 1997; Benbadis et al., 1998; Binder et al., 1996; Desmond et al., 1995; Hertz-Pannier et al., 1997; Lehéricy et al., 2000; Yetkin et al., 1998). In the largest sample reported to date, 91% concordance between IAT and fMRI language lateralization was found in 94 patients with temporal and extratemporal epilepsy (Woermann et al., 2003).

The majority of studies comparing fMRI and IAT language lateralization have relied on word generation tasks as the fMRI language probe, a technique that has been consistently shown to elicit activation in frontal language regions (e.g., Broca's area), and that typically produces LIs concordant with the IAT for subjects with more strongly lateralized language functioning (to either the left or the right hemisphere). For subjects with more bilateral language representation, however, LIs based primarily on the frontal regions activated by word generation tasks have been less consistent with IAT results (i.e., one modality suggesting more bilateral language representation, while the other suggests unilateral language dominance). Activation of temporal language regions has been less reliably demonstrated across individuals than that of frontal areas, likely due to the nature of such fMRI language probes (i.e., word generation), which rely heavily on expressive language functions. For TLE, the advantages of more reliable elicitation of temporal lobe language-related activation are readily evident, given the surgical target. To elicit more posterior language-related activation, and to address the concern regarding accurately identifying individuals with bilateral language representation using fMRI, a few groups have utilized multiple language paradigms.

In one such attempt to utilize multiple fMRI probes to lateralize and localize language functioning, Rutten et al. (2002) used verb generation, verbal fluency, picture naming, and sentence comprehension tasks in a group of 18 patients with TLE, implementing a combined task analysis (CTA) technique they had previously validated in healthy control subjects (Ramsey et al., 2001). These authors (Rutten et al., 2002) achieved more robust results using CTA than with any single task and were able to detect activation in posterior (temporoparietal) language regions in all patients. fMRI achieved concordance with IAT findings in 91% of patients who were left-dominant by IAT, 75% of those with bilateral language representation by IAT, and 67% of those right-dominant by IAT. The investigators concluded that these results offer a more promising approach toward accurate identification of individuals with atypical, particularly bilateral, language representation and suggested that their findings demonstrate a protocol that might effectively be used to obviate the need for IAT evaluation in patients who are strongly left-lateralized for language on fMRI. It should be noted that this group used a fixed, user-independent approach to statistical analysis, which did not allow for individual variability in the threshold set for significant activation, a method that has both strengths and limitations for clinical practice. On one hand, this method provides an objective strategy for analyzing such data in clinical decision making, and use of a less stringent threshold maximizes power to detect task-related activation. On the other hand, as the authors note, the threshold chosen can have a marked effect on the laterality index achieved. More stringent thresholds at times produce more strongly lateralized results, particularly in individuals who demonstrate relative higher degrees of brain activation during fMRI tasks, whereas less stringent thresholds can sometimes allow more effective detection of lateralization in individuals with lesser magnitudes of activation.

Prediction of Postsurgical Language Outcome and Functional Reorganization

In addition to evaluating the potential for supplanting the IAT with fMRI measures of language lateralization and localization, other lines of research have investigated the ability of fMRI language probes to predict postsurgical cognitive deficits, as well as the functional reorganization of language in TLE. As patients undergoing dominant temporal lobectomy to treat epilepsy are at increased risk for acquired cognitive deficits postsurgically, most prominently in language and memory functions, researchers have sought to establish predictive factors that will allow assessment of the likelihood of postsurgical impairment on the level of the individual patient. Previous work has established that individuals who experience a later onset of epilepsy and who have stronger language abilities presurgically are at increased risk for postsurgical language deficits following temporal lobe resection in the language-dominant hemisphere as determined by IAT (Hermann et al., 1994, 1999; Saykin et al., 1995; Stafiniak et al., 1990). Recent work has suggested that fMRI language probes may also prove useful in assessment of risk of postsurgical language deficits.

In a series of 24 patients with epilepsy who underwent left anterior temporal lobectomy (LATL) and 32 patients who underwent right anterior temporal lobectomy (RATL), Sabsevitz et al. (2002, 2003) evaluated the ability of several factors to predict postsurgical confrontation naming (Boston Naming Test) deficits, including preoperative naming performance, age at seizure onset, age at first neurologic event, IAT LI, and fMRI LI on a semantic decision-making task conducted presurgically. The LATL group demonstrated a significant decline in naming performance postsurgically, with more than half of the sample showing a decline greater than 2 standard deviations below the mean of the RATL group. As hypothesized, greater fMRI language lateralization toward the resected hemisphere predicted greater naming decline; this prediction was strongest using a temporal lobe region of interest, but was also significant using a region of interest consisting of the angular gyrus, frontal lobe, and overall left hemisphere. Using a definition of "poor outcome" of a decline in naming performance greater than 2 standard deviations below the RATL group mean, the fMRI temporal lobe LI showed 100% specificity and 73% specificity with the LI threshold set at .25. By comparison, the IAT LI showed 92% sensitivity and 45% specificity. In this sample, preoperative naming performance, age at epilepsy onset, and age at first neurological event showed weak, nonsignificant ($p > .05$) relationships to postsurgical naming outcome. Most significant from a clinical perspective, in this sample of 24 patients who underwent LATL, 16 showed fMRI language activation patterns that clearly demonstrated left-hemisphere dominance. Using the criteria noted above, 81% of these patients showed poor naming outcomes, whereas none of the LATL patients with symmetric or right lateralized language on fMRI showed a poor outcome. Such preliminary studies suggest that presurgical fMRI can be a useful predictor of postsurgical language outcome, a finding potentially of great clinical significance if replicated in future work.

fMRI has demonstrated increased incidence of atypical language lateralization in patients with epilepsy, particularly those with left-hemisphere seizure onset, consistent with prior IAT studies demonstrating higher than expected rates of atypical language lateralization in patients with epilepsy. In recent studies with relatively large sample sizes, atypical fMRI language lateralization was observed in 20–30% of patients with epilepsy (Woermann et al., 2003; Springer et al., 1999). This contrasts with low estimates of atypical language dominance in healthy control samples. In a group of 100 right-handed healthy control subjects, none showed right-hemisphere dominance, and only 6% showed generally symmetrical bilateral representation for language (Springer et al., 1999). In a sample of 50 left-handed and ambidextrous healthy individuals, right-hemisphere language dominance was demonstrated using fMRI in 8% of the sample, and 14% showed symmetric hemispheric activation (Szaflarski et al., 2002). In this sample, atypical language dominance was also related to degree of left-handedness, as well as to family history of left-handedness.

In patients with a left-hemisphere seizure focus, research has demonstrated a higher percentage of subjects with atypical language dominance (Adcock et al., 2003), significant differences in LIs relative to control subjects and patients with right-hemisphere foci (with left-hemisphere focus, patient LIs shifted toward greater right/bilateral language representation) (Adcock et al., 2003; Carpentier et al., 2001; Gaillard et al., 2002), and a significant correlation between presence of a left-hemisphere seizure focus and right-hemisphere language dominance (Sabbah et al., 2003). This trend is demonstrated in a study by Adcock et al. (2003), who used a verbal fluency task to evaluate fMRI language lateralization in right-handed left TLE (LTLE; n = 12), right TLE (RTLE; n = 7), and healthy control (n = 12) subjects. Group contrasts demonstrated that controls showed a strongly left lateralized pattern of activation, with prominent activation of frontal language regions. This pattern was accentuated in the RTLE patients, who showed additional left frontal clusters of activation beyond those shown in the control group. In contrast, relative to the control group, LTLE patients showed diminished left frontal and temporal lobe activation, but increased right temporal activation. Overall, LTLE patients showed a much wider range of LI values than either RTLE or control groups, which were both strongly left lateralized, with little intragroup variability.

Similarly, Thivard et al. (2005) compared brain activation patterns during receptive and expressive language processing in right-handed LTLE and

RTLE patients and healthy comparison subjects. These authors examined frontal and temporal lobe activation patterns during word generation, story listening, and repetition fMRI probes. Strong left-hemisphere dominance was observed in frontal regions during word generation for RTLE and control subjects, but was diminished in LTLE patients, though not to a statistically significant degree. This shift was more pronounced for fMRI tasks linked more strongly to the temporal lobes (story listening, repetition). For these tasks, LTLE patients demonstrated significantly more right-hemisphere lateralization of temporal lobe activation than RTLE or control subjects. Interestingly, neuropsychological performance was stronger in the 19% of this sample who demonstrated atypical language activation patterns on fMRI than in those with typical dominance. Taken together, these findings support previous research demonstrating a reorganization of language functioning away from an epileptic or otherwise neurologically compromised left hemisphere and suggest that such reorganization may convey functional advantages.

In contrast, a preliminary report by Swanson et al. (2002) showed that earlier age of seizure onset is associated with greater atypical language lateralization and that subjects with a left-hemisphere seizure focus whose language skills appear to have undergone reorganization demonstrated poorer naming skills. These findings point to the need for further investigation of the relationship of early risk factors for epilepsy and related abnormalities in neurodevelopment to later brain organization of cognitive functions such as language and memory. fMRI may be an ideal tool to study the reorganization suggested by earlier neuropsychological (Hermann et al., 1995; Saykin et al., 1995) and IAT studies (Glosser et al., 1995).

An important consideration is that fMRI studies have also consistently demonstrated some degree of right-hemisphere language activation in clearly left-hemisphere-dominant healthy control subjects, supporting the argument that language lateralization falls along a continuum of hemispheric dominance. This also highlights a limitation of the hemispheric anesthetization technique implemented in the IAT in understanding language processing; it may be that in some cases functional neuroimaging results may be a more accurate representation of language localization than IAT, a supposition apparently confirmed by surgery in some individual case reports using fMRI (Rutten et al., 2002) and positron emission tomography (PET) (Pardo & Fox, 1993; Hunter et al., 1999). fMRI therefore appears more sensitive than other techniques, such as the IAT, in detecting language-related brain activity in the "nondominant" hemisphere. In addition, several studies have demonstrated apparent dissociation of frontal (expressive) and temporal (receptive) language regions using fMRI (e.g., greater right-hemisphere lateralization for temporal regions but left lateralization for frontal regions, or vice versa) (Lehéricy et al., 2000; Ries et al., 2004; Rutten et al., 2002; Thivard et al., 2005), consistent with previous reports of differential lateralization of receptive and expressive language on the IAT (Kurthen et al., 1992, 1994; Risse et al., 1997). This may explain the discrepancies observed in those studies noting bilateral representation of language using one modality (e.g., IAT or fMRI), but unilateral dominance using the other, particularly when only a single fMRI word-generation task is used, as such tasks are most likely to activate frontal/expressive language regions.

Better understanding of the factors that lead to stronger lateralization of language in favor of one hemisphere over the other will be important in understanding functional outcomes following neurological insult, relevant not only to epilepsy but to other clinical disorders (e.g., brain tumor, traumatic brain injury). In one very small study, correlation of fMRI language activation with diffusion tensor imaging (DTI) data has suggested that white matter abnormalities may be a contributing factor in language reorganization toward the right hemisphere (Briellmann et al., 2003). As atypical dominance and postsurgical language outcome have been associated with earlier age of brain injury and onset of epilepsy (Devinsky et al., 1993; Saykin et al., 1995; Springer et al., 1999; Stafiniak et al., 1990; Woermann et al., 2003), as well as with stronger neuropsychological performance (Thivard et al., 2005), further research will be important to clarify the circumstances under which such language reorganization can improve functionality.

Technical and Analytic Considerations

Multiple studies (e.g., Adcock et al., 2003; Thivard et al., 2005) have demonstrated weaker magnitude of fMRI activation in TLE patients relative to control groups. The reasons for this discrepancy are unclear, but factors related to primary central nervous system (CNS) dysfunction such as refractory epilepsy and its treatment must be considered, including the potential effects of antiepileptic medications on fMRI brain activation patterns. In one study, patients found to have bilateral language representation on IAT showed weaker fMRI activation than those strongly lateralized to either hemisphere (Rutten et al., 2002). These observed differences in the strength of activation among patients with epilepsy and between patient and control groups also highlight the importance of careful consideration of the statistical significance threshold chosen for analysis of both group and individual fMRI activation maps in this population. The use of lower activation thresholds may be appropriate in patient populations to detect weaker levels of activation and assist in lateralization of language. However, the use of lower statistical thresholds has been shown in several studies to weaken LIs and may therefore potentially damage interpretation of laterality categorizations (Adcock et al., 2003; Gaillard et al., 2002; Hertz-Pannier et al., 1997). It may be appropriate to examine a range of thresholds to enhance clinical interpretation. This issue warrants detailed empirical analysis in future studies.

An important consideration is that studies have demonstrated that fMRI language activation patterns are reliable over time, further supporting the potential clinical utility of fMRI for replacing the IAT for language lateralization. In the study noted above, Adcock et al. (2003) examined all subjects at two time points, about 3 mo apart, using the same fMRI verbal fluency probe. They reported that all laterality classifications were in agreement at the two time points (i.e., laterality categorizations were 100% reliable), with good correlation between LIs between the two studies for all study groups (LTLE, RTLE, and controls).

In addition to the issues noted above regarding choice of statistical threshold, it is also important to consider whether laterality conclusions are based on spatial extent of activation (within a whole hemisphere or just a specified region of interest) or magnitude of signal change, as previous work suggests that the magnitude of signal change method may be more reproducible (Adcock et al., 2003). As noted above, this is in part related to the statistical significance threshold chosen, which dictates the spatial extent of observed activation. In addition, LIs calculated on the basis of a region of interest approach may vary significantly depending on the region analyzed, which can include the whole hemisphere or regions of the frontal and temporal cortex, the boundaries of which are typically defined differently by individual investigators. In an attempt to circumvent difficulties with the LI approach, Liégeois et al. (2002) developed a method for direct statistical comparison of task-related activation to ascertain hemispheric language dominance. This method utilized direct comparison of statistical parametric maps of activation in homotopic voxels of each hemisphere, to eliminate the possible confounding effects of statistical threshold and region of interest boundaries. In a sample of eight adolescents with epilepsy, results from this method corresponded entirely with results from invasive language lateralization and localization techniques, including IAT and electrocortical stimulation. These findings are clinically meaningful, as this sample included two patients classified as right-hemisphere dominant for language, and one classified as having bilateral language representation, in addition to five left-hemisphere-dominant patients. Therefore, methods similar to that used by Liégeois et al. (2002) may have good potential for eliminating current concerns regarding relying on fMRI results to determine language lateralization in place of the IAT. As they note, however, review of raw task-induced activation maps remains critical to the accurate clinical interpretation of the data generated by the direct statistical comparison method.

Examples of Clinical Utility of fMRI Language Lateralization and Localization

At Dartmouth–Hitchcock Medical Center (DHMC), fMRI is frequently conducted in candidates for epilepsy surgery for whom an IAT is contraindicated or has been unsuccessful. Patients referred for clinical fMRI language mapping complete one or more language paradigms, including aurally presented verb generation, novelty detection, and semantic–phonemic decision-making tasks. In the verb generation paradigm, patients are presented with blocks of nouns alternating with blocks of tones. For each noun, the patient is asked to mentally generate as many verbs as possible that go with that noun (e.g., for "frog," the patient might think "leap," "croak," or "hop"). With younger individuals, or those with intellectual limitations, the patient is asked simply to think of as many words (of any part of speech) as he or she can that "go with" the target word (e.g., for "frog," such words as "green" or "water"). The patient is asked not to say the words or make any mouth movements. During the control condition (tones), the patient is asked simply to listen and clear his or her mind. Analysis contrasts hemodynamic responses during the two blocked task conditions. The typical pattern of brain activation includes dominant-hemisphere frontal regions, including Broca's area, with more posterior temporal lobe activation observed in some patients. Consistent with the literature, cingulate gyrus activation is also often noted.

Examples of left-, right-, and mixed-dominant activation patterns during word generation are shown in Figure 7.1 (displayed over surface renderings of the patients' own anatomy). The clinical history of each of these patients is illustrative of cases in which fMRI language mapping can be particularly helpful. The left-hemisphere dominant patient is a 19-year-old, right-handed woman with medication-refractory epilepsy thought to be of left temporal lobe origin, and MRI findings consistent with left mesial temporal sclerosis. Neuropsychological assessment demonstrated intact cognitive abilities, with functioning typically at or above the average range across domains. IAT suggested left-hemisphere participation in language, but right-hemisphere participation could not be ruled out because of a persistent trigeminal artery on the right, precluding right-hemisphere injection of sodium amobarbital. In this patient, fMRI language mapping was able to confirm left-hemisphere language dominance.

The right-hemisphere-dominant patient represented in Figure 7.1 is a 13-year-old, left-handed girl with a history of left-sided motor seizures that

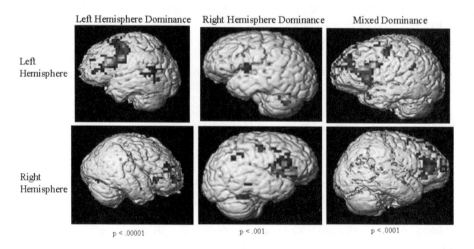

FIGURE 7.1. Word generation task: fMRI activation maps demonstrating left, right, and mixed language dominance.

became medication refractory with the onset of adolescence. EEG demonstrated a right-frontal-lobe seizure focus, and SPECT and MRI studies demonstrated increased activity in a region that appeared to correspond with an area
of cortical dysplasia in the right frontal lobe. Neuropsychological assessment
demonstrated generally intact cognitive abilities, with most functions at or
above the average range, and a significant strength in verbal relative to nonverbal intellect. A mild relative weakness was apparent in susceptibility to distraction. In this patient, fMRI mapping was used to document language
dominance in the epileptogenic right hemisphere. In addition, fMRI motor
mapping was conducted (not shown), which confirmed that peak areas of
activation for the dominant left hand were located proximal to the dysplastic
region thought to represent the epileptic focus. Because of these factors, surgical resection was initially not considered an appropriate option in this case.
Owing to worsening seizures in subsequent years, however, two surgical procedures were later performed. During the first procedure, the resection zone
was limited to preserve dominant motor function. Unfortunately, although
initial improvements were noted, this did not result in satisfactory seizure control, leading to a second resection, which included the primary motor cortex.
Seizure control has been excellent since the second resection, although rehabilitation is ongoing to improve postsurgical deficits in left hand, arm, and leg
functioning. Following the second resection, initial difficulties were also noted
in terms of slurred speech and word-finding problems, which have since
resolved. Of note is that in both of the aforementioned patients, smaller areas
of activation can be seen in the nondominant hemisphere, in homologous
regions. As noted above, this is not an uncommon finding.

For both of these patients, however, clear unilateral hemispheric "dominance" is apparent, in contrast to the case demonstrating mixed dominance.
This is a 20-year-old young man with mixed handedness (writes predominantly with his left hand, but many other activities are typically conducted
with his right) who was diagnosed with a large (Spetzler–Martin grade III–IV)
right posterior temporal/inferior parietal arteriovenous malformation (AVM).
IAT was unsuccessful owing to extensive crossflow resulting from the AVM.
fMRI language mapping was therefore conducted prior to AVM emboli-
zation. Although preoperative neuropsychological data were not available,
this young man also reported a lifelong history of learning and attentional difficulties, including the need for early reading intervention. As can be seen in
Figure 7.1, bilateral frontal activation was apparent. The global peak of brain
activation was observed in the left frontal lobe; however, the presence of such
extensive homologous right-hemisphere activation argued for mixed dominance for language in this case. This is also of interest in relation to the
patient's reported history of learning and attentional problems, given prior
research suggesting a relationship between developmental language and reading disorders and abnormal cerebral lateralization of brain regions related to
language functioning (for review, see Anderson et al., 1993).

Our novelty-detection paradigm is patterned after our single-event word
task (Saykin et al., 1999) and exploits the repetition–suppression memory

phenomena reported in early blocked, visual fMRI studies (Gabrieli et al., 1997; Stern et al., 1996). Its advantage is that it has a minimal cognitive load and requires no response. In addition to its utility for examining memory functioning, this task also allows investigation of regions important for language processing. In this event-related design, the patient initially hears a list of three words that repeat every 2–4 s in a pseudorandom sequence. Following this habituation phase, the patient hears the same three words pseudorandomly interspersed with new words. New words are separated by one to thirteen intervening repeated words. For localization of language-related activation, analysis models the hemodynamic response during listening to words as compared with a resting baseline.

During the semantic–phonemic decision-making task, the patient hears pairs of words. In the semantic condition, the first word in the pair is a category and the second word is either a member of the category or a nonmember (e.g., *beverage–milk* versus *beverage–dog*); the patient is asked to press one button if the second word is a member of the category, and another button if it is not. In the phonemic condition, both words are nonsense words, created by rearranging the letters of target words in the task; the patient is asked to press one button if the two nonsense words are the same (e.g., *scumi–scumi*), and another button if they are not (e.g., *scumi–grabe*). For localization of language-related activation, analysis models the hemodynamic response during semantic versus phonemic processing, or during semantic processing as compared with a resting baseline. For both of these tasks, activation of the posterior superior temporal gyrus in the vicinity of Wernicke's area can typically be observed.

The combined use of the word generation and novelty detection paradigms is demonstrated in Figures 7.2 and 7.3. This patient is a 9-year-old, right-handed boy who has evidenced left hemiparesis and epilepsy since infancy. Neuroimaging has demonstrated an atrophic right hemisphere, as well as extensive polymicrogyria and possible cortical dysplasia in the right frontal and parietal lobes, findings that have been interpreted in part to represent the results of a prenatal stroke. Neuropsychological assessments have demonstrated global impairment in cognition, with findings consistent with functioning in the mild-to-moderate range of mental retardation, and similar impairment across neuropsychological domains. As hemispherectomy was under consideration to treat his seizures and IAT was thought unfeasible in this patient, he was referred for fMRI mapping of language functioning. As shown in Figures 7.2 and 7.3, left-hemisphere dominance was apparent using both the word-generation and novelty-detection tasks, with activation of regions thought to represent Broca's and Wernicke's areas in this patient. These can be visualized on the surface rendering of the patient's brain (Figure 7.2) and as displayed over a high-resolution anatomical volume image (Figure 7.3).

The similarity between the temporal regions activated in this patient during language processing in the novelty detection task and in the semantic–phonemic decision-making task can be seen by comparing Figures 7.3 and 7.4. The patient whose activation is demonstrated in Figure 7.4 is a 48-year-old, right-handed man who experienced seizures for several years prior to undergoing neuroimag-

Verb Generation Task (p = .00001)

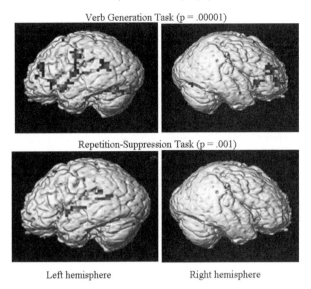

Left hemisphere   Right hemisphere

FIGURE 7.2. Combined use of expressive and receptive fMRI language probes: Surface rendering.

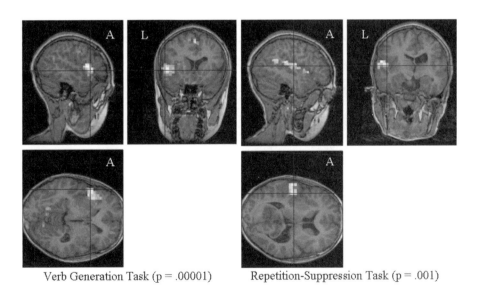

Verb Generation Task (p = .00001)   Repetition-Suppression Task (p = .001)

FIGURE 7.3. Combined use of expressive and receptive fMRI language probes: Anatomical visualization.

ing. Brain MRI then revealed a nonenhancing lesion with abnormal expansion and T2-weighted signal throughout most of the anterior and inferior left temporal lobe. Left-hemisphere dominance was demonstrated in this patient, using both the word generation paradigm (not shown) and the semantic–phonemic decision-making task, in which posterior superior temporal gyrus activation was observed in regions very similar to those observed in Figure 7.3 during the novelty detection task, and thought to approximate Wernicke's area in both patients. These clinical examples, as well as those found elsewhere (e.g., McDonald et al., 2006), demonstrate the power of fMRI as a noninvasive technique for accurate lateralization and localization of regions critical to language functioning prior to surgical intervention.

As noted above, however, the most consistently demonstrated finding in the literature has been lateralization and localization of language functioning in frontal regions approximating Broca's area, as these regions have proved easiest to reliably activate using language generation paradigms. Reliable activation of temporal language regions across subjects is best obtained through use of multiple fMRI language paradigms, which typically include receptive language tasks involving semantic processing, reading, or other language-processing activities more likely to activate posterior language regions. In a study directly designed to assess the reproducibility of fMRI activation patterns during language processing within and between subjects and scanning sessions, Fernandez et al. (2003) demonstrated good within-test and test–retest reliability of task-related activation patterns for a semantic judgment probe. Similar reliability was demonstrated regardless of language dominance, though reliability was somewhat greater for frontal versus temporoparietal language regions.

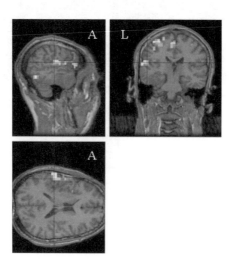

Semantic-Phonemic Decision-Making Task (p = .01)

FIGURE 7.4. Receptive language regions visualized using semantic decision making.

fMRI of Memory Processing in TLE

Research on assessment of memory processing in epilepsy using fMRI has emphasized the development of task paradigms with the potential to replace the IAT. Such studies have approached this goal from various perspectives, including assessment of the relationship of hemispheric differences in memory activation to side of seizure focus, evaluation of potential reorganization of memory functions away from the epileptogenic MTL, and prediction of postsurgical seizure and memory outcome using presurgical fMRI activation patterns. Particular emphasis has been placed on assessing memory functioning in left (or language dominant) TLE, given the well-documented increased risk of postsurgical verbal memory deficits in this group, although nonverbal deficits have also been reported following right temporal lobe (TL) resection. Relative to the body of work regarding fMRI assessment of language processing in epilepsy, that investigating memory functioning is comparatively limited, although preliminary findings have provided important insights.

Relationship of Side of Seizure Focus to fMRI Brain Activation during Memory Processing

Studies examining memory functioning in TLE using fMRI have demonstrated a relationship between side of seizure focus and brain activation. In the first published fMRI study directly examining memory processing in TLE, Detre et al. (1998) used a complex visual scene encoding task to assess functional asymmetry in comparison with IAT memory lateralization, based on a paradigm previously shown to activate bilateral MTL structures in healthy controls (Stern et al., 1996). This fMRI memory probe, which has now been used in several studies by this group (Killgore et al., 1999; Rabin et al., 2002, 2004; Casasanto et al., 2001), involved evaluation of MTL activation during memorization of novel complex scenes relative to a control condition involving viewing of a degraded version of one of the encoding stimuli. In this initial study (Detre et al., 1998), TLE patients ($n = 7$ LTLE, 3 RTLE) demonstrated markedly more asymmetric MTL activation during novel scene encoding than controls ($n = 8$), who showed generally symmetric MTL activation, with a slight right-hemisphere predominance. The direction of hemispheric asymmetry was concordant with IAT memory findings in all patients. The investigators concluded that this pattern could not be attributed to epilepsy-related structural abnormalities alone, as two patients demonstrated greater fMRI activation and better IAT memory performance ipsilateral to the seizure focus.

Jokeit et al. (2001) were likewise able to detect alterations in lateralization of activation during memory processing in TLE patients using a mental spatial navigation task. This paradigm asked patients to visualize walking between preselected destinations in their hometown, interspersed with blocks of a counting control condition. MTL structures were reliably activated in both TLE patients ($n = 16$ LTLE, 14 RTLE) and control subjects ($n = 17$); activation was observed primarily in the parahippocampal gyri. Although controls did not show systematic hemispheric asymmetry of activation, inter-hemispheric laterality differences correctly identified the side of seizure focus in 90% of TLE patients (mean LI higher contralateral to side of seizure focus). This discrepancy was largely due to reduced MTL activation ipsilateral to sei-zure focus, with patients with hippocampal sclerosis showing significantly fewer activated voxels than patients with extrahippocampal–temporal lobe pathology. These findings were thought to be directly related to memory func-tioning rather than general visuospatial abilities, given the positive correla-tions between right MTL fMRI activation and out-of-scanner performance on neuropsychological tests of nonverbal memory, but not tests of more general visuoconstruction skills. Left MTL fMRI activation was also correlated with left-hemisphere IAT memory performance for visually presented objects, though not with scores on out-of-scanner verbal memory measures.

Although the memory probes described above were primarily visuo-spatial in nature, differential lateralization of fMRI activation based on side of seizure focus has also been demonstrated using verbal task paradigms. Using a semantic decision-making task, Bellgowan et al. (1998) were able to discrimi-nate carefully matched groups of LTLE and RTLE patients (n = 14 in each group) based on their fMRI activation patterns. Participants heard a list of animal names and were asked to press a button for animals that they judged to be both "found in the United States" and "used by people." Activation dur-ing semantic processing was contrasted with that during a tone discrimination condition. Whereas frontal and parietal lobe activation was similar in the LTLE and RTLE groups, RTLE patients showed predominant task-related left MTL activation in the hippocampus, parahippocampal gyrus, and collateral sulcus, while LTLE patients demonstrated little significant activation in these regions. This task did not elicit right MTL activation in either TLE group, a not unexpected finding given that such semantic tasks would not typically be predicted to generate right-hemisphere activation. These findings suggest that semantic task paradigms are potentially useful for preferential activation of the left MTL. This also highlights the difference in this fMRI probe from other tasks discussed here, which tend to focus on encoding versus retrieval of infor-mation, or "novelty detection," rather than the encoding via semantic pro-cessing employed in the task used by Bellgowan et al. The authors hypothe-sized that the lack of left MTL activation in LTLE patients in spite of relatively intact episodic memory functioning may result from structural abnormalities, but may also indicate intra- or interhemispheric reorganization of memory functions in this group, potentially related to factors such as age at seizure onset.

In another study using fMRI to lateralize memory functions in TLE, Golby et al. (2002) examined encoding in six patients with LTLE and three with RTLE, using four types of stimuli (patterns, faces, scenes, and words). All subjects showed MTL activation (hippocampus, parahippocampal gyrus, entorhinal cortex) during novel stimulus processing, and fMRI lateralization of memory was concordant with IAT in eight of nine cases, with greater MTL activation observed contralateral to the side of seizure focus. In general, RTLE patients demonstrated relatively greater left than right MTL activation during novel stimulus encoding across stimulus types, whereas the reverse was true for LTLE patients. In previous work, this group had demonstrated material specificity of memory encoding lateralization in healthy young adults using fMRI, with verbal stimuli preferentially engaging the left MTL, and nonverbal stimuli preferentially activating the right MTL (Golby et al., 2001). In TLE patients (Golby et al., 2002), group analysis demonstrated a tendency toward a material-specific interaction between side of seizure focus and stimulus type, such that LTLE patients showed right MTL activation for novelty encoding of words (normally a strongly left-lateralized task), while RTLE subjects showed left MTL activation for novel patterns (normally strongly right-lateralized). These data may therefore demonstrate functional reorganization of memory circuitry in TLE.

Along these lines, Dupont et al. (2000) investigated differences in the neural substrate of memory processing between TLE patients and healthy control subjects. Using a verbal encoding task, these investigators demonstrated that during encoding control subjects showed increased activation in a temporo–parieto–occipital network, which was predominant in the left hemisphere and included prominent activation of the ventrolateral frontal region. During word retrieval controls showed increased activation in the above regions, with additional activation in bilateral parahippocampal regions. Parahippocampal activation was more prominent in the right hemisphere. In contrast, during both encoding and retrieval LTLE patients demonstrated decreased activation in regions active in controls, but showed a marked increase in dorsolateral prefrontal cortex activation, which was not evident in the control group. During retrieval, bilateral parahippocampal activation was also noted, though diminished relative to that in controls. As the TLE group also showed significant deficits in task performance accuracy relative to controls, the authors hypothesized that this increased frontal activation in the patients relative to controls might be suggestive of dysfunctional reorganization of memory networks in TLE, due either to hippocampal dysfunction or to the broader epileptogenic process.

In an effort to understand the changes in memory circuitry involved in delayed retrieval in LTLE, this group (Dupont et al., 2001) conducted the same fMRI retrieval task in the same group of patients and controls 24 h after the initial study. As in the prior study (Dupont et al., 2000), memory retrieval at 24 h following initial assessment was significantly poorer in LTLE patients than in controls, with control performance remaining generally stable at the 24-h delay, and patient performance declining slightly, though not significantly (Dupont et al., 2001). In the control group, brain activation during delayed retrieval demonstrated a somewhat similar pattern to immediate retrieval, though decreases were evident in parahippocampal, occipitotemporal, and ventrolateral frontal activation, and increased activation was apparent in the right posterior hippocampus and bilateral parietal cortex. In the LTLE group, activation in neocortical brain regions observed during immediate retrieval was dramatically decreased at delayed retrieval, and no MTL activation was apparent. The authors concluded that these findings demonstrate the critical role of MTL structures in verbal memory, particularly in retrieval of learned material, and surmised that dysfunction of MTL structures in TLE likely underlies the memory deficits and alterations in fMRI activation they observed in patients relative to controls.

Richardson et al. (2003) likewise examined the putative reorganization of verbal memory functions in a homogeneous group of LTLE patients with clear radiologically defined hippocampal sclerosis. In this study, MTL fMRI activation patterns during verbal encoding were examined in 12 control subjects and 24 LTLE patients. The LTLE group was further subdivided into patients with and without amygdalar sclerosis in addition to hippocampal sclerosis. In the combined patient group, greater activity was observed in the right hippocampus and parahippocampal gyrus during successful encoding relative to the control group. During successfully encoded emotional relative to neutral words, the patient group with left amygdalar and hippocampal sclerosis showed greater right amygdalar activation relative to patients with left hippocampal sclerosis only.

In another study (Richardson et al., 2004a) this group demonstrated a relationship between hippocampal pathology (segmented hippocampal volume, gray matter density as measured by voxel-based morphometry, and sclerosis as assessed by T2 signal) and MTL fMRI activation. In a sample of 16 LTLE patients, a greater degree of left hippocampal volume loss was related to decreased encoding-related fMRI activation in the left hippocampus for neutral words, but increased activation in the right hippocampus. The converse was evident in subjects with less left hippocampal volume loss, who showed enhanced left hippocampal activation and diminished right hippocampal activity. This shift toward right hippocampal activation was also evident with increased abnormal left hippocampal T2 signal. A similar shift toward greater right MTL activation was observed related to left amygdalar pathology (abnormal T2 signal) for encoding of emotional stimuli. Interdependence was demonstrated between hippocampal and amygdalar pathology and this presumed functional reorganization of encoding-related activation for emotional stimuli, with greater left MTL pathology related to increased right MTL activation. Interaction analyses showed that with greater left amygdalar pathology, less left hippocampal and greater right hippocampal activation was observed during encoding of emotional stimuli. With greater left hippocampal pathology, diminished left amygdalar activation and increased right amygdalar activation were noted. Taken together, these findings from Richardson et al. (2003, 2004a) support the argument for reorganization/reallocation of verbal encoding functionality to homologous regions in the nonepileptic right MTL and suggest that such reorganization may become more likely in cases where the left MTL demonstrates more severe structural pathology. Key findings from the studies discussed above are summarized in Table 7.1.

TABLE 7.1. Comparison of fMRI MTL Memory Activation in Healthy Controls and Left and Right TLE Patients

Authors	Sample (age range, yr)	fMRI memory tasks	Control findings	Left TLE findings	Right TLE findings
Detre et al. (1998)	Controls: n = 8 (18–40) LTLE: n = 7 (17–48) RTLE: n = 3 (18–37)	Complex scene encoding (visually presented stimuli)	Slight R hemispheric predominance of MTL activation.	4/7 showed R hemispheric predominance > 2 SD from HC mean. 1/7 showed R hemispheric predominance < 2 SD from HC mean. 1/7 had no hemispheric asymmetry. 1/7 had L hemispheric predominance.	2/3 showed L hemispheric predominance. 1/3 showed R hemispheric predominance.
Bellgowan et al. (1998)	Controls: N/A LTLE: n = 14 (20–57) RTLE: n = 14 (28–69)	Semantic decision making (aurally presented stimuli)	N/A	Little significant activation of L hippocampus, parahippocampal gyrus, and collateral sulcus.	Extensive activation of L hippocampus, parahippocampal gyrus, and collateral sulcus.
Dupont et al. (2000)	Controls: n = 10 (23–30) LTLE: n = 7 (18–53) RTLE: N/A	Encoding and retrieval of a supraspan word list (visually presented stimuli)	Encoding: Activation in bilateral occipital cortex, ventrolateral frontal cortex, and fusiform gyrus, left parietal and superior temporal cortex. Retrieval: Broadly similar to encoding, but slight decrease in occipital activation, and increase in spatial extent of left superior temporal and ventrolateral frontal cortex activation. New appearance of activation in left occipitotemporal regions, bilateral inferomedial temporal cortices, and left frontal medial cingular cortex.	Activation seen in bilateral parietal, medial frontal, and dorsolateral frontal cortex, and left superior temporal and ventrolateral frontal cortex. Relative to controls, showed decreases in occipital (encoding), occipitotemporal (retrieval), left temporal (retrieval), and MTL (retrieval) activation, and increased frontal activation (encoding/retrieval).	N/A

(continued)

TABLE 7.1. (continued)

Authors	Sample (age range, yr)	fMRI memory tasks	Control findings	Left TLE findings	Right TLE findings
Dupont et al. (2001)	Controls: n = 10 (23–31) LTLE: n = 7 (18–53) RTLE: N/A (same subjects as Dupont et al., 2000, 24 h later)	Retrieval of a supraspan word list (visually presented stimuli)	Decreased activation relative to 24 h prior in bilateral MTL and occipitotemporofrontal regions, but increase in bilateral parietal activation.	No activation observed in MTL, activation noted in bilateral lingual gyrus, left posterior cingulate, DLPFC, and medial frontal cortex, but overall reduction in activation relative to 24 h prior.	N/A
Jokeit et al. (2001)	Controls: n = 17 (7–63) LTLE: n = 16 (13–55) RTLE: n = 14 (14–54)	Visualization of familiar environments (Roland's hometown walking task)	Mean MTL asymmetry not significantly different from zero.	Mean MTL asymmetry showed tendency toward R hemispheric predominance.	Mean MTL asymmetry showed tendency toward L hemispheric predominance.
Golby et al. (2002)	Controls: N/A LTLE: n = 6 (26–33) RTLE: n = 3 (42–54)	Encoding of faces, words, scenes, and patterns (visually presented stimuli)	N/A	Relatively greater novelty-associated activation in the R MTL across tasks.	Relatively greater novelty-associated activation in the L MTL across tasks.
Richardson et al. (2003)	Controls: n = 12 (19–48) LTLE: n = 24 (18–54) RTLE: N/A	Semantic decision making with emotional component (visually presented stimuli)	During successful encoding MTL activation observed in L hippocampus; no R MTL activation.	During successful encoding activation in L MTL inferior to hippocampus; significant activation in R MTL. All patients had L hippocampal	N/A

204

				N/A
			sclerosis; those who also had L amygdala sclerosis showed greater R amygdala activation than patients with a normal-appearing L amygdala for successfully encoded emotional, as compared with neutral, words.	
Richardson et al. (2004a)	Controls: $n = 12$ (19–48) (apparently same controls as in Richardson et al., 2003) LTLE: $n = 16$ (18–54) RTLE: N/A	Semantic decision making with emotional component (visually presented stimuli)	Main effect of encoding in L hippocampus	
			More severe L hippocampal pathology correlated with decreased L hippocampal encoding-related activation, but enhanced R hippocampal activity. More severe L amygdalar pathology correlated with decreased L hippocampal encoding-related activation for emotional stimuli, but enhanced R hippocampal activity. More severe L hippocampal pathology correlated with decreased L amygdalar encoding-related activation for emotional stimuli, but enhanced R amygdalar activity.	

Note. fMRI, functional MRI; MTL, medial temporal lobe; TLE, temporal lobe epilepsy; HC, healthy control; DLPFC, dorsolateral prefrontal cortex.

In a novel approach to examination of the ability of fMRI MTL activation patterns to lateralize TLE (i.e., correctly identify side of seizure focus), Schacher et al. (2006) utilized a fearful faces paradigm to elicit amygdalar activity (i.e., activation of MTL structures without relying on memory processing). They studied 12 TLE patients (6 RTLE, 6 LTLE), 5 patients with epileptic foci outside the MTL, and 17 control subjects. In addition to the fearful faces paradigm, subjects also completed the hometown walking task described above to allow examination of memory-related MTL activation, as well as a verbal fluency paradigm to determine language lateralization. Reproducibility of activation patterns for the fearful faces paradigm was demonstrated through repeat imaging of 12 of the control subjects. For the control group, the fearful faces paradigm elicited bilateral superior amygdala activation across subjects, which was reproduced on repeat imaging. Similarly, for epilepsy patients with a non-MTL seizure focus, asymmetry of amygdala activation was not significantly different from zero. In contrast, for TLE patients, amygdala activation was typically lateralized contralateral to side of seizure onset. This pattern was observed in 11 of 12 patients, most of whom showed only unilateral amygdala activation. In addition, lateralization of amygdalar activation was in agreement with asymmetries in parahippocampal activation as demonstrated by the hometown walking task for 9 of 12 TLE patients. Three TLE patients showed dissociated amygdalar and parahippocampal activation. A combination of MTL activation data gained from the two fMRI paradigms successfully discriminated TLE patients from healthy controls and non-MTL epilepsy patients. These findings provide exciting insights into the ability of fMRI activation of MTL structures to lateralize TLE; future studies integrating such data with postsurgical cognitive and seizure outcomes may be helpful in developing clinically viable fMRI probes for presurgical assessment of the MTL in TLE.

Prediction of Postsurgical Memory and Seizure Outcome and Functional Reorganization

Another line of research evaluating memory functioning in TLE using fMRI has demonstrated a utility for fMRI memory probes in predicting postsurgical outcome following temporal lobectomy in terms of seizure freedom and cognitive integrity. Previous research has demonstrated that postsurgical memory outcome can be predicted by several variables. Predictive brain structural factors include presurgical hippocampal volume (Richardson et al., 2004b) and severity of hippocampal sclerosis on presurgical structural MRI images (Trennery et al., 1993) and on pathology of the resected tissue (Hermann et al., 1992; Sass et al., 1994), while functional predictors of postsurgical memory outcome include presurgical performance on neuropsychological assessment (Richardson et al., 2004b; Helmstaedter & Elger, 1996; Jokeit et al., 1997) and presurgical IAT memory performance (Jokeit et al., 1997; Bell et al., 2000; Loring et al., 1995). Predictors of seizure outcome following MTL resection have included interictal brain hypometabolism on functional imaging (Manno et al., 1994; Weinand & Carter, 1994) as well as IAT abnormalities (Sperling et al., 1994; Loring et al., 1994). Demonstration of fMRI predictors of postsurgical seizure and cognitive outcome will further strengthen the utility of this technique as a clinical tool, and a few studies have provided valuable data toward this goal.

Killgore et al. (1999) reported that presurgical fMRI memory lateralization predicted postsurgical seizure status as effectively as IAT in a sample of eight TLE patients (5 LTLE, 3 RTLE). These patients were included in the sample studied in Detre et al. (1998), in which they completed the scene-encoding task described above. Seizure freedom 1 yr postsurgery demonstrated an association with presurgical asymmetry of MTL fMRI activation, such that higher activation in the nonepileptogenic hemisphere was positively related to seizure freedom. Comparison of the predictive power of fMRI and IAT results revealed that both methods correctly classified the seizure outcome of 75% of subjects when used alone, but classification improved to 100% when information from fMRI and IAT LIs was combined. These findings point to the potential predictive utility of fMRI memory activation patterns in predicting seizure freedom, but also suggest that fMRI and the IAT provide complementary information.

This group has also demonstrated a relationship between MTL fMRI activation and postsurgical recognition memory changes (Rabin et al., 2002, 2004; Casasanto et al., 2001). In a sample of 11 TLE patients (8 LTLE, 3 RTLE) who underwent anteromesial temporal lobectomy, Casasanto et al. (2001) demonstrated a significant positive correlation between presurgical fMRI memory LI in the MTL during scene encoding and change in recognition memory performance pre- to postsurgery. In all but one subject, patients with greater presurgical MTL memory task-related activation in the non-surgical hemisphere showed improved memory performance after surgery, whereas those with greater MTL activation ipsilateral to the seizure focus showed a postsurgical memory decline. These findings were then replicated in larger samples (Rabin et al., 2002, 2004). In these subsequent studies MTL LI from presurgical fMRI again correlated significantly with postsurgical recognition memory change. In addition, absolute MTL activation ipsilateral to seizure focus showed a significant negative correlation with memory change, whereas contralateral activation showed no correlation. In contrast, no significant correlation was observed between IAT laterality and memory outcomes. These results are consistent with previous neuropsychological and pathology findings suggesting that greater presurgical structural and functional integrity of the epileptogenic MTL is related to increased postsurgical functional deficits.

Szaflarski et al. (2004) present data from 19 healthy control subjects and 6 TLE patients (3 LTLE, 3 RTLE) who later underwent temporal lobectomy. This study used a somewhat different scene-encoding paradigm from that described above, designed to mimic the stimuli in use in the center's IAT protocol. Consistent with prior research, healthy controls demonstrated bilateral MTL activation during scene encoding, and greater lateralization of activation was observed in the TLE group. The degree of concordance between IAT and presurgical fMRI memory lateralization was lower than that described by other studies, however, with agreement observed in only 50% of patients, all of whom were seizure-free postsurgery. In two of the cases with disagreement between IAT and fMRI results, fMRI demonstrated symmetric MTL activation, whereas IAT demonstrated impaired memory functioning in the epileptogenic hemisphere; both of these subjects had persistent seizures postsurgery (Engel class III). In the remaining case, fMRI lateralized MTL dysfunction to the right hemisphere, and IAT lateralized dysfunction to the left. Differences in the concordance between IAT and fMRI data in this study and that found in other similar work may be attributable to differences in activation task and/or method of construction and interpretation of LIs. Comparison of memory performance pre- and postsurgery in the TLE group was not available.

Richardson et al. (2004b) examined the relationship of presurgical fMRI activation patterns to postoperative memory functioning in a subset of 10 of the right-handed patients with LTLE and mesial–temporal sclerosis reported in (Richardson et al., 2003, 2004a), all of whom were seizure-free postsurgery. Their data demonstrated that postsurgical memory decline was strongly predicted by a multiple regression model including left hippocampal volume, presurgical verbal memory, and an LI comparing left and right hippocampal fMRI activation during successful encoding of neutral words. Overall, presurgical fMRI assessment of verbal memory encoding was in fact the strongest independent predictor of postoperative memory performance, above preoperative verbal memory on neuropsychological testing and left hippocampal volume. Consistent with prior work suggesting that greater functional integrity of tissue ipsilateral to seizure focus leads to greater postsurgical cognitive decline, these authors found that greater fMRI activation during verbal memory encoding in the left, relative to the right, hippocampus was correlated with a higher degree of postsurgical verbal memory decline. It is important to note that the positive predictive value of fMRI data for memory decline was meaningful at the individual level, using standard clinical memory measures as the dependent variable, providing early evidence that fMRI memory probes can show clinical utility.

In RTLE, Janszky et al. (2005) examined the ability of presurgical fMRI activation patterns to predict postsurgical nonverbal memory outcome in 16 patients. Using the mental navigation task discussed above (hometown walk), they found a correlation between presurgical fMRI lateralization and postsurgical memory outcome (change in nonverbal memory retention score pre- to postsurgery), with relatively reduced MTL activation in the epileptogenic hemisphere (greater activation in the nonepileptic MTL) correlating with better memory outcome. Although memory change pre- to postsurgery was not significant at the overall group level, it is interesting to note that in this sample all patients with greater activation in the MTL ipsilateral to seizure focus or symmetric MTL activation demonstrated decreased memory performance after surgery. These findings provide useful data to support the clinical utility of fMRI in presurgical evaluation of RTLE patients. As some epilepsy surgery centers do not routinely perform IAT in patients with RTLE, particularly those who are right-handed (presuming left-hemisphere language dominance), or who have an apparent right-hemisphere lesion on structural MRI, the ability to use fMRI to predict postsurgical memory outcome may prove to be a very valuable clinical tool.

Theoretical and Clinical Implications

It is of great theoretical interest to examine the ways in which the fMRI studies reviewed above support or refute prior models of cognitive outcome following temporal lobectomy. Two mechanisms for explaining memory changes following temporal lobectomy have previously been proposed: that of functional reserve and that of functional adequacy (Chelune, 1995). The functional reserve model puts forth that postoperative memory functioning is dependent on the ability of the nonepileptic MTL to support memory (i.e., greater support of memory in the MTL contralateral to seizure focus presurgically should predict better memory outcome). In contrast, the functional adequacy model supposes that postsurgical memory deficits are related to the extent to which the epileptic MTL supports memory preoperatively (i.e., greater memory support ipsilateral to seizure focus predicts poorer memory outcome). These two hypotheses are not mutually exclusive, and the data presented above appear to offer some support for both theories.

Demonstration of the reliability of techniques for evoking MTL activation in TLE patients at the level of the individual may in the future allow fMRI to replace the IAT for memory assessment. In a recent study examining relational versus novelty processing in healthy control subjects, Binder et al. (2005) demonstrated a dissociation between anterior and posterior hippocampal activation in response to stimulus-processing demands. In prior work, Saykin et al. (1999) likewise demonstrated a dissociation between anterior and posterior MTL regions for memory processing of novel versus familiar stimuli. Such findings suggest that fMRI probes can be designed not only to target the hippocampus, but to elicit activation in specific hippocampal subregions, a feature that could be of great clinical utility in TLE, in which the anterior hippocampus has been most implicated in epileptogenesis. Data from pathological and lesion studies and functional neuroimaging (PET, fMRI) have provided conflicting conclusions regarding the anterior–posterior division of encoding and retrieval processes in the MTL (see Saykin, 1999, for further discussion), however, and as yet there has not been sufficient replication of consistent activation patterns in hippocampal subregions using fMRI probes to provide data of certain clinical validity.

Overall then, stronger lateralization of fMRI memory task-related activation has been shown to be related to side of seizure focus (greater activation contralateral to seizure focus), as well as to postsurgical seizure and cognitive outcome (better outcome when presurgical fMRI memory LI favors the nonsurgical hemisphere). These findings suggest sensitivity of fMRI to brain dysfunction within the epileptogenic zone, which has great potential utility for surgical planning. Taken together, the above studies suggest that some fMRI memory paradigms may be suitable for assessment of memory lateralization at the level of the individual patient, leading to the eventual replacement of the IAT, following replication of the findings described above in larger samples. Given the evidence for material specificity of hemispheric MTL functioning in memory encoding in TLE, it will be beneficial for future studies to include assessment of memory across multiple stimulus modalities in the same patients. This will allow the development of fMRI paradigms with increased sensitivity to lateralize and localize brain regions critical for memory functioning, which can then be used to assist in forecasting likely postsurgical outcomes in TLE.

Conclusion

fMRI of language and memory processing has provided important insights in TLE that may prove informative in other neurological and neurodevelopmental disorders. Research to date has demonstrated that fMRI language and memory probes are available that will likely one day serve to replace the IAT for presurgical lateralization and localization of cognitive functions. In addition, a recent cost analysis has demonstrated considerable savings of total direct costs for fMRI over IAT (Medina et al., 2004). At present, based on the simple criteria of language lateralization, fMRI appears essentially capable of assuming the functions of the IAT, and has been shown to reliably lateralize language with similar effectiveness. However, fMRI language mapping does not yet have the proven reliability and validity of other presurgical assessment techniques used to set the surgical margin (e.g., direct cortical stimulation) to prevent acquired deficits, and must therefore still be considered part of a comprehensive presurgical assessment battery. Here it is also important to acknowledge that although fMRI is thought to demonstrate activation of regions important for a given cognitive process, some regions may be active that are not directly related to the "core" function being assessed, and still other regions underlying the target cognitive process may not demonstrate significant activation at the chosen threshold. This further underscores the importance of direct cortical stimulation at the stage of setting the surgical margin.

In terms of memory, the cumulative body of research is not yet sufficient to allow fMRI to supplant the IAT in terms of predicting postsurgical functional outcome. In this respect, then, the IAT remains the "gold standard" for presurgical evaluation. It is important to recognize, however, that neither the IAT nor fMRI procedures have been subjected to the rigorous research standards currently required by evidenced-based medicine practices. That is, neither the IAT nor fMRI mapping techniques have been implemented in the context of randomized, controlled clinical trials to examine the effectiveness of outcome predictions. Although the clinical and ethical rationale for the lack of such studies is evident, it is important to recognize that thorough, systematic assessment of postsurgical outcome data in relation to presurgical localization data for language and memory localization has not been adequately completed either for the IAT or for fMRI. fMRI paradigms likely to successfully replace the IAT will almost certainly include multiple language and memory tasks, in order to elicit activation of broad neural networks that include both frontal and temporal language and memory circuitry. Some studies have begun to examine such combined task approaches (e.g., Deblaere et al., 2002), though no consensus on the tasks to be used is apparent from the available literature as yet. In addition to the potential ability of fMRI to replace the IAT, fMRI research has provided important information regarding potential reorganization of cognition away from the epileptogenic MTL, as well as preliminary data suggesting utility for predicting postsurgical seizure freedom and cognitive outcome.

It is important to recognize the technical and clinical considerations that remain critical when using fMRI both in clinical research and in direct clinical applications, some of which have been alluded to in this chapter, and which are discussed in more detail elsewhere (McDonald et al., 2006). Technical considerations include the choice of brain regions to be imaged (e.g., whole brain versus region of interest approach), as well as the specific scan parameters (imaging plane, slice thickness, positioning) chosen. The effects of brain anatomy on fMRI activation data can also be significant, including both problems common across subjects (e.g., signal dropout in important brain regions of interest, such as the temporal lobes) and those resulting from individual anatomic variation, which may affect fMRI activation patterns (e.g., arteriovenous malformations, large-space-occupying lesions).

The statistical significance threshold chosen for a given analysis can also critically affect the conclusions drawn from fMRI data, a particularly important issue for data that are to be used in making surgical decisions. As discussed above, manipulation of statistical thresholds can increase or decrease observed activation, thereby potentially affecting LI values. Consideration of the threshold to be used is particularly important in clinical populations, including epilepsy, as some studies have described global differences in the number of significantly activated voxels between patient groups and healthy control subjects. Similarly, as the overall level of activation may vary with age, consideration must be given to varying statistical thresholds for younger versus older subjects. This issue will become increasingly important as consideration is given to the use of fMRI in setting surgical margins in the future.

Specifically with regard to epilepsy, few studies to date have explicitly addressed the potential effects of antiepileptic medications on fMRI activation patterns, despite the known or presumed direct effects of anticonvulsants on cerebral blood flow and metabolism (Ketter et al., 1999; Matheja et al., 2000; Theodore, 1988, 2000; Theodore et al., 1989). In addition, few studies to date have had adequate power to address such potentially confounding issues as sex differences in language lateralization, which have the potential to affect the interpretation of findings for fMRI language mapping. It is also important to recognize the difficulty inherent in attempts to compare directly the data gathered from fMRI with that from IAT, given the differences in aspects of cognitive functioning typically assessed using these techniques.

Finally, implementation of fMRI protocols and data analysis remain quite time-consuming, even though many preprocessing steps and procedures can be automated. This amount of professional time and expertise may preclude the routine use of fMRI for clinical purposes in some centers, particularly in the absence of insurance reimbursement procedures for the efforts of professional staff members, unless clinical studies are being conducted under the auspices of a research protocol. The issue of reimbursement for clinical fMRI will, we hope, soon be resolved. In early 2006, new current procedural terminology (CPT) codes for fMRI were being evaluated by the Centers for Medicare and Medicaid Services (CMS). A survey was recently conducted to determine the relative value units (RVUs) that will be associated with this procedure. When fMRI becomes a more routine, reimbursable diagnostic and treatment planning procedure, significant growth and evolution in approaches for the use of fMRI in epilepsy and other disorders can be expected. At the same time, more research is warranted to examine the sensitivity and specificity of various available fMRI probes of language and memory for diagnostic and prognostic applications.

ACKNOWLEDGMENTS

This work was funded in part by members of the Partnership for Pediatric Epilepsy Research, which includes the American Epilepsy Society, the Epilepsy Foundation, the Epilepsy Project, Fight against Childhood Epilepsy and Seizures, and Parents against Childhood Epilepsy. Aspects of this work were also supported by the National Alliance for Medical Image Computing (National Institutes of Health Grant No. U54 EB005149), as well as the Hitchcock Foundation and the Ira DeCamp Foundation. We thank our colleagues in the Department of Diagnostic Radiology and the Epilepsy Center and Epilepsy Surgery Program at Dartmouth–Hitchcock Medical Center for their contributions to the data presented in this chapter.

REFERENCES

Adcock, J. E., Wise, R. G., Oxbury, J. M., et al. (2003). Quantitative fMRI assessment of the differences in lateralization of language-related brain activation in patients with temporal lobe epilepsy. *NeuroImage, 18,* 423–438.

American Academy of Neurology. (1996). Assessment: Neuropsychological testing of adults. Considerations for neurologists. Report of the Therapeutics and Technology Assessment Subcommittee of the American Academy of Neurology. *Neurology*, *47*, 592–599.

Anderson, K. C., Brown, C. P., & Tallal, P. (1993). Developmental language disorders: Evidence for a basic processing deficit. *Current Opinion in Neurology and Neurosurgery*, *6*, 98–106.

Babb, T., & Brown, W. J. (1987). Pathological findings in epilepsy. In J. Engel (Ed.), *Surgical treatment of the epilepsies* (pp. 511–540). New York: Raven Press.

Baciu, M., Kahane, P., Minotti, L., et al. (2001). Functional MRI assessment of the hemispheric predominance for language in epileptic patients using a simple rhyme detection task. *Epileptic Disorders*, *3*, 117–124.

Bahn, M. M., Lin, W., Silbergeld, D. L., et al. (1997). Localization of language cortices by functional MR imaging compared with intracarotid amobarbital hemispheric sedation. *American Journal of Roentgenology*, *169*, 575–579.

Bell, B. D., Davies, K. G., Haltiner, A. M., et al. (2000). Intracarotid amobarbital procedure and prediction of postoperative memory in patients with left temporal lobe epilepsy and hippocampal sclerosis. *Epilepsia*, *41*, 992–997.

Bell, G. S., & Sander, J. W. (2001). The epidemiology of epilepsy: The size of the problem. *Seizure*, *10*, 306–314.

Bellgowan, P. S., Binder, J. R., Swanson, S. J., et al. (1998). Side of seizure focus predicts left medial temporal lobe activation during verbal encoding. *Neurology*, *51*, 479–484.

Benbadis, S. R., Binder, J. R., Swanson, S. J., et al. (1998). Is speech arrest during Wada testing a valid method for determining hemispheric representation of language? *Brain and Language*, *65*, 441–446.

Benson, R. R., Fitzgerald, D. B., LeSueur, L. L., et al. (1999). Language dominance determined by whole brain functional MRI in patients with brain lesions. *Neurology*, *52*, 798–809.

Binder, J. R., Bellgowan, P. S., Hammeke, T. A., et al. (2005). A comparison of two FMRI protocols for eliciting hippocampal activation. *Epilepsia*, *46*, 1061–1070.

Binder, J. R., Swanson, S. J., Hammeke, T. A., et al. (1996). Determination of language dominance using functional MRI: A comparison with the Wada test. *Neurology*, *46*, 978–984.

Briellmann, R. S., Mitchell, L. A., Waites, A. B., et al. (2003). Correlation between language organization and diffusion tensor abnormalities in refractory partial epilepsy. *Epilepsia*, *44*, 1541–1545.

Carpentier, A., Pugh, K. R., Westerveld, M., et al. (2001). Functional MRI of language processing: Dependence on input modality and temporal lobe epilepsy. *Epilepsia*, *42*, 1241–1254.

Casasanto, D. J., Glosser, G., Killgore, W. D. S., et al. (2001). Presurgical fMRI predicts memory outcome following anterior temporal lobectomy. *Journal of the International Neuropsychological Society*, *7*, 183.

Chelune, G. J. (1995). Hippocampal adequacy versus functional reserve: Predicting memory functions following temporal lobectomy. *Archives of Clinical Neuropsychology*, *10*, 413–432.

Deblaere, K., Backes, W. H., Hofman, P., et al. (2002). Developing a comprehensive presurgical functional MRI protocol for patients with intractable temporal lobe epilepsy: A pilot study. *Neuroradiology*, *44*, 667–673.

Desmond, J. E., Sum, J. M., Wagner, A. D., et al. (1995). Functional MRI measurement of language lateralization in Wada-tested patients. *Brain*, *118*, 1411–1419.

Detre, J. A., Maccotta, L., King, D., et al. (1998). Functional MRI lateralization of memory in temporal lobe epilepsy. *Neurology*, *50*, 926–932.

Devinsky, O., Perrine, K., Llinas, R., et al. (1993). Anterior temporal language areas in patients with early onset of temporal lobe epilepsy. *Annals of Neurology*, *34*, 727–732.

Dupont, S., Samson, Y., Van de Moortele, P. F., et al. (2001). Delayed verbal memory retrieval: A functional MRI study in epileptic patients with structural lesions of the left medial temporal lobe. *NeuroImage*, *14*, 995–1003.

Dupont, S., Van de Moortele, P. F., Samson, S., et al. (2000). Episodic memory in left temporal lobe epilepsy: A functional MRI study. *Brain*, *123*, 1722–1732.

Fernandez, G., Specht, K., Weis, S., et al. (2003). Intrasubject reproducibility of presurgical language lateralization and mapping using fMRI. *Neurology*, *60*, 969–975.

Gabrieli, J. D., Brewer, J. B., Desmond, J. E., et al. (1997). Separate neural bases of two fundamental memory processes in the human medial temporal lobe. *Science*, *276*, 264–266.

Gaillard, W. D., Balsamo, L., Xu, B., et al. (2002). Language dominance in partial epilepsy patients identified with an fMRI reading task. *Neurology*, *59*, 256–265.

Gleissner, U., Helmstaedter, C., Schramm, J., et al. (2002). Memory outcome after selective amygdalohippocampectomy: A study in 140 patients with temporal lobe epilepsy. *Epilepsia*, *43*, 87–95.

Glosser, G., Saykin, A., Deutsch, G., et al. (1995). Patterns of reorganization of memory functions within and between cerebral hemispheres as assessed by the intracarotid amobarbital test. *Neuropsychology*, *9*, 449–456.

Golby, A. J., Poldrack, R. A., Brewer, J. B., et al. (2001). Material-specific lateralization in the medial temporal lobe and prefrontal cortex during memory encoding. *Brain*, *124*, 1841–1854.

Golby, A. J., Poldrack, R. A., Illes, J., et al. (2002). Memory lateralization in medial temporal lobe epilepsy assessed by functional MRI. *Epilepsia*, *43*, 855–863.

Goldstein, L. H., & Polkey, C. E. (1993). Short-term cognitive changes after unilateral temporal lobectomy or unilateral amygdalo-hippocampectomy for the relief of temporal lobe epilepsy. *Journal of Neurology, Neurosurgery and Psychiatry*, *56*, 135–140.

Hamandi, K., Salek-Haddadi, A., Fish, D. R., et al. (2004). EEG/functional MRI in epilepsy: The Queen Square Experience. *Journal of Clinical Neurophysiology*, *21*, 241–248.

Hauser, A. W. (1998). Incidence and prevalence. In H. J. Engel & T. A. Pedley (Eds.), *Epilepsy: A comprehensive textbook* (pp. 47–57). Philadelphia: Lippincott-Raven.

Helmstaedter, C., & Elger, C. E. (1996). Cognitive consequences of two-thirds anterior temporal lobectomy on verbal memory in 144 patients: A three-month follow-up study. *Epilepsia*, *37*, 171–180.

Helmstaedter, C., Elger, C. E., Hufnagel, A., et al. (1996). Different effects of left anterior temporal lobectomy, selective amygdalohippocampectomy, and temporal cortical lesionectomy on verbal learning, memory, and recognition. *Journal of Epilepsy*, *9*, 39–45.

Helmstaedter, C., Grunwald, T., Lehnertz, K., et al. (1997). Differential involvement of left temporolateral and temporomesial structures in verbal declarative learning and memory: Evidence from temporal lobe epilepsy. *Brain and Cognition, 35,* 110–131.

Hermann, B. P., Perrine, K., Chelune, G. J., et al. (1999). Visual confrontation naming following left anterior temporal lobectomy: A comparison of surgical approaches. *Neuropsychology, 13,* 3–9.

Hermann, B. P., Seidenberg, M., Haltiner, A., et al. (1995). Relationship of age at onset, chronologic age, and adequacy of preoperative performance to verbal memory change after anterior temporal lobectomy. *Epilepsia, 36,* 137–145.

Hermann, B. P., Wyler, A. R., Somes, G., et al. (1994). Dysnomia after left anterior temporal lobectomy without functional mapping: Frequency and correlates. *Neurosurgery, 35,* 52–56.

Hermann, B. P., Wyler, A. R., Somes, G., et al. (1992). Pathological status of the mesial temporal lobe predicts memory outcome from left anterior temporal lobectomy. *Neurosurgery, 31,* 652–656.

Hertz-Pannier, L., Gaillard, W. D., Mott, S. H., et al. (1997). Noninvasive assessment of language dominance in children and adolescents with functional MRI: A preliminary study. *Neurology, 48,* 1003–1012.

Hunter, K. E., Blaxton, T. A., Bookheimer, S. Y., et al. (1999). (15)O water positron emission tomography in language localization: A study comparing positron emission tomography visual and computerized region of interest analysis with the Wada test. *Annals of Neurology, 45,* 662–665.

Janszky, J., Jokeit, H., Kontopoulou, K., et al. (2005). Functional MRI predicts memory performance after right mesiotemporal epilepsy surgery. *Epilepsia, 46,* 244–250.

Jokeit, H., Ebner, A., Holthausen, H., et al. (1997). Individual prediction of change in delayed recall of prose passages after left-sided anterior temporal lobectomy. *Neurology, 49,* 481–487.

Jokeit, H., Okujava, M., & Woermann, F. G. (2001). Memory fMRI lateralizes temporal lobe epilepsy. *Neurology, 57,* 1786–1793.

Ketter, T. A., Kimbrell, T. A., George, M. S., et al. (1999). Baseline cerebral hypermetabolism associated with carbamazepine response, and hypometabolism with nimodipine response in mood disorders. *Biological Psychiatry, 46,* 1364–1374.

Killgore, W. D., Glosser, G., Casasanto, D. J., et al. (1999). Functional MRI and the Wada test provide complementary information for predicting post-operative seizure control. *Seizure, 8,* 450–455.

Kurthen, M., Helmstaedter, C., Linke, D. B., et al. (1994). Quantitative and qualitative evaluation of patterns of cerebral language dominance: An amobarbital study. *Brain and Language, 46,* 536–564.

Kurthen, M., Helmstaedter, C., Linke, D. B., et al. (1992). Interhemispheric dissociation of expressive and receptive language functions in patients with complex-partial seizures: An amobarbital study. *Brain and Language, 43,* 694–712.

Lehéricy, S., Cohen, L., Bazin, B., et al. (2000). Functional MR evaluation of temporal and frontal language dominance compared with the Wada test. *Neurology, 54,* 1625–1633.

Lemieux, L. (2004). Electroencephalography-correlated functional MR imaging studies of epileptic activity. *Neuroimaging Clinics of North America, 14,* 487–506.

Liégeois, F., Connelly, A., Salmond, C. H., et al. (2002). A direct test for lateralization of language activation using fMRI: Comparison with invasive assessments in children with epilepsy. *NeuroImage, 17,* 1861–1867.

Loring, D. W., Meador, K. J., Lee, G. P., et al. (1994). Wada memory performance predicts seizure outcome following anterior temporal lobectomy. *Neurology, 44,* 2322–2324.

Loring, D. W., Meador, K. J., Lee, G. P., et al. (1995). Wada memory asymmetries predict verbal memory decline after anterior temporal lobectomy. *Neurology, 45,* 1329–1333.

Manno, E. M., Sperling, M. R., Ding, X., et al. (1994). Predictors of outcome after anterior temporal lobectomy: Positron emission tomography. *Neurology, 44,* 2331–2336.

Matheja, P., Weckesser, M., Debus, O., et al. (2000). Drug-induced changes in cerebral glucose consumption in bifrontal epilepsy. *Epilepsia, 41,* 588–593.

McDonald, B. C., Saykin, A. J., Williams, J. M., et al. (2006). MRI Wada test: Prospects for presurgical mapping of language and memory. In S. H. Faro & F. B. Mohamed (Eds.), *Functional MRI: Basic principles and clinical applications* (pp. 279–315). New York: Springer-Verlag.

Medina, L. S., Aguirre, E., Bernal, B., et al. (2004). Functional MR imaging versus Wada test for evaluation of language lateralization: Cost analysis. *Radiology, 230,* 49–54.

National Institutes of Health. (1990). Surgery for epilepsy. *NIH Consensus Statement Online, 8,* 1–20.

Paglioli, E., Palmini, A., Portuguez, M., et al. (2006). Seizure and memory outcome following temporal lobe surgery: Selective compared with nonselective approaches for hippocampal sclerosis. *Journal of Neurosurgery, 104,* 70–78.

Pardo, J. V., & Fox, P. T. (1993). Preoperative assessment of the cerebral hemispheric dominance for language with CBF PET. *Human Brain Mapping, 1,* 57–68.

Rabin, M. L., Narayan, V. M., Kimberg, D. Y., et al. (2004). Functional MRI predicts post-surgical memory following temporal lobectomy. *Brain, 127,* 2286–2298.

Rabin, M. L., Salvucci, A. E., Tang, K., et al. (2002). Functional magnetic resonance imaging predicts postsurgical memory outcome in temporal lobe epilepsy patients. *Epilepsia, 43,* 90.

Ramsey, N. F., Sommer, I. E. C., Rutten, G. J., et al. (2001). Combined analysis of language tasks in fMRI improves assessment of hemispheric dominance for language functions in individual subjects. *NeuroImage, 13,* 719–733.

Rausch, R. (1992). Role of the neuropsychological evaluation and the intracarotid sodium amobarbital procedure in the surgical treatment for epilepsy. *Epilepsy Research Supplement, 5,* 77–86.

Richardson, M. P., Strange, B. A., & Dolan, R. J. (2004a). Encoding of emotional memories depends on amygdala and hippocampus and their interactions. *Nature Neuroscience, 7,* 278–285.

Richardson, M. P., Strange, B. A., Duncan, J. S., et al. (2003). Preserved verbal memory function in left medial temporal pathology involves reorganisation of function to right medial temporal lobe. *NeuroImage, 20*(Suppl. 1), S112–S119.

Richardson, M. P., Strange, B. A., Thompson, P. J., et al. (2004b). Pre-operative verbal memory fMRI predicts post-operative memory decline after left temporal lobe resection. *Brain, 127,* 2419–2426.

Ries, M. L., Boop, F. A., Griebel, M. L., et al. (2004). Functional MRI and Wada determination of language lateralization: A case of crossed dominance. *Epilepsia*, *45*, 85–89.

Risse, G. L., Gates, J. R., & Fangman, M. C. (1997). A reconsideration of bilateral language representation based on the intracarotid amobarbital procedure. *Brain and Cognition*, *33*, 118–132.

Rutten, G. J., Ramsey, N. F., van Rijen, P. C., et al. (2002). fMRI-determined language lateralization in patients with unilateral or mixed language dominance according to the Wada test. *NeuroImage*, *17*, 447–460.

Sabbah, P., Chassoux, F., Leveque, C., et al. (2003). Functional MR imaging in assessment of language dominance in epileptic patients. *NeuroImage*, *18*, 460–467.

Sabsevitz, D. S., Swanson, S. J., Hammeke, T. A., et al. (2002). Predicting naming deficits following left anterior temporal lobectomy using fMRI. *Journal of the International Neuropsychological Society*, *8*, 317.

Sabsevitz, D. S., Swanson, S. J., Hammeke, T. A., et al. (2003). Use of preoperative functional neuroimaging to predict language deficits from epilepsy surgery. *Neurology*, *60*, 1788–1792.

Sander, J. W., Hart, Y. M., Johnson, A. L., et al. (1990). National general practice study of epilepsy: Newly diagnosed epileptic seizures in a general population. *Lancet*, *336*, 1267–1271.

Sander, J. W. A. S., & Shorvon, S. D. (1996). Epidemiology of the epilepsies. *Journal of Neurology, Neurosurgery and Psychiatry*, *61*, 433–443.

Sass, K. J., Westerveld, M., Buchanan, C. P., et al. (1994). Degree of hippocampal neuron loss determines severity of verbal memory decrease after left anteromesiotemporal lobectomy. *Epilepsia*, *35*, 1179–1186.

Saykin, A. J., Johnson, S. C., Flashman, L. A., et al. (1999). Functional differentiation of medial temporal and frontal regions involved in processing novel and familiar words: An fMRI study. *Brain*, *122*, 1963–1971.

Saykin, A. J., Stafiniak, P., Robinson, L. J., et al. (1995). Language before and after temporal lobectomy: Specificity of acute changes and relation to early risk factors. *Epilepsia*, *36*, 1071–1077.

Schacher, M., Haemmerle, B., Woermann, F. G., et al. (2006). Amygdala fMRI lateralizes temporal lobe epilepsy. *Neurology*, *66*, 81–87.

Sperling, M. R., Saykin, A. J., Glosser, G., et al. (1994). Predictors of outcome after anterior temporal lobectomy: The intracarotid amobarbital test. *Neurology*, *44*, 2325–2330.

Springer, J. A., Binder, J. R., Hammeke, T. A., et al. (1999). Language dominance in neurologically normal and epilepsy subjects: A functional MRI study. *Brain*, *122*, 2033–2046.

Stafiniak, P., Saykin, A. J., Sperling, M. R., et al. (1990). Acute naming deficits following dominant temporal lobectomy: Prediction by age at first risk for seizures. *Neurology*, *40*, 1509–1512.

Stern, C. E., Corkin, S., Gonzalez, R. G., et al. (1996). The hippocampal formation participates in novel picture encoding: Evidence from functional magnetic resonance imaging. *Proceedings of the National Academy of Sciences of the United States of America*, *93*, 8660–8665.

Swanson, S. J., Binder, J. R., Possing, E. T., et al. (2002). fMRI language laterality during a semantic task: Age of onset and side of seizure focus effects. *Journal of the International Neuropsychological Society*, *8*, 222.

Szaflarski, J. P., Binder, J. R., Possing, E. T., et al. (2002). Language lateralization in left-handed and ambidextrous people: fMRI data. *Neurology, 59,* 238–244.

Szaflarski, J. P., Holland, S. K., Schmithorst, V. J., et al. (2004). High-resolution functional MRI at 3T in healthy and epilepsy subjects: Hippocampal activation with picture encoding task. *Epilepsy and Behavior, 5,* 244–252.

Tatum, W. O., IV, Benbadis, S. R., & Vale, F. L. (2000). The neurosurgical treatment of epilepsy. *Archives of Family Medicine, 9,* 1142–1147.

Theodore, W. H. (1988). Antiepileptic drugs and cerebral glucose metabolism. *Epilepsia, 29,* S48–S55.

Theodore, W. H. (2000). Therapeutics: Pharmacologic. In J. C. Mazziotta, A. W. Toga, & R. S. J. Frackowiak (Eds.), *Brain mapping: The disorders* (pp. 599–612). San Diego: Academic Press.

Theodore, W. H., Bromfield, E., & Onorati, L. (1989). The effect of carbamazepine on cerebral glucose metabolism. *Annals of Neurology, 25,* 516–520.

Thivard, L., Hombrouck, J., du Montcel, S. T., et al. (2005). Productive and perceptive language reorganization in temporal lobe epilepsy. *NeuroImage, 24,* 841–851.

Trenerry, M. R., Jack, C. R., Jr., Ivnik, R. J., et al. (1993). MRI hippocampal volumes and memory function before and after temporal lobectomy. *Neurology, 43,* 1800–1805.

Weinand, M. E., & Carter, L. P. (1994). Surface cortical cerebral blood flow monitoring and single photon emission computed tomography: Prognostic factors for selecting temporal lobectomy candidates. *Seizure, 3,* 55–59.

Wiebe, S., Blume, W. T., Girvin, J. P., et al. (2001). Effectiveness and efficiency of surgery for temporal lobe epilepsy study group: A randomized, controlled trial of surgery for temporal-lobe epilepsy. *New England Journal of Medicine, 345,* 311–318.

Williamson, P. D., Weiser, H. G., & Delgado-Escueta, A. (1987). Clinical characteristics of partial seizures. In J. Engel (Ed.), *Surgical treatment of the epilepsies* (pp. 101–120). New York: Raven Press.

Woermann, F. G., Jokeit, H., Luerding, R., et al. (2003). Language lateralization by Wada test and fMRI in 100 patients with epilepsy. *Neurology, 61,* 699–701.

Worthington, C., Vincent, D. J., Bryant, A. E., et al. (1997). Comparison of functional magnetic resonance imaging for language localization and intracarotid speech amytal testing in presurgical evaluation for intractable epilepsy: Preliminary results. *Stereotactic and Functional Neurosurgery, 69,* 197–201.

Yetkin, F. Z., Swanson, S., Fischer, M., et al. (1998). Functional MR of frontal lobe activation: Comparison with Wada language results. *American Journal of Neuroradiology, 19,* 1095–1098.

CHAPTER 8

Functional Neuroimaging of Impaired Language in Aphasia

Bruce Crosson

This chapter focuses on imaging of language in patients with acquired aphasia, specifically in patients whose aphasias are caused by stroke. Aphasia, of course, is an impairment of language functions caused by brain damage or disease. Aphasia is associated with roughly 25% of strokes, and only 21% of stroke patients with acute aphasia eventually recover normal language function (Kertesz & McCabe, 1977; Mayo, 1993; Paolucci et al., 1996). Even subtle aphasia substantially limits the employability of stroke survivors and degrades quality of life by limiting intellectual activity. More severe aphasia poses a major obstacle to communication with friends, family, and caregivers and profoundly degrades the role of affected patients in family life. The study of aphasia with functional imaging can help us not only to understand how language functions are organized after dominant-hemisphere damage, but also to determine how brain mechanisms reorganize during rehabilitation. Moreover, functional imaging can be used as a tool to develop conceptually driven aphasia treatments. When a therapeutic strategy is based on a theoretical model of how treatment changes the neural substrates of language, functional imaging can be used to assess the conceptual underpinnings of treatment. In other words, functional imaging can help assess whether a treatment engages or suppresses activity in different neural components of the language system, as the conceptual treatment model predicts. Treatment strategies then can be modified to address discrepancies between the theoretical model and findings. Addressing such questions demands that functional imaging be used early in treatment development so that treatments can be adequately refined based on the feedback obtained from functional imaging studies before proceeding to large-scale, multicenter trials of treatment effectiveness. Used in this way, functional imaging can enhance the efficiency of treatment development, ultimately saving research and health care dollars and leading to more effective treatments to mitigate the effects of aphasia. Such utilization of functional imaging is a paradigm shift from the more academic exercise of describing impaired language systems, or even changes in brain organization from pre- to posttreatment. It will require that aphasia researchers aggressively set about optimizing imaging techniques to meet this challenge.

To address these issues, this chapter is divided into two sections. The first section seeks to define the critical issues in functional neuroimaging studies of aphasia. It reviews and assesses currently available literature on recovery from and rehabilitation of aphasia, and discusses potential directions for future research that not only will enhance our knowledge of how the language system is organized in patients with aphasia but also will contribute to effective treatment development. The second section addresses the substantial technical challenges for imaging language functions in aphasia. In particular, some attention is paid to how to image spoken language in patients with aphasia using functional magnetic resonance imaging (fMRI). Because of the wide availability of magnetic resonance imaging (MRI) scanners and the presence of an endogenous contrast, blood-oxygen-level-dependent (BOLD) contrast, fMRI has become the most widely used functional imaging technique for the study of cognition. It has enormous potential to contribute to the field of aphasia, but technical problems must be overcome before this potential can be fully realized. Most particularly, most fMRI studies of language production to date have used silent production to study language output in aphasia because of the technical challenges involved in the spoken generation of language. Silent generation has a number of disadvantages, including an inability to monitor accuracy of responses and adherence to instructions, and an inability to fully measure activity related to speaking, the final act in the sequence of events leading to language production. Finally, a few concluding remarks are offered that look toward future research in functional neuroimaging of aphasia.

Review and Evaluation of Literature on Functional Imaging in Aphasia

In this section, currently available functional neuroimaging literature on language processes in patients with aphasia is reviewed. There are two major topics. The first is what functional imaging tells us about recovery in aphasia. A critical issue is whether language reorganizes to cortex surrounding the lesion or other cortex in the damaged hemisphere, or whether it reorganizes to the previously nondominant, usually right, hemisphere. A review of the literature indicates that the answer to this question is that in cases of substantial, chronic aphasia, it is not a question of a wholesale reorganization of language to the dominant or previously nondominant hemisphere. Rather, for specific areas of damage, functions may shift to the right hemisphere, but even this principle is complicated, as discussed below. The second major topic is what functional imaging research can tell us about the reorganization of language during rehabilitation. Again, a critical issue is whether successful rehabilitation in chronic aphasia involves the reorganization of functions to the previously nondominant hemisphere or recruitment of perilesional cortex in the dominant hemisphere. Once both issues have been addressed, the findings from the diverse literature on functional neuroimaging in aphasia are integrated into a coherent summary of our current knowledge.

Functional Imaging of Recovery in Aphasia

The question of the role of the right hemisphere in recovery from aphasia did not begin with functional imaging. Debate on this topic has endured for more than a century. In 1877 Barlow noted a 10-year-old boy who regained language after a lesion of Broca's area and who lost language function again after lesion of the right hemisphere. In 1887 Gowers noted that some patients who recovered from aphasia after left-hemisphere stroke lost speech again after a right-hemisphere lesion, suggesting that some language functions reorganize to the right hemisphere. Although some dichotic listening literature in the late 1900s provided equivocal evidence regarding left- versus right-hemisphere functions in aphasia (Dobie & Simmons, 1971; Schulhoff & Goodglass, 1969; Shanks & Ryan, 1976; Sparks et al., 1970), other dichotic listening studies suggested the transfer of language comprehension functions to the right hemisphere for both Wernicke's and Broca's aphasias (Crosson & Warren, 1981; Johnson et al., 1977). More definitive evidence of right-hemisphere participation in recovery from aphasia (in at least some patients) has come from studies showing that patients with aphasia lost language function when the right, but not the left, hemisphere was anesthetized during Wada tests (Kinsborne, 1971) or when patients who had partially recovered from aphasia after left-hemisphere lesion showed worsening of language functions during objective testing after subsequent right-hemisphere lesions (Basso et al., 1989).

Application of functional neuroimaging techniques to the study of language functions in aphasia has led to a reexamination of left- and right-hemisphere contributions to language functions. Yet such studies have not resolved the controversy regarding left- versus right-hemisphere participation in language functions in recovery from aphasia. Some studies suggest that language functions in aphasia are primarily the product of right-hemisphere activity (Abo et al., 2004; Gold & Kertesz, 2000; Weiller et al., 1995). Other studies have indicated that language functions in aphasia are subserved primarily by the reorganization of functions in perilesional regions of the language-dominant hemisphere (Breier et al., 2004; Duffau et al., 2001; Léger et al., 2002; Miura et al., 1999; Seghier et al., 2001; Warburton et al., 1999).

Extending the focus on the left hemisphere in aphasia recovery, Zahn et al. (2004) have advocated the concept of "redundancy recovery," which is well worth considering. In redundancy recovery, impairments can be compensated for to some extent by intact areas of the language network normally subserving closely related functions. Thus, in this concept, recovery mechanisms extend beyond perilesional regions to other areas that are normally involved in the language network, perhaps even to some in the right hemisphere. In this regard, some investigators have emphasized the importance of participation of left posterior perisylvian cortices in recovery and rehabilitation after aphasia (e.g., Cato et al., 2004b; Heiss et al., 1999), and Crosson et al. (2005) suggested shared code that is encoded in this region of cortex could be used to leverage rehabilitation.

Problems in functional neuroimaging of aphasia recovery are particularly evident in studies advocating exclusively for left- or right-hemisphere recovery mechanisms. Such methodological problems are discussed in detail in the next section, "Reorganization of Language during Rehabilitation." Briefly, these problems include the following. Group analyses that obscure important individual differences in perilesional or right-hemisphere activity have sometimes been used. Some investigators ignore important data from their own studies suggesting that activity in the opposite hemisphere is important in some individuals. Others use tasks, such as word repetition, that may only partially reveal mechanisms relevant to everyday functional language.

Indeed, a growing number of studies indicate that the recovery of function in aphasia is a more complex process than a simple reversal of normal left-hemisphere lateralization (i.e., transferring language functions as a whole to the right hemisphere) or exclusive recruitment of left-perilesional and other language areas. Some studies indicate that a shift of language functions to the right hemisphere occurs primarily in regions homologous to damaged areas of the left hemisphere (Calvert et al., 2000; Lazar et al., 2000; Thulborn, 1999). For example, Weiller et al. (1995) showed reorganization of activity to the right-hemisphere homologue of Wernicke's area in patients who had lesions of Wernicke's area and had recovered from Wernicke's aphasia. In another study, patients with aphasia, with lesions of the left pars opercularis (the posterior part of Broca's area), showed right pars opercularis activity during narrative language production, whereas this area did not demonstrate activity in patients with aphasia without lesions in the pars opercularis or in neurologically normal controls (Blank et al., 2003).

Still other investigations indicate that good recovery of language functions in aphasia is accompanied by greater perilesional than right-hemisphere reorganization, whereas poorer recovery of language functions is accompanied by greater right-hemisphere than perilesional reorganization (Cao et al., 1999; Heiss et al., 1997, 1999; Karbe et al., 1998; Perani et al., 2003; Rosen et al., 2000). Indeed, the data of Heiss et al. (1997) indicate that larger lesions are associated with poor recovery of language functions and reorganization to the right hemisphere. Thus, level of recovery may be one important variable accounting for some of the variability in findings regarding the role of left- versus right-hemisphere mechanisms in recovery. In studies of chronic apha- sia, subject samples are more likely to be heavily weighted with patients with limited recovery and, therefore, greater right-hemisphere activity. Further, it is important to note that although patients with good recovery generally use left- hemisphere mechanisms for language, this does not mean that in patients with persistent aphasia, therapeutic strategies should focus exclusively on engaging left-hemisphere mechanisms. In chronic aphasias, the left-hemisphere mecha- nisms that might support language recovery may be too severely compromised to engage in rehabilitation, whereas in patients with good recovery, these mechanisms may still be intact enough to support significant recovery.

Naeser et al. (2004) have given a somewhat more complex viewpoint regarding the degree of right-hemisphere activity during language production in patients with chronic aphasia. Their work is also of interest because they are one of the few research groups to do overt (oral) narrative language pro- duction in a sample of patients with aphasia during functional neuroimaging. Such a paradigm was made possible by the use of dynamic susceptibility con- trast with gadolinium to measure differences in relative regional cerebral blood flow (see below for more extended discussion). Their four patients with chronic nonfluent aphasia showed significantly higher activity in right than left supplementary motor area (SMA) during narrative language attempts, whereas their four neurologically normal controls showed greater activity in left than right SMA during narrative language. (The investigators' methodol- ogy did not allow for separation of SMA from pre-SMA; thus, "SMA" in this study subsumes both divisions of medial Brodmann's area 6.) The aphasia group also showed higher activity in right perisylvian regions of interest (ROIs) than the control group during narrative production, but this difference was not specific to language production and apparently occurred to some degree for silent viewing of visual patterns as well. These authors have inter- preted their findings as indicative of poor modulation and overactivation of right-hemisphere language homologues, perhaps due to loss of transcallosal inhibition from the left to the right hemisphere. Some support for this position comes from a study by the same group in which repetitive transcranial mag- netic stimulation (rTMS) was used, ostensibly to inactivate the right pars triangularis (the anterior portion of Broca's area homologue) during language therapy. Each of four patients given this treatment had improved language performance at 2 mo posttreatment, suggesting that inactivating the right pars triangularis had a beneficial effect on language (Martin et al., 2004). Yet, as noted earlier in this chapter, there is good reason to believe that right- hemisphere language areas make a contribution to language recovery in some patients with aphasia. Although Naeser et al.'s data suggested that activity in the right pars triangularis could interfere with reorganization of language in their patients, they do not exclude the possibility that other right-hemisphere mechanisms are contributing to language production. Clearly, fMRI studies pre- and posttreatment would contribute to our understanding of the impact of this rTMS treatment on the organization of language systems.

In a recent study, Kim et al. (2002) presented a provocative finding that may shed more light on the issue of variability of right-hemisphere activity during language production in nonfluent aphasia. Their data showed that nonfluent patients with a left basal ganglia lesion in addition to left frontal damage demonstrated bilateral lateral frontal activity during language production and that nonfluent patients with left frontal, but no left basal ganglia damage demonstrated primarily right lateral frontal activity during language production. In an fMRI study of reorganization during treatment, Crosson et al. (2005) found the same pattern during word production in two patients: The patient with a left frontal and basal ganglia lesion showed bilateral lateral frontal activity, whereas in the patient with a left frontal lesion but an intact left basal ganglia, lateral frontal activity was completely lateralized to the right hemisphere during word production. The latter authors suggested that the right pre-SMA may use an intact left basal ganglia to suppress left lateral frontal activity, making it easier for right frontal mechanisms to take over language production. This conjecture was based on an earlier study by Crosson et al. (2003) that showed the opposite pattern during word generation in neurologically normal participants: widespread activity in the right basal ganglia in almost a total absence of right frontal activity. At the same time, the left pre-SMA, the left basal ganglia, and varying regions of left lateral frontal cortex were also active during word generation. The authors suggested that in normal word generation, the left pre-SMA uses the right basal ganglia to suppress right frontal activity, thereby keeping it from interfering with left frontal activity during word production. This interpretation is in keeping with the known bilateral connections of pre-SMA to the basal ganglia (Inase et al., 1999) and with the concept that one function of the basal ganglia is to suppress undesired activity (e.g., Mink, 1996; Nambu et al., 2002). It also is consistent with the positron emission tomography (PET) study of Blank et al. (2003), who showed that in neurologically normal subjects, the right pars opercularis shows a decrease in activity during narrative language production, as compared with a resting baseline, whereas the left pars opercularis shows an activity increase in the same comparison.

This interpretation of the findings of Kim et al. (2002) and Crosson et al. (2005) would explain why Brunner et al. (1982) found that aphasia was more persistent in cases with frontal plus basal ganglia lesion than in cases with either cortical or basal ganglia lesion alone. That is, when the basal ganglia are damaged in cases of large left frontal lesion, there is no mechanism for suppressing inadequate and noisy left-hemisphere activity, which can compete with right frontal activity and prevent reorganization to more capable, though not entirely optimal, right-hemisphere mechanisms. This interpretation is also consistent with a recent dissertation study performed in our laboratory in which Parkinson (2005) found the degree of basal ganglia intactness to predict improvement in treatment and to modulate frontal influences, with greater basal ganglia intactness predicting greater improvement. A further finding was that when basal ganglia contributions were controlled in patients with moderate to severe aphasia, larger frontal lesions actually predicted greater improvement. On the surface, this finding of greater lesion predicting more improvement during treatment seems counterintuitive. However, larger frontal lesions also may prevent noisy left frontal activity from competing with right frontal attempts to reorganize language production in more severely impaired patients.

A complicating factor in the functional imaging studies reviewed above is how to interpret right-hemisphere or perilesional activity when it is present. When significant right-hemisphere activity has been present during language production tasks in aphasia, investigators have commonly characterized this right-hemisphere activity as supporting language production. However, it should be noted that Rosen et al. (2000) questioned the right-hemisphere contribution to language functions in aphasia, suggesting that increased right-hemisphere activity merely represents the release of right-hemisphere mechanisms from inhibition by the damaged left hemisphere. Crosson et al. (2005), however, have questioned whether some perilesional activity may represent noisy processing with inadequate resolution for language tasks. Both of these interpretations may have some validity under different circumstances.

Finally, Fernandez et al. (2004) demonstrated the power of imaging patients across the course of recovery. They imaged a patient who had a lesion of Wernicke's area, the left inferior supramarginal gyrus, and left posterior insula, and who had conduction aphasia both 1 mo and 12 mo after stroke, with significant recovery occurring across the interval. In the early phases of recovery, the main difference from normal controls was greater activity in the right supramarginal gyrus. Increased activity in the right supramarginal gyrus continued in the chronic scan, but increased activity in perilesional areas of the left hemisphere were also evident at this time, suggesting that the perilesional activity may have played some role in recovery. In eight patients with aphasia, given PET scans of word generation an average of 2 and then 11 mo poststroke, Cardebat et al. (2003) found increased activity in both the right and left hemispheres. Positive correlations with language improvement were shown with activity in the superior temporal cortex bilaterally. In short, activity in both hemispheres may have contributed to recovery. Thus, longitudinal studies may offer some ability to resolve the question of when activity in an area represents a contribution to recovery. Repeated scans have been used in studies of neuroplasticity during treatment, which is the topic of the next section.

Reorganization of Language during Rehabilitation

Functional imaging studies of neural substrates underlying successful aphasia treatment are rare, and like studies of recovery of function, they have not resolved the question of whether treatment effects are due to engaging left-hemisphere perilesional or right-hemisphere mechanisms. Belin et al. (1996) studied seven patients with "nonfluent" aphasia who had received Melodic Intonation Therapy (MIT), assumed by many to develop right-hemisphere language abilities. When repetition without MIT strategies was compared with listening to words, increased activity was seen in the right sensorimotor mouth region, the right-hemisphere homologue of Wernicke's area, right prefrontal cortex, and the right anterior superior temporal gyrus. Taken by themselves, these results might suggest engagement of right-hemisphere compensatory mechanisms during repetition. However, when repetition invoking MIT strategies was compared with repetition without invoking MIT strategies, a significant increase in activity in (left) Broca's area and a decrease in several right-hemisphere regions occurred. Although Belin et al.'s study can be criticized because it did not measure change in language production mechanisms from pre- to posttreatment status, the findings do suggest that it is important to measure the mechanisms responsible for therapeutic change.

Cornelissen et al. (2003) administered a contextual priming treatment for naming to three patients with largely posterior perisylvian lesions and moderately severe anomia. All patients improved from the treatment. Changes in neural substrates for naming were assessed with magnetoencephalography (MEG)/magnetic source imaging (MSI). Although strong areas of right-hemisphere activity were noted in pre- and posttreatment imaging for each patient, the only area to show a consistent activity increase in each patient was in the left inferior parietal cortex. Thus, like the study of Belin et al. (1996), the Cornelissen study suggested that activation of the left-hemisphere cortex can be an important substrate for treatment.

However, a study by Musso et al. (1999) yielded much clearer results regarding the recruitment of right-hemisphere mechanisms during aphasia treatment. These investigators gave four patients with Wernicke's aphasia and left temporoparietal lesions short-term language training, emphasizing comprehension, between 12 PET scans imaging language comprehension. Improvement on language comprehension measures correlated with increased activity in the right superior temporal gyrus and the left precuneus. These data support the idea that the right-hemisphere region homologous to damaged left-hemisphere mechanisms can be recruited to support the reorganization of language mechanisms during rehabilitation.

Crosson et al. (2005) analyzed pre- and posttreatment fMRI data from two patients with mild-to-moderate chronic nonfluent aphasia who had received an intention treatment designed to change lateralization of language production mechanisms from the left to the right frontal cortex. Basically, the treatment consisted of initiating picture-naming trials with a complex left-hand movement (opening a box and pushing a specific button on a joy port inside the box, with the left hand in the left hemispace). Errors were corrected by having patients repeat the correct item while making a nonsymbolic gesture with the left hand (see Richards et al., 2002, or Crosson et al., 2005, for a more detailed description). The conceptual rationale behind the treatment was that the complex left-hand movement or nonsymbolic left-hand gesture would prime an intentional mechanism (specifically right pre-SMA) in the right hemisphere, which in turn would activate the right frontal cortex, which could support language production, thereby facilitating transfer of language production to this cortex. Both patients also received an attention treatment, during which they directed their attention 45 degrees to their left to view pictures, which they named. Because the attention treatment was not believed to activate the intention mechanism that interacts with lateral frontal mechanisms used in language production, it was hypothesized that these nonfluent patients would benefit from the intention treatment, but not the attention treatment. Patients received fMRI of an event-related category-member generation task before and after treatment. This word retrieval task was selected for fMRI sessions because Crosson et al. (2001) had shown that category-member generation demonstrated greater sensitivity to pre-SMA activity than object naming and because it was assumed that any shifts in activity to the right hemisphere would generalize from picture naming to this form of word retrieval. The first patient, whose lesion involved both the left frontal cortex and the basal ganglia, showed significant improvement on the intention treatment, but not on the attention treatment, consistent with the experimental hypothesis. Right pre-SMA activity and right lateral frontal cortex showed substantial increases in extent of activation from pre- to posttreatment imaging, which also was consistent with the experimental hypothesis. The second patient, whose lesion involved left lateral frontal cortex but spared the basal ganglia, showed significant improvement on the intention treatment, as expected, but she also improved during the attention treatment. During fMRI prior to the intention treatment, lateral frontal activity was already 100% lateralized to the right lateral frontal cortex and remained so after treatment. Both left and right pre-SMA were active both before and after treatment. It also is of interest that posterior perisylvian activity emerged on posttreatment fMRI scans for both patients. Neither patient had such activity during pretreatment fMRI; this posterior perisylvian activity was not lateralized in the first patient, and was lateralized to the left hemisphere in the second patient. As noted above, the pretreatment data of these patients was consistent with the data of Kim et al. (2002), indicating that frontal activity reorganizes to the right hemisphere for language production when the left basal ganglia are intact, but bilateral frontal activity occurs when the left basal ganglia are severely compromised. When language production has not lateralized to right frontal cortex before treatment, it appears that the intention treatment can trigger such reorganization, at least in some patients. Finally, the data suggested that both the right frontal and left perisylvian cortex provided neural substrates important to the recovery of word retrieval.

Using fMRI, Peck et al. (2004a) studied the relationship between hemodynamic response (HDR) peaks in right-hemisphere areas and response latencies in a word generation task. In word generation, they found that the delay in HDR peaks between the right primary auditory cortex and the mouth sensorimotor cortex were highly correlated with the delay between hearing a category and generating a category member for pre- and posttreatment images. This finding indicated entrainment of right-hemisphere activity to the task and suggests involvement of the right hemisphere in this language task for patients with aphasia.

Making Sense of Functional Imaging Data in Aphasia

On the surface, the literature on functional neuroimaging in aphasia can be quite confusing. The major question regarding whether recovery is supported by the perilesional cortex of the left hemisphere or by the homologous right-hemisphere regions has generated little consensus. Evidence can be cited for either left- or right-hemisphere mechanisms providing the neural substrate for rehabilitation. Yet if one reads the literature carefully and more critically, and at the same time applies a little logic, the findings in aggregate do suggest a likely scenario. On this basis, the following discussion is offered as a heuristic that can guide future research.

One might start by stating that it seems highly likely that both left- and right-hemisphere mechanisms are important in recovery and rehabilitation and that the importance of the mechanisms within each hemisphere varies, depending on a number of factors. The reasons for variability in right- and left-hemisphere activity in the aphasia functional neuroimaging literature are many. Among the most likely reasons for this variability are differences in tasks used to assess the neural substrates of language, differences in patient samples that are studied, and differences in the homogeneity or heterogeneity of lesions in the sample under study. In addition, the way in which questions are asked affects the methods used to gather and to analyze the data and therefore can affect results. Finally, the viewpoint of a particular group of investigators may affect the way in which data are interpreted.

In clarifying this confusing picture, it should also be stated at the outset that there is little evidence that language functions are transferred to the right hemisphere in a wholesale fashion. If this were the case, severe global aphasia would be a very rare phenomenon because the right hemisphere would simply assume language functions and mitigate the effects of a left-hemisphere lesion. At the same time, compromised language production in patients with aphasia during Wada testing when the right, but not the left, hemisphere is anesthetized (Kinsborne, 1971) and loss of language function in patients with aphasia after right-hemisphere lesion (Barlow, 1877; Gowers, 1887; Basso et al., 1989) provide compelling evidence for right-hemisphere participation in language functions in aphasia. On this basis alone, it seems that recovery, with or without rehabilitation, is likely to use residual left-hemisphere language functions as a platform for recovery, using homologous areas of the right hemisphere to substitute for left-hemisphere mechanisms when necessary (Heiss et al., 1999). Thus, the search for global transfer of language functions to the right hemisphere or the global maintenance of left-hemisphere language functions should be abandoned in favor of methods that interrogate specific areas of left and right hemisphere participation in recovery. The degree of left- versus right-hemisphere participation in language appears to depend on a number of factors, including the degree of compromise to various left -hemisphere mechanisms, the availability of left-hemisphere mechanisms that can substitute for damaged areas, and the nature of intervening speech and language therapy. Further, as noted above, the data of Kim et al. (2002) suggest that the integrity of mechanisms governing lateralized processing may also determine how recovery plays out. Finally, Finger et al. (2003) pointed out that the capability of the right hemisphere to assume language functions probably varies considerably among patients.

As noted above, some studies have suggested that global lesion size is important in both the quality of recovery and the lateralization of language functions in aphasia. Larger lesions tend to lead to poorer recovery and greater right-hemisphere activity (Cao et al., 1999; Heiss et al., 1997, 1999; Karbe et al., 1998; Perani et al., 2003; Rosen et al., 2000). This gross correlation probably occurs in heterogeneous samples because larger left-hemisphere lesions generally compromise a larger number of language structures than smaller left-hemisphere lesions. The more structures that are compromised, the less are the residual language skills and knowledge on which recovery can be based. The best studies for demonstrating right-hemisphere lateralization of specific mechanisms are those in which relatively homogeneous lesions of specific areas occur, for example, the studies showing that consistent damage to Wernicke's area can lead to increased activity of its right-hemisphere homologue during language tasks (Musso et al., 1999; Weiller et al., 1995) or the study showing that the right pars opercularis activates during narrative language only when the left pars opercularis is damaged (Blank et al., 2003). In studies with more heterogeneous samples, right-hemisphere mechanisms participating in recovery can be obscured, especially if group analyses are emphasized, because the location and degree of right-hemisphere participation may vary with the location and degree of a left-hemisphere lesion. For example, Breier et al. (2004) relied mainly on group analyses in a more heterogeneous sample to conclude that recovery was mainly supported by left-hemisphere activity, but they also noted that some individual subjects did show regions of right-hemisphere activity. This finding suggests that, especially in heterogeneous samples, individual subject analysis should be the primary methodology. Otherwise, variations in lesion location may lead to underestimates of both perilesional and right-hemisphere activity.

Damage to mechanisms that control lateralization of brain activity during language also has the potential to impact the degree of right- versus left-hemisphere participation in recovery and probably accounts for some of the variability in reorganization of activity to the right hemisphere. Evidence suggests that lateralization of language is not simply a passive function of language-related cortex, but it is actively regulated. For example, as noted above, Crosson et al. (2003) suggested that the right basal ganglia suppress right frontal activity during word generation to keep it from interfering with left frontal processes for neurologically normal subjects. Crosson et al. (2005) also suggested that a reversal of this process, that is, suppression of noisy and dysfunctional left frontal activity through the left basal ganglia, could account for why Kim et al. (2002) found reorganization of activity to right frontal cortex during word generation in nonfluent aphasia only when the left basal ganglia were undamaged. The fact that Parkinson (2005) found that the degree of integrity of the basal ganglia predicts positive treatment outcome in a sample of patients dominated by nonfluent aphasia suggests that the right frontal activity found in such patients has a positive functional significance. This interpretation implies that the damaged left frontal cortex will attempt to perform language production functions in nonfluent aphasia even when it is potentially less functional than its right-hemisphere counterpart and that suppression of this tendency will reduce interference with right-hemisphere mechanisms.

As noted above, another mechanism potentially contributing to lateralization of language production in aphasia is the size of the left-hemisphere lesion. In a sample of patients dominated by nonfluent aphasia, Parkinson (2005) found that larger left frontal lesions actually predict better treatment outcome. One should keep in mind that the patients in Parkinson's study had chronic aphasias with significant anomias and that their lesions were generally of moderate size or larger. Thus, the interpretation was offered that when lesions of left frontal mechanisms are large enough to significantly compromise language production on a chronic basis, very large frontal lesions prevent noisy language production processes, leaving the right frontal mechanisms free to assume language production to the degree to which they are capable. In contrast, in moderately large lesions, remaining left frontal mechanisms continue to generate noisy output that can interfere with right frontal attempts to assume production. It should be noted that the Parkinson (2005) data were lacking in patients with small lesions showing good recovery; those patients would not have qualified for the treatment study from which he drew his cases. Thus, the cases of more circumscribed left-hemisphere lesions, in which recovery relies primarily on left-hemisphere mechanisms (e.g., Cao et al., 1999; Heiss et al., 1997; Karbe et al., 1998; Perani et al., 2003; Rosen et al., 2000), were not represented in his sample.

There is an additional layer of complexity in these cases in which right frontal activity seems to assume language production functions. Two considerations are important. First, once a lesion is large enough to severely and permanently compromise language production mechanisms in the left hemisphere, right frontal mechanisms may provide a more functional substrate for recovery and rehabilitation than the remaining left frontal mechanisms. Even so, the right frontal mechanisms are likely to be considerably less skilled than previously intact left frontal ones, which provides limitations to the degree of recovery. Second, it appears that optimal recovery in such cases is facilitated by posterior persylvian mechanisms of the left hemisphere. Cato et al. (2004a, 2004b) found that in a treatment designed to facilitate the shift of production mechanisms to the right frontal cortex, the degree of intactness of posterior mechanisms (as well as higher auditory–verbal comprehension scores) predicted a positive treatment outcome. Crosson et al. (2005) found evidence that this left-hemisphere cortex was active after, but not before, the same treatment. Heiss et al. (1999) also implicated the posterior perisylvian left-hemisphere cortex in recovery from aphasia. Zahn and colleagues' (2004) concept of redundancy recovery may be relevant here. In other words, recovery is optimized when treatment facilitates the recruitment of the left posterior perisylvian cortex. Although this cortex may not normally participate in the type of word generation being imaged (Crosson et al., 2003), it may contribute a lexical–semantic code that can facilitate word production processes in the right frontal cortex during recovery from or treatment for nonfluent aphasia.

To summarize, attempts to establish an inviolable canon that either perilesional or right-hemisphere activity is exclusively responsible for language recovery in aphasia are not likely to be fruitful. There is ample evidence that both mechanisms can account for language recovery in different circumstances and, indeed, can even work together to facilitate language recovery in some cases. Further, it is possible that both left- and right-hemisphere activity can impede optimal functioning under some circumstances, that is, when it competes with a more functional substrate for recovery in the opposite hemisphere. The challenge for future research is to develop an understanding of when and how various left- and right-hemisphere mechanisms contribute to recovery and rehabilitation. Meeting this challenge will be no small task, as multiple influences are likely to determine how recovery progresses and what is the optimal substrate for recovery. It will require several generations of building, assessing, and modifying conceptual models of recovery and treatment before we have a viable means of understanding the phenomena that currently plague the functional neuroimaging literature in aphasia. Nonetheless, the importance of this endeavor cannot be overestimated. It is necessary to acquire the scientific knowledge base for developing the most effective treatments for aphasia.

Techniques for Imaging Language Systems in Aphasia

Making progress in understanding neural substrates for recovery in and rehabilitation of aphasia depends on the adequacy of techniques and strategies used to image relevant neural systems. There is no shortage of technical challenges in imaging language systems in aphasia, and dealing effectively with these challenges is necessary to obtain useful information. Functional magnetic resonance imaging (fMRI) is clearly the most widely available technology that can be applied to this endeavor; thus, it will be the predominant technology used by researchers to study neural systems in aphasia. Hence, this discussion focuses primarily on fMRI technology.

There are several problems that must be addressed to obtain the most accurate and complete understanding of neural activity in aphasia. Briefly, a few of these are as follows:

1. Data analyses must take into account variations in lesion boundaries between subjects to accurately assess perilesional activity.

2. When language production is an issue, it is highly desirable to use spoken as opposed to silent language production during functional imaging sessions. However, speaking during scanning sessions creates artifacts that can be mistaken for brain activity in BOLD contrast fMRI, currently the most common form of fMRI. Use of spoken language allows investigators to image structures involved in the realization of spoken output that may differ from those used in silent generation. Further, spoken responses can be used to track the accuracy of task performance.

3. Response latencies of patients with aphasia to stimuli in imaging paradigms are usually longer and more variable than in normal persons. This variability must be addressed in event-related paradigms, where analyses are timed to the cognitive activities one is studying.

4. Analyses performed on data from different sessions can be differentially sensitive to brain activity in various cognitive paradigms. It is necessary to address this problem so that changes in sensitivity are not mistaken for changes in activity of neural systems.

5. The selection of a cognitive paradigm to image language systems in patients with aphasia must take into consideration both the nature of the cognitive inquiry and the sensitivity of the paradigm to activity in the neural substrates of interest at the individual subject level.

In the following paragraphs, each of these issues is discussed.

Variable Lesion Boundaries between Patients

In the overwhelming majority of cognitive neuropsychology studies, the use of group statistics that average fMRI or PET images across subjects on a voxel-by-voxel basis is the analysis of choice. The reason for the popularity of this technique is simple: Averaging images across subjects substantially increases sensitivity to small, incremental changes in cognitive activity, which allows investigators to explore the brain structures responsible for specific cognitive functions with great precision. However, as noted above, the issue of perilesional activity is critical in addressing neural substrates of language in aphasia, and much of the debate regarding reorganization of language systems in aphasia has centered on the participation of perilesional versus homologous right-hemisphere regions. If group analyses were used, perilesional activity in some patients would be averaged with an absence of activity in lesioned tissue of other patients, resulting in a gross underestimate of perilesional activity. Further, when the activation of right-hemisphere homologues of language cortex depends on the degree of damage to their specific left-hemisphere counterparts, then the boundaries of the left-hemisphere lesion may affect which right-hemisphere structures are active as well. If Blank et al. (2003) had averaged images of patients with and without lesions of the left pars opercularis, the activity in the right pars opercularis for patients with lesions of its left-hemisphere homologue would have been averaged with the absence of right pars opercularis activity for patients without lesions to its left-hemisphere homologue. Had this been done, little consistent activity would have been seen in the right pars opercularis, and Blank et al. never would have discovered the relationship between damage to the left pars opercularis and activity in its right-hemisphere counterpart. For this reason, images from patients with aphasia must be analyzed at the individual subject level because the varying sizes, shapes, and locations of lesions makes it impossible to obtain valid statistical parametric maps of activity in perilesional locations or even in right-hemisphere homologues of language areas with data averaged across subjects. This caveat can be applied to PET as well as to fMRI images. The one exception to the necessity of using individual subject analyses is that when the lesions are extremely homogeneous between patients in an experimental sample, averaging across subjects may be used to increase sensitivity, especially to right-hemisphere activity. However, in this circumstance, it should still be remembered that even seemingly small variations in lesion size between patients can lead to an underestimation of perilesional activity.

Imaging during Spoken Language

As noted above, optimal imaging of language production systems requires patients with aphasic to produce spoken responses during functional imaging of language production. Speaking during BOLD contrast fMRI acquisition creates signal intensity artifacts that, in large part, appear related to inhomogeneities in the magnetic field caused by changes in the pressure of air containing paramagnetic oxygen and by movement of the jaw and tongue. (See Kemeny et al., 2005, for a discussion of BOLD artifacts during overt speech.) These artifacts can be mistaken for brain activity if the images are not properly analyzed. Although Barch et al. (1999, 2000) used group analyses of uncorrected fMRI images to average out these artifacts, they recommended that individual subject analyses not be performed on uncorrected data because of the speech-related artifacts during overt language output. As just noted, fMRI data analyses in aphasia must be carried out at the individual subject level because variations in lesion topography between subjects would result in a gross underestimation of perilesional or even right-hemisphere activity if fMRI images were averaged across subjects. There are two basic ways of dealing with speech-related artifacts: use of alternative imaging techniques or removing the artifacts during image analysis.

Regarding alternative imaging techniques, there are three possibilities. The first is the use of PET. For example, Blank et al. (2003) used ^{15}O labeled water to image activity in patients with and without left pars opercularis lesions during overt continuous speech. Although PET is not subject to the susceptibility artifacts present in BOLD contrast fMRI during overt speech, PET does have several disadvantages.

1. PET technology is not as generally available as MRI. Thus, the number of centers with access to the technology is limited.
2. Because of the short half-life of ^{15}O, the most commonly used isotope in functional imaging of cognition, a cyclotron must be located proximal to the PET camera. The expenses of acquiring and maintaining this capability are high.
3. The technique is invasive, in the sense that it requires intravenous administration of the tracer and involves exposure to radiation. Thus, there is some degree of risk involved.
4. PET is not amenable to event-related paradigms, which can provide greater cognitive precision under some circumstances.

The second alternative technology is dynamic susceptibility contrast fMRI. Naeser et al. (2004) imaged continuous overt speech in patients with this technique. Dynamic susceptibility contrast fMRI requires intravenous injection of a bolus of gadolinium. Because gadolinium is paramagnetic, it disturbs the homogeneity of the magnetic field as it passes through the vasculature, causing loss of signal. Because the signal loss is proportional to the amount of tracer in a region, it can be used to determine regional cerebral blood volume. Because regional cerebral blood volume and regional cerebral blood flow are correlated, the technique is sensitive to activity changes that trigger changes in regional cerebral blood flow and can be used to monitor activity across time on a voxel-by-voxel basis. This method provides a high contrast-to-noise ratio and, therefore, is less likely to be affected by speech-related artifacts. Although it does not use a radioactive isotope, like PET, and can be used during overt speech, it does have some drawbacks.

1. It is invasive in the sense that it requires administration of a bolus of gadolinium.
2. It is not as amenable to event-related paradigms as is BOLD contrast fMRI.

A third alternative technique, arterial spin labeling (ASL) fMRI has recently been tested during overt speech in neurologically normal subjects (Kemeny et al., 2005). In ASL techniques, the spins of protons in water in the blood are inverted, or "tagged," as they pass through the carotid artery on their way to the brain (Buxton, 2001). After a time sufficient to allow the tagged water molecules to pass into brain tissue, tagged images of various slices are acquired. To obtain a measure of cerebral blood flow, the tagged images are subtracted from untagged images of the same slices. In this way, changes in regional cerebral blood flow can be monitored across time on a voxel-by-voxel basis. Kemeny et al. (2005) demonstrated that bilateral–temporal–polar speech-related artifacts that appear in BOLD contrast fMRI images acquired during overt speech do not occur in ASL fMRI images. Although ASL fMRI is noninvasive and can be used in event-related fMRI paradigms, some caveats should be noted.

1. Some ASL techniques do not allow for whole-brain acquisitions, including the technique used by Kemeny et al. (2005). At the time this chapter was written, a comparison of whole-brain ASL to whole-brain BOLD contrast fMRI during overt speech had not been performed. Thus, a comparison of the sensitivity of the two techniques across a large number of brain regions had not been made.

2. ASL has a lower temporal resolution than BOLD contrast fMRI when a large number of slices are acquired. For example, Kemeny et al. collected one image every 30 s.

3. Kemeny et al. (2005) relied primarily on group analyses to compare ASL and BOLD contrast fMRI in overt speech. Barch et al. (1999) had shown that speech-related artifacts can be mitigated largely by averaging them out in a group analysis. Thus, to evaluate their usefulness for imaging in aphasia, the presence of artifacts should be evaluated at the individual subject level because that is the level of analysis appropriate to most aphasia studies.

Nonetheless, further development and investigation of ASL techniques for use in aphasia imaging should be accomplished, and the technique appears promising as an answer to speech-related artifacts.

Regarding the removal of speech-related artifacts during image processing in BOLD contrast fMRI, there are several methods for accomplishing this goal. The first is to drop the images affected by artifacts from the analysis. BOLD fMRI is based on regional hemodynamic responses, which last on the order of 10–12 s for a single event. Speech-related artifacts do not extend significantly beyond the few seconds it takes to complete a verbal response (Plate 8.1a). Thus, in event-related paradigms, much of the hemodynamic response is normally available for analysis even after dropping those images affected by speech-related artifacts. For example, Carter et al. (2000) analyzed data collected during verbal responses to a Stroop paradigm in neurologically normal subjects after dropping the first 2.5 s of images. The remaining images were quite adequate to define differences between conditions in a group analysis. Likewise, in fMRI paradigms where multiple events are clustered into a single block, increased signal from the more extended hemodynamic response is evident after speech during the block ends, when the signal from the hemodynamic response is returning to baseline. Martin et al. (2004) used this part of the hemodynamic response to image brain systems in patients with aphasia during a naming paradigm. This method of analysis has the advantage of simplicity, but it also loses some data and may suffer some loss of sensitivity to activity as a result.

A second method for dealing with speech-related artifacts in BOLD contrast fMRI is called motion–parameter regression. Most fMRI analyses involve the application of algorithms to correct for global head motion. As a result of applying these algorithms, translational and angular deviations from the base image are calculated, and these parameters can be used along with multiple linear regression techniques to remove motion artifacts from the time series on a voxel-by-voxel basis (Bullmore et al., 1999; Friston et al., 2000). However, speech-related artifactual signal changes seem to be more dependent on local changes in the magnetic field caused by movement of the tongue and jaw and by the density of paramagnetic oxygen within the vocal cavity than they are dependent on global head motion. This being the case, local signal artifacts may not always correlate highly with global head motion, and the usefulness of motion–parameter regression may be limited accordingly. Further, most algorithms that correct for global motion are not sensitive to motions of more than an acquisition voxel, and thus residual large motions remain uncorrected and unmeasured by these algorithms.

Fortunately, Birn et al. (1999) developed a detrending technique to reduce motion artifacts from fMRI images obtained during overt language production in normal participants. Gopinath (Gopinath, 2003; Gopinath et al., 2003) devised an elaboration of this technique, called "selective detrending," to deal with speech-related signals. Essentially, this procedure uses protypical artifacts from nonbrain voxels in an initial deconvolution analysis to ascertain which voxels have signal changes that correlate with the artifacts. Voxels correlated with protypical artifacts can then be detrended for the artifact with which they correlate most highly in the following manner. Detrending is applied only to those voxels that correlate with a protypical artifact. If a voxel's signal change correlates with prototypical hemodynamic responses obtained from brain voxels as well as with prototypical artifacts, only the first three time points after a correct response are detrended to minimize the effect of detrending on the hemodynamic response; but for voxels that correlate only with a protypical artifact and not with a hemodynamic response, the entire time series is detrended.

Data from spoken word production of a patient with aphasia, are shown in Plate 8.1. As noted above, Plate 8.1a shows the relatively fast time course of a speech-related artifact superimposed on the time course for a true hemodynamic response. It is this temporal difference in the time courses that allows separation and mitigation of the speech-related artifact from the hemodynamic response. Plate 8.1b shows activity before the motion artifact was removed. Functional activity in the voxels represents the correlation between the acquired time series and the convolution of the deconvolved hemodynamic response with the temporal sequence for events. Red represents $R^2 \geq .16$; yellow represents $R^2 \geq .20$. Note the false-positive activity within the sylvian fissure, which is enlarged secondary to the lesion. Activity should not occur within the sylvian fissure, because there is no gray matter within the fissure to generate this activity. Plate 8.1c shows activity when the first two time points of each time series were dropped from deconvolution analysis to mitigate speech-related artifact, and Plate 8.1d shows activity when time courses were selectively detrended for speech-related signal artifact. Note that in Plate 8.1c and 8.1d, the false-positive activity in the sylvian fissure disappeared. Gopinath (2003) showed that when both sensitivity and specificity are considered, the selective detrending procedure performs superiorly to simply dropping two images for each response from the analysis, to motion–parameter regression, and to a technique in which every voxel is detrended for speech-related signal change without regard to its correlation with protypical artifacts.

Variability in Response Latencies for Patients with Aphasia

In any analysis of fMRI time series, the investigator must somehow feed into the analysis information about where in the time series a hemodynamic response should begin if it is present. In experiments with neurologically normal subjects, the latency between stimulus presentation and spoken response is short and relatively uniform in most paradigms. In this case, stimulus onset can be used to mark the beginning of hemodynamic responses for analyses. However, long and variable response latencies for participants with aphasia raise issues regarding when during the time series a hemodynamic response should begin. Analyses can be timed to stimulus onset (stimulus-locked analyses) or timed to response onset (response-locked analyses). In our laboratory, we have assessed both methods. Which method is better depends on the paradigm used to elicit spoken responses. In some instances, each method provides information not provided by the other (Wabnitz et al., 2005). In other words, some voxels meet the statistical threshold in the response-locked but not the stimulus-locked analysis, and other voxels meet the statistical threshold in the stimulus-locked but not the response-locked analysis. Cognitive processes involved in language production paradigms include analysis of the stimulus that elicits the response (e.g., picture, category member), retrieval or generation of the response, and actual production of the response once it has been retrieved or generated. Thus, some processes for such paradigms may be more closely associated with stimulus onset and others may be more closely associated with response onset. In instances in which both stimulus-locked and response-locked analyses provide unique information, a union of the voxels active in either analysis can be used to determine all voxels active in the task. It is not always obvious which analysis provides the best representation of the underlying activity in which the investigator is interested or whether the union analysis should be used. Investigators are encouraged to use empirical methods to determine the type of analysis that best represents the system in which they are interested.

Equating for Sensitivity between fMRI Sessions

Investigating changes in the neural substrates of language across aphasia treatment involves imaging patients' language systems before and after treatment. Pre- and posttreatment fMRI images can show large differences in the distribution of significant voxels throughout the brain. Such differences in sensitivity raise substantive questions for interpretation. For example, when pre- and posttreatment images are thresholded with the same statistical values, are regional differences in activity between pre- and posttreatment images due to changes in neural substrates for the fMRI task, that is, to neuroplastic changes induced by rehabilitation, or are they simply due to the fact that the images are differentially sensitive to BOLD responses? Gopinath (2004) developed a procedure to equate images from two different fMRI sessions for sensitivity. Essentially, the procedure equates images for sensitivity to BOLD responses across sessions on a voxel-by-voxel basis. In brief, the residual variance from a deconvolution analysis in each voxel is used as a basis to estimate the noise structure of the two image sets. After making adjustments for non-Gaussian noise, signal curves approximating BOLD responses are added to the adjusted residual noise bed at the same points at which the actual responses occurred in the time series for both image sets. Different known amplitudes of signal are used, and detection probability curves (fraction of voxels in the data set "activated" as a function of the chosen statistical threshold) are generated for each data set for each of the different levels of signal added. These detection probability curves then are used to equate the statistical values in the two image sets for sensitivity. Gopinath (2004) evaluated instances in which only correct responses were used in pre- and posttreatment data for subjects with aphasia. He found that differences in number of correct responses from pre- to posttreatment image sessions was a key factor contributing to differences in sensitivity. However, other paradigmatic factors also contribute to differences in sensitivity and can be addressed by the technique.

Selection of a Cognitive Paradigm

An extensive discussion of cognitive paradigms for use with aphasia is beyond the scope of this chapter and would provide the material for a lengthy chapter by itself. Nonetheless, this crucial methodological consideration deserves some mention. The cognitive paradigm that is selected for aphasia experiments is a crucial determinant of what information is gleaned from an experiment. Thus, cognitive paradigms must be carefully selected with the experimental question and the likely limitations of alternative strategies in mind. What has become standard fare for the majority of cognitive neuroscience research in neurologically normal subjects is to isolate specific subcomponents of cognitive processes to a single, or at least a small number of brain structures. However, Newman et al. (2001) demonstrated that activity often is greater in specific components of the language system when language tasks are compared to rest than when they are compared to other language tasks. Essentially, these authors warned that lower absolute levels of activation can result when baseline and experimental tasks share processes. Thus, paradigms that attempt to image the neural substrate for a single cognitive element by using closely related tasks could jeopardize the ability to image relevant activity at the individual subject level.

For example, Peck et al. (2004b) discussed the design of a sentence generation task for use in fMRI studies of aphasia. In preparation for this usage, the sentence generation task (generating a passive-voice sentence, given a picture) was piloted with normal subjects using two different baseline tasks: picture naming and passive viewing of nonsense objects. One criterion for choosing a paradigm was that it demonstrate activity in Broca's area during sentence generation inasmuch as this area has shown involvement in syntax processing in both imaging and lesion studies. Although activity in Broca's area was shown when passive viewing of nonsense objects was used as a baseline task for sentence generation, this activity was not evident in group analyses when picture naming was used as the baseline task. At the individual subject level, the extent of activity in Broca's area was significantly less when picture naming was used as the baseline than when nonsense object viewing was used as the baseline task. The authors suggested that Broca's area was used both in word retrieval and in syntax generation and, therefore, participation of Broca's area was obscured when word retrieval was used as a baseline task for sentence generation. Because the authors wished to see activity in Broca's area during sentence generation in patients with aphasia when it was not damaged, they selected nonsense object viewing as the baseline task. From a purely cognitive standpoint, picture naming would have been the preferred baseline task because it would have isolated syntax generation from word retrieval. However, this design would have compromised the ability to detect activity in a critical structure in patients undergoing rehabilitation for syntax generation. Another consideration is whether the purpose of the imaging activity in patients with aphasia is to isolate one cognitive component from another or to image all potential system elements that might be compromised. Finally, when imaging recovery in aphasia, the relationship of the experimental task to the concept of recovery should be considered. For example, some studies have used repetition as a task to gauge recovery in aphasia. However, repetition is rarely performed in everyday attempts at communication. Because word finding is a skill used in everyday communication, word-finding paradigms have more of a relationship to functional recovery of language skills. Thus, no single principle for selecting one design over another can be offered. Both the purpose of the study from a cognitive standpoint and the sensitivity of the paradigm to activity in the relevant neural substrates should be considered. Generally, sensitivity should be considered at the individual subject level for reasons already discussed.

Methodology Caveats and Needs

A few concluding remarks focus on caveats and needs in functional imaging of aphasia. Because the quality of the data we get is dependent on our methodological choices, it is important to consider methodological options carefully with the purpose of the experiment in mind. It is abundantly clear that in all but the most homogeneous lesion samples, group methodologies that average functional images across subjects are inappropriate. Although a few examples of homogeneous lesion samples exist (e.g., Blank et al., 2003; Musso et al., 1999; Weiller et al., 1995), these are exceptions. When lesion samples are heterogeneous, as is usually the case in functional imaging studies of aphasia, group averaging of functional images will obscure perilesional activity and, many times, even right-hemisphere activity homologous to lesioned areas of the left hemisphere. Variations in lesion location and functional activity between patients with aphasia are important clues that can be deciphered only at the individual subject level of analysis in heterogeneous lesion samples. Thus, the most of our remarks have concerned methodological issues that affect individual subject analyses.

Another caveat concerns evaluation of activity changes when changes in neural systems as a result of recovery or treatment are the topic of interest. To the best of my knowledge, studies that compare the stability of functional imaging findings during the same language task across multiple sessions with patients with aphasia did not exist at the time this chapter was written. Clearly, such studies are needed. For example, the choice of techniques for analyzing change could be affected by such knowledge. Studies using various cognitive paradigms in neurologically normal subjects (Machielsen et al., 2000; Maldjian et al., 2002; Wei et al., 2004; Swallow et al., 2003) can give some guidance in this matter. In general, these studies determined that if a voxel in an individual subject is activated during a task in one session, the probability of its being activated during the same task in a second session is about 1 in 3. This finding suggests that voxel-by-voxel analyses across sessions within individual subjects are not stable enough to separate simple session-to-session variability from changes related to treatment or recovery. However, using larger regions of interest (ROIs) appears promising as far as stability is concerned. Generally, within larger ROIs known to be relevant to a specific task, the percentage of a volume active from one session to the next appears to range from 60 to 85% (Machielsen et al., 2000; Maldjian et al., 2002; Wei et al., 2004; Swallow et al., 2003). Thus, for individual subjects, reproducibility is much better at the ROI level than at the individual voxel level. Such ROI approaches have been successfully used in the imaging of language (e.g., Naeser et al., 2004) and treatment change (e.g., Crosson et al., 2005) for patients with aphasia.

Regarding the lack of voxel-to-voxel correspondence of activity between fMRI sessions, there are some parallels in microelectrode stimulation mapping of animals. The point-to-point correspondence can vary considerably between sessions, and the total area of cortex or the percent of the total area mapped that is occupied by a specific function (e.g., motor representation for a specific digit in primates) is used as a measure of plasticity from pre- to post-intervention (e.g., Nudo et al., 1996). Indeed, Kleim et al. (2003) have proposed that this underlying variability in cortical maps is a necessary substrate for learning. Although it is uncertain as to how such observations in the motor cortex of rats and monkeys might scale to human fMRI, the existence of this variability in the mapping of animal cortex suggests that variability in voxel-to-voxel correspondence of fMRI maps from one time to another may to some degree be a function of the variability in the underlying map and not a function of the reliability of the technique. Further, the use of the total volume of activity within a region has a parallel in the animal literature (Nudo et al., 1996; Kleim et al., 2003). The reliability and stability of various fMRI measures of activity in specific ROIs from one time to another deserve further attention in patients with aphasia so that routine changes in maps can be distinguished from neuroplastic changes induced by recovery or rehabilitation.

A final caveat is that in planning fMRI or other functional imaging experiments in aphasia, methodological considerations must be carefully weighed. In addition to the considerations of experimental question and sensitivity of technique, investigators also should take into account the potential bias that an experimental paradigm or method of analysis might produce in their data. The use of fMRI and other functional imaging techniques such as PET or magnetic source imaging has tremendous potential to inform us about the nature and limitations of neuroplasticity in recovery from and rehabilitation for aphasia. Whether or not this potential is realized in our studies depends on how carefully we apply the various techniques that are available. Although convergence across experimental paradigms and/or platforms (fMRI, PET, magnetic source imaging) can be useful in assessing the validity of findings, careful application of methodology will be the foundation of replication and validation of inferences.

Concluding Remarks

There is a significant degree of variability in findings and interpretations in the currently available functional imaging literature on aphasia. Nonetheless, a careful evaluation of this literature indicates that perilesional activity, activity in other structures of the language-dominant hemisphere, and activity in areas of the right hemisphere homologous to damaged regions of the left hemisphere can all contribute to recovery and rehabilitation. The degree to which each contributes will vary from case to case and is dependent on the degree of damage to language structures, the degree of damage to structures controlling lateralization of function, the total number of language structures that are damaged, the variable capacity, between individuals, of the right hemisphere for assuming language functions of the damaged cortex, the nature of the treatment a patient has received, and other factors. Given the number of potential factors involved, it is important to remember that individual variability in the neural substrates of recovery and rehabilitation is likely to be considerable. This being the case, individual subject analyses should be used, unless a group of patients with highly homogeneous lesions and symptoms can be assembled. The methodological considerations for this research can be daunting and must be kept in mind when using such data for theorizing and model building . Nonetheless, such problems cannot deter us from this realm of inquiry. The data and conceptual understanding of neural substrates gleaned from this research will be essential for designing maximally effective treatments and mitigating the deficits caused by aphasia.

REFERENCES

Abo, M., Senoo, A., Watanabe, S., et al. (2004). Language-related brain function during word repetition in post-stroke aphasics. *NeuroReport*, *15*, 1891–1894.

Barch, D. M., Braver, T. S., Saab, F. W., et al (2000). Anterior cingulate and the monitoring of response conflict: Evidence from an fMRI study of overt verb generation. *Journal of Cognitive Neuroscience*, *12*, 298–309.

Barch, D., Sabb, F., Carter, C., et al. (1999). Overt verbal responding during fMRI scanning: Empirical investigations of problems and potential solutions. *NeuroImage*, *10*, 642–657.

Barlow, T. (1877). On a case of double cerebral hemiplegia, with cerebral symmetrical lesions. *British Medical Journal*, *2*, 103–104.

Basso, A., Gardelli, M., Grassi, M. P., et al. (1989). The role of the right hemisphere in recovery from aphasia: Two case studies. *Cortex*, *25*, 555–566.

Belin, P., Van Eeckhout, P., Zilbovicius, M., et al. (1996). Recovery from nonfluent aphasia after melodic intonation therapy: A PET study. *Neurology*, *47*, 1504–1511.

Birn, R. M., Bandettini, P. A., Cox, R. W., et al. (1999). Event-related fMRI of tasks involving brief motion. *Human Brain Mapping*, *7*, 106–114.

Blank, S. C., Bird, H., Turkheimer, F., et al. (2003). Speech production after stroke: The role of the right pars opercularis. *Annals of Neurology*, *54*, 310–320.

Breier, J. I., Castillo, E. M., Boake, C., et al. (2004). Spatiotemporal patterns of language-specific brain activity in patients with chronic aphasia after stroke using magnetoencephalography. *NeuroImage*, *23*, 1308–1316.

Brunner, R. J., Kornhuber, H. H., Seemuller, E., et al. (1982). Basal ganglia participation in language pathology. *Brain and Language*, *16*, 281–299.

Bullmore, E. T., Brammer, M. J., Rebe-Hesketh, S., et al. (1999). Methods for diagnosis and treatment of stimulus-correlated motion in generic brain activation studies using fMRI. *Human Brain Mapping*, *7*, 38–48.

Buxton, R. B. (2001). *Introduction to functional magnetic resonance imaging: Principles and techniques*. New York: Cambridge University Press.

Calvert, G. A. Brammer, M. J., Morris, R. G., et al. (2000). Using fMRI to study recovery from acquired aphasia. *Brain and Language*, *71*, 391–399.

Cao, Y., Vikingstad, E. M., George, K. P., et al. (1999). Cortical language activation in stroke patients recovering from aphasia with functional MRI. *Stroke, 30*, 2331–2340.

Cardebat, D., Demonet, J.-F., De Boissezon, et al. (2003). Behavioral and neurofunctional changes over time in healthy and aphasic subjects: A PET language activation study. *Stroke, 34*, 2900–2906.

Carter, C. S., MacDonald, A. M., Botvinick, M., et al. (2002). Parsing executive processes: Strategic vs. evaluative functions of the anterior cingulate cortex. *Proceedings of the National Academy of Sciences of the United States of America, 97*, 1944–1948.

Cato, M. A., Parkinson, R. B., Wierenga, C., et al. (2004a). Predicting rehabilitative treatment success in chronic nonfluent aphasia: Lesion and performance characteristics. *International Neuropsychological Society: 32nd Annual Meeting Program and Abstracts, 32*, 92–93.

Cato, M. A., Parkinson, R. B., Wierenga, C. E., et al. (2004b). Lesion pattern relates to rehabilitative treatment success in chronic nonfluent aphasia. Program No. 665.13. *Society for Neuroscience 2004 abstract viewer/itinerary planner*. Washington, DC: Society for Neuroscience. Available online at *www.sfn.org*.

Cornelissen, K., Laine, M., Tarkiainen, A., et al. (2003). Adult brain plasticity elicited by anomia treatment. *Journal of Cognitive Neuroscience, 15*, 444–461.

Crosson, B., Bacon Moore, A., Gopinath, K., et al. (2005). Role of the right and left hemispheres in recovery of function during treatment of intention in aphasia. *Journal of Cognitive Neuroscience, 17*, 392–406.

Crosson, B., Benefield, H., Cato, M. A., et al. (2003). Left and right basal ganglia and frontal activity during language generation: Contributions to lexical, semantic, and phonological processes. *Journal of the International Neuropsychological Society, 9*, 1061–1077.

Crosson, B., Sadek, J. R., Maron, L., et al. (2001). Relative shift in activity from medial to lateral frontal cortex during internally versus externally guided word generation. *Journal of Cognitive Neuroscience, 13*, 272–283.

Crosson, B., & Warren, R. L. (1981). Dichotic ear preference for C-V-C words in Wernicke's and Broca's aphasias. *Cortex, 17*, 249–258.

Dobie, R., & Simmons, B. (1971). A dichotic threshold test: Normal and brain damaged subjects. *Journal of Speech and Hearing Research, 14*, 71–81.

Duffau, H., Bauchet, L., Lehéricy, S., et al. (2001). Functional compensation of the left dominant insula for language. *NeuroReport, 12*, 2159–2163.

Fernandez, B., Cardebat, D., Demonet, J.-F., et al. (2004). Functional MRI follow-up study of language processes in healthy subjects and during recovery in a case of aphasia. *Stroke, 35*, 2171–2176.

Finger, S., Buckner, R.L., & Buckingham, H. (2003). Does the right hemisphere take over after damage to Broca's area? The Barlow case of 1877 and its history. *Brain and Language, 85*, 385–395.

Friston, K. J., Williams, S., Howard, R., et al. (2000). Movement-related effects in fMRI time-series. *Magnetic Resonance in Medicine, 35*, 346–355.

Gold, B. T., & Kertesz, A. (2000). Right hemisphere semantic processing of visual words in an aphasic patient: An fMRI study. *Brain and Language, 73*, 456–465.

Gopinath, K. S. (2003). *Reduction of noise associated with stimulus correlated motion in event related overt word generation paradigms*. Unpublished doctoral dissertation, University of Florida, Gainesville.

Gopinath, K. S., Crosson, B., White, K. D., et al. (2004). *Sensitivity compensation method for improved comparisons between pre- and post-treatment fMRI scans of aphasia patients.* Unpublished manuscript.

Gopinath, K., Peck, K., Soltysik, D., et al. (2003). A selective detrending method for reduction of noise associated with event-correlated motion in fMRI time-series for an event-related overt word generation paradigm. *Proceedings of the International Society for Magnetic Resonance in Medicine, 11,* 388.

Gowers, W. R. (1887). *Lectures on the diagnosis of diseases of the brain.* London: Churchill.

Heiss, W.-D., Karbe, H., Weber-Luxenburger, G., et al. (1997). Speech-induced cerebral metabolic activation reflects recovery from aphasia. *Journal of the Neurological Sciences, 145,* 213–217.

Heiss, W.-D., Kessler, J., Thiel, A., et al. (1999). Differential capacity of left and right hemispheric areas for compensation of poststroke aphasia. *Annals of Neurology, 45,* 430–438.

Inase, M., Tokuno, H., Nambu, A., et al. (1999). Corticostriatal and cortico-subthalamic input zones from the presupplementary motor area in the macaque monkey: Comparison with the input zones from the supplementary motor area. *Brain Research, 833,* 191–201.

Johnson, J., Sommers, R., & Weidner, W. (1977). Dichotic ear preference in aphasia. *Journal of Speech and Hearing Research, 20,* 116–129.

Karbe, H., Thiel, A., Weber-Luxenburger, G., et al. (1998). Brain plasticity in postroke aphasia: What is the contribution of the right hemisphere? *Brain and Language, 64,* 215–230.

Kemeny, S., Ye, F. Q., Birn, R., et al. (2005). Comparison of continuous overt speech fMRI using BOLD and arterial spin labeling. *Human Brain Mapping, 24,* 173–183.

Kertesz, A., & McCabe, P. (1977). Recovery patterns and prognosis in aphasia. *Brain, 100,* 1–18.

Kim, Y.-H., Ko, M.-H., Parrish, T. B., et al. (2002). Reorganization of cortical language areas in patients with aphasia: A functional MRI study. *Yonsei Medical Journal, 43,* 441–445.

Kinsborne, M. (1971). The minor cerebral hemisphere as a source of aphasic speech. *Archives of Neurology, 25,* 302–306.

Kleim, J. A., Bruneau, R., Calder, K., et al. (2003). Functional organization of adult motor cortex is dependent upon continued protein synthesis. *Neuron, 40,* 167–76.

Lazar, R. M., Marshall, R. S., Pile-Spellman, J. et al. (2000). Interhemispheric transfer of language in patients with left frontal cerebral arteriovenous malformation. *Neuropsychologia, 38,* 1325–1332.

Léger A, Démonet, J.-F., Ruff, S., et al. (2002). Neural substrates of spoken language rehabilitation in an aphasic patient: An fMRI study. *NeuroImage, 17,* 174–183.

Machielsen, W. C. M., Rombots, S. A. R. B., Barkhof, F., et al. (2000). FMRI of visual encoding: Reproducibility of activation. *Human Brain Mapping, 9,* 156–164.

Maldjian, J. A., Laurienti, P. J., Driskill, L., et al. (2002). Multiple reproducibility indices for evaluation of cognitive functional MR imaging paradigms. *American Journal of Neuroradiology, 23,* 1030–1037.

Martin, P. I., Naeser, M. A., Theoret, H., et al. (2004). Transcranial magnetic stimulation as a complementary treatment for aphasia. *Seminars in Speech and Language*, 25, 181–191.

Mayo, N. E. (1993). Epidemiology and recovery. In R. W. Teasell (Ed.), *Long-term consequences of stroke: State of the art reviews in physical medicine* (pp. 1–25). Philadelphia: Hanley and Belfast.

Mink, J. W. (1996). The basal ganglia: Focused selection and inhibition of competing motor programs. *Progress in Neurobiology*, 50, 381–425.

Miura, K., Nakamura, Y., Miura, F., et al. (1999). Functional magnetic resonance imaging to word generation task in a patient with Broca's aphasia. *Journal of Neurology*, 246, 939–942.

Musso, M., Weiller, C., Kiebel, S., et al. (1999). Training-induced brain plasticity in aphasia. *Brain*, 122, 1781–1790.

Naeser, M. A., Martin, P. I., Baker, E. H., et al. (2004). Overt prepositional speech in chronic nonfluent aphasia studied with the dynamic susceptibility contrast fMRI method. *NeuroImage*, 22, 29–41.

Nambu, A., Tokuno, H., & Takada, M. (2002). Functional significance of the cortico-subthalamo-pallidal "hyperdirect" pathway. *Neuroscience Research*, 43, 111–117.

Newman, S. D., Twieg, D. B., & Carpenter, P. A. (2001). Baseline conditions and subtractive logic in neuroimaging. *Human Brain Mapping*, 14, 228–235.

Nudo, R. J., Milliken, G. W., Jenkins, W. M., et al. (1996). Use-dependent alterations of movement representations in primary motor cortex of adult squirrel monkeys. *Journal of Neuroscience*, 16, 785–807.

Paolucci, S., Antonucci, G., Gialloretti, L. E., et al. (1996). Predicting stroke inpatient rehabilitation outcome: The prominent role of neuropsychological disorders. *European Neurology*, 36, 385–390.

Parkinson, R. B. (2005). *Object and action naming in aphasic stroke patients: Lesion characteristics related to treatment improvement.* Unpublished doctoral dissertation, University of Florida, Gainesville.

Peck, K. K., Moore, A. B., Crosson, B., et al. (2004a). Pre and post fMRI of an aphasia therapy: Shifts in hemodynamic time to peak during an overt language task. *Stroke*, 35, 554–559.

Peck, K. K., Wierenga, C. E., Bacon Moore, A., et al. (2004). Comparison of baseline conditions to investigate syntactic production using functional magnetic resonance imaging. *NeuroImage*, 23, 104–110.

Perani, D., Cappa, S. F., Tettamanti, M., et al. (2003). A fMRI study of word retrieval in aphasia. *Brain and Language*, 85, 357–368.

Richards, K., Singletary, F., Rothi, L. J. G., et al. (2002). The activation of intentional mechanisms through utilization of nonsymbolic movements in aphasia rehabilitation. *Journal of Rehabilitation Research and Development*, 39, 445–454.

Rosen, H. J., Petersen, S. E., Linenweber, M. R., et al. (2000). Neural correlates of recovery from aphasia after damage to left inferior frontal cortex. *Neurology*, 55, 1883–1894.

Schulhoff, C., & Goodglass, H. (1969). Dichotic listening, side of brain injury, and cerebral dominance. *Neuropsychologia*, 7, 149–160.

Seghier, M., Lazeyras, F., Momjian, S., et al. (2001). Language representation in a patient with a dominant right hemisphere: fMRI evidence for an intrahemispheric reorganisation. *NeuroReport*, 12, 2785–2790.

Shanks, J., & Ryan, W. (1976). A comparison of aphasic and non-brain-injured adults on a dichotic CV-syllable listening task. *Cortex*, *12*, 100–112.

Sparks, G., Goodglass, H., & Nickel, B. (1970). Ipsilateral versus contralateral extinction in dichotic listening resulting from hemisphere lesions. *Cortex*, *6*, 249–260.

Swallow, K. M., Braver, T. S., Snyder, A. Z., et al. (2003). Reliability of functional localization using fMRI. *NeuroImage*, *20*, 1561–1577.

Thulborn, K. R., Carpenter, P. A., & Just, M. A. (1999). Plasticity of language-related brain function during recovery from stroke. *Stroke*, *30*, 749–754.

Wabnitz, A., Jasper, B. W., Moore, A. B., et al. (2005). fMRI reveals subcortical activations bridge the stimulus–response interval during word generation by nonfluent aphasics. *International Neuropsychological Society: 33rd Annual Meeting Program and Abstracts*, *33*, 118.

Warburton, E., Price, C. J., Swinburn, K., et al. (1999). Mechanisms of recovery from aphasia: Evidence from positron emission tomography studies. *Journal of Neurology, Neurosurgery, and Psychiatry*, *66*, 155–161.

Wei, X., Yoo, S.-S., Dickey, C. C., et al. (2004). Functional MRI of auditory verbal working memory: Long-term reproducibility analysis. *NeuroImage*, *21*, 1000–1008.

Weiller, C., Isensee, C., Rijntjes, M., et al. (1995). Recovery from Wernicke's aphasia: A positron emission tomographic study. *Annals of Neurology*, *37*, 723–732.

Zahn, R., Drews, E., Specht, K., et al. (2004). Recovery of semantic word processing in global aphasia: A functional MRI study. *Cognitive Brain Research*, *18*, 322–336.

CHAPTER 9

Functional Neuroimaging of Traumatic Brain Injury

Helen M. Genova
Neal M. Fitzpatrick
Frank G. Hillary

An estimated 1.5 million people sustain traumatic brain injury (TBI) in the United States each year (Guerrero et al., 2000). On average, 230,000 people are hospitalized with a TBI, 80,000–90,000 people sustain long-term disabilities, and 50,000 of these TBI incidences are fatal (Jager et al., 2000; Sosin et al., 1989, 1995; Thurman et al., 1999). The consequences of TBI are widespread, affecting any areas of cognitive, emotional, sensory, or motor functioning, and the long-term disabilities associated with TBI are often permanent.

Trauma-related brain damage has traditionally been conceptualized as having two forms: primary injury and secondary injury. Primary injury is nonreversible damage to neural tissue occurring during periods of significant acceleration/deceleration or head-versus-obstacle contact, often taking the form of cerebral contusion, hemorrhage, and/or axonal shear injury. Extensive work examining primary injury in animal models has established the biomechanical thresholds for the various injury subtypes observed following TBI (Ommaya & Hirsch, 1971; Gennarelli et al., 1982; McIntosh et al., 1996). Secondary injury is associated with the pathophysiological processes occurring hours to days after the trauma, including a host of interrelated factors such as blood–brain barrier disruption, mitochondrial dysfunction, and metabolic crisis (for a comprehensive review, see Unterberg et al., 2004). In brief, immediately following brain trauma, excessive neuronal firing in the absence of appropriate O_2 metabolism leads to dependence on anaerobic cellular respiration, which may result in lactate elevations and ischemia (Katayama et al., 1990) and is associated with poor prognosis (Yamaki et al., 1996b). In addition, stimulation of glutamate receptors results in an influx of water-binding ions, such as Ca^{+2}, into the cell body, resulting in widespread edema, increased intracranial pressure, and further ischemic cell death (glutamate and hyperglycolysis are discussed again when this chapter focuses on neurometabolism). Early disruption of basic neurophysiology has long-term implications for baseline cerebral blood flow and oxygen metabolism following TBI. Taken together, these early factors have proven crucial for understanding both the acute and long-term consequences of TBI, and several imaging techniques discussed in this chapter offer critical insights into the basic pathophysiology associated with acute and chronic TBI.

As noted, the disabilities caused by TBI range from mild to severe and symptoms can be physical, cognitive, and/or psychiatric in nature. These varied and often overlapping deficits have widespread implications for a patient's everyday functioning and often affect both the individual sustaining the injury as well as family members/caregivers providing support. Functional neuroimaging provides a unique opportunity to examine and characterize the influences of TBI on basic alterations in neurophysiology and the associated changes in neural networks accounting for the myriad of behavioral deficits evident following TBI in humans.

Overview of Functional Imaging and TBI

Functional neuroimaging has been used to investigate both metabolic and functional alterations in the brain and provide insight into the neural substrates of the behavioral deficits observed following TBI (Ricker et al., 2001a). Positron emission tomography (PET), single-photon emission tomography (SPECT), functional magnetic resonance imaging (fMRI), and proton magnetic resonance spectroscopy (pMRS) have all been employed to varying degrees over the past two decades to study the effects of TBI. To a lesser extent, electroencephalography (EEG) and magnetoencephalography (MEG) have also been employed in the examination of TBI. An important goal of this chapter is to examine how functional neuroimaging has influenced our understanding of the pathophysiology of trauma, the basic changes in neural networks responsible for brain functioning in TBI, and the behavioral deficits associated with adult TBI. In addition, we focus on studies of *adult* TBI for two reasons. First, the functional imaging literature examining infant, child, and adolescent TBI is quite extensive, and an exhaustive review of adult and child TBI is therefore not possible here. Second, because TBI at younger ages occurs in a developing brain, the goals and methods of examination and models predicting brain function are often quite different. For a review of functional imaging in child and adolescent TBI, we refer the interested reader to Munson et al. (2006). Moreover, although animal models of TBI have proven invaluable for understanding the pathophysiology and recovery mechanisms following TBI, this chapter predominantly reflects the work in humans over the past two decades.

We first consider the applications of resting/baseline studies. Resting or baseline studies will include those providing a measurement of an identifiable neurophysiological parameter at a given moment in time, or a "snapshot" of brain functioning. We then review dynamic functional imaging or "time series" measurements and how such methods have been used to examine a variety of deficits associated with TBI. Finally, we consider the methodological issues facing researchers using functional imaging to examine TBI and the future directions for this form of research.

pMRS in TBI

A technique providing a "snapshot" of neurometabolic status that has proven useful in characterizing acute and chronic TBI is pMRS. pMRS is based on the same basic physical principles as conventional MRI sequences; however, the signal comes from larger macromolecules that have distinct local magnetic properties. Each of these larger nuclei maintains a discrete orientation when placed within the MR field and can be localized and quantified. The data collected through the use of pMRS do not create a contrast image, but instead appear as a spectrum, and individual signals, or metabolites, can be found at predictable locations in the spectrum (see Plate 9.1). The primary signals of interest in pMRS arise from N-acetylaspartate (NAA), creatine/phosphocreatine (Cre), choline-containing compounds (Cho), glutamate (GLU), and lactate. NAA is found only in the central nervous system, it is the second most abundant compound in the brain (only GLU is more abundant), and it is produced in the neuron's mitochondria. Although its role in neural recovery following injury remains a topic of investigation, NAA is thought to be involved in a variety of neurometabolic processes, and it has been the focus of brain injury literature because it is a marker for axonal repair, mitochondrial dysfunction, and cell death. The choline peak (which is elevated when concentrations of phosphocholine, glycerophosphocholine, and choline increase) has been shown to be elevated for weeks following injury in areas of local tissue breakdown and edema or repair. For a comprehensive review of pMRS and its use in the study of neurotrauma, see Brooks et al. (2001).

As noted above, a host of neurometabolic alterations exist following brain trauma, and pMRS provides the unique opportunity to examine baseline alterations in neurometabolism noninvasively. For example, diminished cerebral NAA concentrations have been documented using pMRS and correlated with brain injury in both animals (Smith et al., 1998) and humans

(Brooks et al., 2000; Garnett et al., 2000; Friedman et al., 1999). Research using pMRS has shown NAA reductions following TBI as early as 1 h postinjury (Smith et al., 1998), and examination of metabolism in humans has revealed that NAA depression may continue for months prior to metabolic rebound (Brooks et al., 2001; Friedman et al., 1999). Examiners have used pMRS to document altered neurometabolism in both acute (Ross et al., 1998) and chronic TBI (Friedman et al., 1998, 1999) and there is evidence of significant correlation with injury severity and cognitive outcome (Friedman et al., 1998, 1999, Garnett et al., 2000). For example, in the case of chronic TBI, concentrations of metabolic markers such as NAA and Cho have been shown to be predictive of cognitive performance and outcome at 1.5, 3, and 6 mo following the injury (Friedman et al., 1999). Moreover, research acquiring pMRS data within the first 2 wk of injury and at 6 mo following injury revealed it to be sensitive to neurometabolic changes over time (Garnett et al., 2000). For many of these studies, diminished NAA and elevations in Cho have been the most common findings following moderate and severe TBI, and these metabolic alterations have shown the greatest relationship to clinical outcome variables. Researchers have also used pMRS methods to characterize persistent vegetative state (PVS) following TBI. For example, Carpentier and colleagues (2006) recently examined the influence of "invisible" brainstem lesions on PVS by combining spectroscopy and structural MRI data (T2* and FLAIR). Other examiners have used pMRS to document metabolic alterations in thalamic nuclei in individuals in a PVS at the time of scanning (Uzan et al., 2003). It is important to note that structural MRI detected no thalamic abnormality, yet NAA/Cre values in the thalamus discriminated between individuals emerging from PVS (n = 6) and individuals remaining in PVS (n = 8). Taken together, these findings reveal the sensitivity of pMRS in detecting altered neurometabolism following severe TBI and the potential for characterizing general brain status even when sampling discrete areas of tissue via region of interest (ROI) analysis.

An important area of future exploration is the use of pMRS to examine glutamate as a catalyst for secondary injury (e.g., hyperglycolysis). As noted above, the term *hyperglycolysis* has been used to describe neuronal firing during periods of metabolic crisis resulting in reliance on anaerobic respiration and the potential for further neuronal death. In experimental TBI, regional hyperglycolysis has been observed within hours of the injury and may occur regardless of the pathophysiology (e.g., subdural hematoma, cerebral contusion) (Inglis et al., 1992; Sunami et al., 1989; Katayama et al., 1990; for review, see Hovda et al., 1992). Therefore, GLU has repeatedly been observed to play a critical role in the exacerbation of primary injury, and, recently, through the use of noninvasive pMRS methods, investigators have examined the relationship between early GLU elevations and patient outcome. For example, Shutter et al. (2004) examined glutamate/glutamine (Glx) and Cho elevations in 42 patients at approximately 7 d postinjury, finding a significant relationship between these values and patient outcome at 6–12 mo postinjury. Related work examined Glx in children, and although Glx in occipital regions was elevated, these examiners failed to detect a relationship between Glx and outcome (Ashwal et al., 2004). The authors noted that data collection may not have occurred early enough during time periods postinjury when Glx would be peaking in this sample.

The role of GLU in secondary injury early following moderate and severe TBI is critical to understand, yet to date there has been little examination of GLU using pMRS during the first days following injury in severe TBI. This gap in the literature is most likely attributable to previous software limitations for pMRS data analysis, the use of low-field magnets, and difficulty in isolating GLU in the spectra (glutamate and glutamine, another amino acid, are very difficult to distinguish). However, an understanding of the role of GLU in human neurotrauma may now be advanced through the serial application of pMRS at high magnetic field strength and the measurement of absolute, as opposed to relative, metabolic concentrations during acute recovery.

Overall, pMRS has proven to be a promising technique for examining neurometabolic disruption following TBI. It is noninvasive and can be used repeatedly over a protracted recovery course to document basic brain changes following TBI. As noted, however, there remains little application of pMRS to very acute TBI (i.e., within 24–48 h of injury), and the findings in adult populations have come from somewhat small samples and occasionally have been interpreted in conjunction with results for children (Ross et al., 1998). Further work employing pMRS to examine TBI is required to standardize the optimal postinjury time period for data acquisition; there remains surprisingly little longitudinal work documenting the evolution of neurometabolism over the recovery course following TBI. Finally, in the case of severe TBI, investigations using pMRS should include analyses of important neurometabolites (e.g., glutamate, lactate), which have not been the focus of examinations to date, yet may aid in characterizing the progression of secondary injury in TBI and associated cognitive and functional outcomes.

Imaging Baseline Functioning following TBI

Because TBI disrupts a host of basic metabolic processes, examiners have worked to develop novel methods that allow for whole-brain analysis of trauma-induced alterations in neurometabolism. Compared with other functional imaging techniques, PET is the gold standard for examining baseline neurometabolism and has been used most extensively to quantify the cerebral metabolic rate of oxygen ($CMRO_2$) and cerebral metabolic rate of glucose (CMRglc) following TBI. There is an extensive literature using PET to examine baseline neurometabolic phenomena after TBI; the following review is not

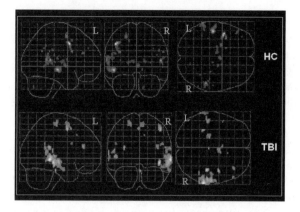

FIGURE 9.1. An image revealing the greater right-hemisphere activation in individuals with TBI during a demanding task of working memory. Adapted from Christodoulou et al. (2001). Copyright 2001 by BMJ Publishing Group. Adapted by permission.

exhaustive, but attempts to integrate the major findings occurring over the past two decades.

Like pMRS, baseline PET measurements of neurometabolism require no overt response by patients and, for this reason, can be used during the very early stages of recovery from TBI. The primary focus of early PET studies in TBI was to determine if information about brain metabolism provided additional information about brain injury that was not available with traditional structural imaging techniques such as computed tomography/magnetic resonance imaging (CT/MRI). Examiners were able to verify that metabolic abnormalities documented via PET were more extensive than the focal areas apparent on structural imaging (Langfitt et al.,1986; Jansen et al., 1996) and sensitive to injury in mild TBI (mTBI) where no focal injury was evident (Ruff et al., 1994; Gross et al., 1996). These early studies confirmed that PET was capable of detecting TBI-related brain changes and demonstrated the importance of examining the neurometabolic markers of injury associated with observable alterations in brain structure.

Because of the baseline differences in neurometabolism observed using PET, other examiners set out to investigate the relationship between cognitive deficits and neurometabolic alterations. For example, using PET, Ruff et al. (1994) examined whole-brain glucose metabolism and correlated findings with cognitive performance outside the scanner. Ruff and colleagues (1994) demonstrated a relationship between cognitive deficits and metabolic disturbance in the frontal and anterior temporal areas. Similar methods were used by Fontaine and colleagues (1996) to demonstrate the relationship between cognitive deficits and metabolic derangements in prefrontal and cingulate areas using (18F)-fluorodeoxyglucose. Although there are important method-ological shortcomings in these early studies, the most salient being the tempo-ral disconnect between PET measurement and cognitive assessment (which was performed outside the scanner, and in the case of Ruff et al., separated by up to a month of scanning), these findings are important for two reasons. First, they further established that PET is sensitive to detecting abnormalities in brain areas outside visible lesion sites typically visible on conventional structural imaging. Second, these studies represent the first work to connect the metabolilc alterations evident in using PET with the behavioral conse-quences of TBI.

An important contribution by Bergsneider and colleagues (2001) repre-sented the first work using PET to document hyperglycolysis in humans. These examiners employed fluorodeoxyglucose-PET (FDG-PET) to examine glucose utilization as a marker for hyperglycolysis, when similar investigation of secondary injury had been previously relegated to animal models of TBI. This seminal research was a precursor to a decade of widespread application of PET to examine the metabolic alterations associated with TBI.

Over the past two decades, PET has been used in a variety of ways to examine pathophysiology following TBI, including changes in cerebrovascular parameters in acute neurotrauma. By using PET, examiners have been able to verify, in humans and animals, a host of cerebrovascular abnormalities, including decoupling of $CMRO_2$ and CMROglc, diminished cerebral blood flow (CBF), and compensatory increases in oxygen extraction fraction (OEF). For example, a critical research application using PET to study TBI has been the examination of ischemia during secondary injury. Because of widespread disruption in basic cerebrovascular parameters, ischemic cell death has been thought to be common following severe TBI, but the physiological parameters for ischemia have proven difficult to establish. However, baseline ^{15}O PET measurements have been used successfully to examine ischemic thresholds fol-lowing TBI (Cunningham et al., 2005; Diringer et al., 2002; Steiner et al., 2003), and in one study examiners observed that persistent metabolic crisis and "classic" indicators of ischemia (e.g., elevated lactate/pyruvate ratio) may actually occur in the absence of frank ischemic cell death (Vespa et al., 2005). Similarly, using ^{15}O PET, Coles et al. (2004) investigated mechanisms of cere-bral ischemia and the relationship between ischemic cell death and outcome following severe TBI. Data from this work showed that within 24 h of severe TBI, ischemic brain volume correlated with poorer outcome at 6 mo post-injury, as indicated by a poor Glasgow Outcome Score (Coles et al., 2004).

Other work has shown that PET compares favorably to invasive surgical procedures when examining basic neurometabolic parameters. For example, research by Hutchinson et al. (2002) revealed that ^{15}O PET can be used to complement invasive measurements such as jugular bulb oximetry and micro-dialysis for examining cerebrovascular reactivity in severe TBI. It is important to note that this study showed that PET imaging was more sensitive in detecting ischemia than bedside monitoring procedures, such as jugular bulb oximetry.

In parallel with work using functional imaging techniques to investigate acute TBI, other researchers have used imaging to explore the influence of brain trauma on chronic metabolic functioning. For example, PET has been used to investigate altered neurometabolism in the cerebral white matter of individuals sustaining TBI. In this study, investigators noted pervasive abnormalities across subjects, allowing them to conclude that cases of moderate and severe TBI are likely most accurately conceptualized as diffuse or focal and diffuse (Wu et al., 2004). That is, irrespective of what is observable on traditional structural MRI (i.e., contusion, subdural hematoma), these PET findings indicate that the pathophysiology following more severe neurotrauma rarely results in an isolated focal injury.

Other examiners have focused on both acute and chronic alterations in cerebrovascular parameters following TBI, such as CBF and $CMRO_2$. Reduced baseline CBF has been well documented in both humans and animal models of TBI (Bouma et al., 1991; Kochanek et al., 2002; Schroder et al., 1996; Yamaki, 1996a) and, near lesion sites, reduced CBF is evident at 1 yr following the injury (Kochanek et al., 2002). Based on this literature, PET has proven invaluable for examining the baseline alterations in CBF, the relationship between CBF and oxygen utilization, and the association between cerebrovascular parameters and injury severity and outcome (for a comprehensive review of this literature, see Golding, 2002).

Using a combination of FDG-PET and whole-brain MEG during presentation of sensory stimulation, other examiners have been able to characterize baseline neurometabolism and brain response in patients in a persistent vegetative state (PVS) (Schiff et al., 2002). This study provided important evidence that brain activity in this small sample of individuals in PVS ($n = 5$) was not random neural activity. These functional imaging findings instead characterized discrete and identifiable neural networks indicative of organized brain function.

PET methods have been used more recently to examine the efficacy of clinical interventions designed to minimize the influence of secondary injury following severe TBI. For example, PET methods afford the ability to track neurometabolism following clinical interventions such as hyperventilation (Coles et al., 2002; Diringer et al., 2002), cerebral perfusion pressure (CPP), manipulation (Steiner et al., 2003; Johnston et al., 2005), and the influence of medications on glucose uptake (Kraus et al., 2005). For example, using ^{15}O PET, Steiner and colleagues (2003) investigated the efficacy of elevating CPP to treat hypoperfusion in areas surrounding cerebral contusions. This study successfully increased CBF in perilesional areas by manipulating CPP and highlighted the use of PET to examine the efficacy of interventions designed to treat ischemia following TBI.

Finally, although quite dissimilar from PET in its method (see Bagic & Sato, Chapter 3, this volume), MEG has also been used to examine aberrant resting activity following mTBI. Lewine and colleagues (1991) used MRI and MEG methods in combination to examine postconcussive symptomatology in a sample of individuals with mTBI. These examiners successfully demonstrated the sensitivity of combining structural MRI and MEG data in order to discriminate among healthy adults, individuals with resolved mTBI, and individuals with ongoing symptomatology following mTBI. These data revealed the sensitivity and specificity in using MEG to detect symptoms following even mild brain injuries. Although it maintains several important methodological advantages compared with other imaging techniques (the most significant being its superior temporal resolution) there remains a paucity of work using MEG to examine the behavioral deficits associated with TBI. The very limited MEG literature in this area is attributable to its expense and the limited number of current MEG facilities for conducting this work.

Activation Studies in TBI

Functional neuroimaging techniques now provide researchers with an opportunity to study changes in the neural networks associated with the behavioral deficits observed following TBI. Clinical researchers have emphasized that dynamic neuroimaging techniques hold significant promise for assessing outcomes and the success of novel TBI treatments and interventions (Levin, 1992; Ricker et al., 2001a). For example, fMRI has recently enjoyed widespread application in clinical studies, primarily owing to the accessibility of magnetic resonance (MR) technology, its noninvasiveness, and its low cost as compared with PET. The application of fMRI to the study of TBI is still novel, however, and much work remains to be done before its potential can be realized.

With the exception of work examining finger oscillation (Prigatano et al., 2004) and hand-grasp movements (Jang et al., 2005) in chronic TBI and a serial MRI study of early motor recovery (Lotze et al., 2006), there has been little work using functional imaging to examine motor and sensory impairment. For this reason, the following several sections focus on the literature examining discrete areas of cognitive dysfunction typically observed following TBI. Much of the work discussed herein represents cross-sectional data in which comparisons have been made between a prototypical response (i.e., healthy control sample) and the response provided by individuals with TBI. Although such designs have limitations, these studies represent the important first work using functional imaging techniques to characterize behavioral deficits following TBI.

Executive Dysfunction

The term "executive dysfunction" is used to describe a constellation of cognitive deficits in the areas of reasoning, planning, mental flexibility, concept formation, and other higher-order cognitive processes. Because of the link between executive functions and frontal lobe connections, and in particular the dorsolateral–prefrontal circuits (see Cummings, 1993) and the ubiquity of frontal lobe injury in TBI, impairments in executive functioning are nearly universal following TBI (Brooks et al., 1999; Gentilini et al., 1985; Leon-Carrion et al., 1998; Gutentag et al., 1998; Shallice & Burgess, 1991; Rieger & Gauggel, 2002; McDonald et al., 2002; Cicerone & Giacino, 1992).

Investigators are now using functional imaging techniques to examine the neural correlates of executive dysfunction following TBI. One of the most well-studied neuropsychological tests for the assessment of executive functioning is the Wisconsin Card Sorting Task (WCST) (Berg, 1948; Grant & Berg, 1948). The WCST requires subjects to decipher a set of rules in order to accurately sort a deck of cards. The task instructions for the WCST provide minimal structure and, throughout the test, the rules change, requiring the subject to inhibit previously learned responses. Thus, the WCST demands significant mental flexibility and problem-solving skills. Executive dysfunction in TBI has been substantiated, using the WCST, by multiple investigators (Martzke et al., 1991; Leon-Carrion et al., 1998).

Using ^{15}O PET during WCST performance, Kirkby et al. (1996). examined executive dysfunction in a single case of moderately severe TBI. To control for genetic determinants of baseline cerebral blood flow, the subject with TBI was compared with his monozygotic twin, who had not sustained a brain injury. Also included were 10 pairs of monozygotic twins to serve as additional controls. The investigators found that during performance of the WCST, the subject with TBI showed reduced regional cerebral blood flow in the inferior portion of the left inferior frontal gyrus and increased regional cerebral blood flow in the left hippocampus, as compared with the uninjured twin. Because performance was comparable between the twins, the authors interpreted the increased hippocampal involvement of the injured twin as compensatory and perhaps engaging long-term memory networks because of the disruption of prefrontal working memory networks. Although these data are difficult to generalize to other samples, this case study represents an early example of the potential for using functional imaging to document basic brain changes responsible for executive dysfunction in TBI.

More recently, Lombardi et al. (1999) examined the relationship between regional brain metabolism and performance on the WCST in a group of eight individuals with mixed TBI severity. These examiners did not directly examine WCST performance during PET data collection; they used an auditory continuous performance test in the scanner and correlated the relationship between PET activation on this test and perseverative responses on the WCST performed within 1 mo of PET imaging. The results indicated that perseverative errors were negatively correlated with right (but not left) dorsolateral prefrontal cortex (PFC) and caudate nucleus activation. The authors concluded that this dorsolateral frontal-caudate circuit was critical for performance of the WCST. Although there are clear shortcomings to the method used by Lombardi and colleagues (1999), including the temporal disconnect between behavioral and functional data, this study represents an important early attempt to examine perseveration following TBI and may serve as the basis for more specific hypothesis testing in future studies of perseveration in TBI. For example, future work may include ROI analysis of the right dorsolateral PFC and caudate nucleus, as well as other neural substrates in this network, in order to clarify the nature of these deficits in TBI.

Attention/Concentration and Inhibition

It is well established that individuals with TBI often show impairments on tasks of attention and concentration (Oddy et al., 1985; van Zomeren & van den Burg, 1985; Ponsford & Kinsella, 1992; Stuss et al., 1989), and functional neuroimaging has recently been used to examine basic deficits in attention and concentration following TBI. Early work by Humayun and colleagues (1989) employed FDG-PET to examine visual vigilance following mild to moderate TBI. The study included three individuals with TBI between 3 and 12 mo postinjury and three matched healthy adults. The study findings indicate that, on average, the TBI sample showed increased regional CMRglc in the anterior temporal and anterior frontal cortices relative to controls. Decreased glucose metabolism in the posterior temporal cortex, posterior frontal cortex, and left caudate nucleus was also observed in subjects with TBI. Although the sample size was small, these early PET findings are consistent with the traditional experimental models of head injury and what is observed clinically in TBI; the frontal and temporal systems are the most commonly affected areas in cases of closed-head trauma.

Recently, Soeda et al. (2005) adapted the Stroop task (Stroop, 1935) to the fMRI environment in order to investigate impairments in attention and response inhibition in individuals with TBI. These investigators were specifically interested in the role of the anterior cingulate cortex (ACC) in mediating attentional resources following TBI. Findings indicated that healthy controls showed activation in the anterior cingulate, replicating findings of other neuroimaging tasks utilizing the Stroop, and individuals with TBI exhibited less activation in the ACC, specifically in the ACed, or the "affective division" of the ACC. The ACed has been linked to attention switching and the deficits specific to attention-deficit/hyperactivity disorder (ADHD) during this task. Because of its hypothesized role in attention, the authors concluded that the observed deficits were due to deficiencies in the neuronal network responsible for attention, as opposed to difficulty with response inhibition or other related cognitive deficits. Interestingly, the TBI group performed worse but not significantly worse than healthy controls (HCs) ($p = .51$). Even so, the authors concluded that failure to integrate the anterior cingulate into the neural network on the part of individuals with TBI resulted in poorer attentional performance. These findings appear to corroborate what has been known of the ACed on tasks of attention in a sample of individuals with TBI; the cingulate thus appears to provide critical resources in this neural network, allowing for controlled responses to stimuli. This is apparent in the healthy adults sample and in the individuals with TBI specifically showing diminished activity in the ACC on this task. It should be noted that the relationship between activation and performance in this study remains somewhat unclear, and this has important implications for interpreting the meaning of the differential brain activation observed between individuals with TBI and healthy adults (discussed in greater detail later).

Working Memory

Working memory (WM) is considered to be a fundamental component that influences most areas of general cognitive functioning (Courtney, 2004), and basic information-processing efficiency in human cognition is influenced by the interaction between processing speed and the size and flexibility of the WM buffer (Demaree et al., 1999; Salthouse, 1996; Salthouse & Coon, 1993). Because working memory functioning is largely mediated by networks in the lateral prefrontal cortex and these same areas are highly susceptible to disruption following TBI, WM impairment is one of the single most common deficits following TBI (Hamm et al., 1996; McDowell et al., 1997; Stuss et al., 1985; Levin et al., 1990). Because it is so often disrupted, WM is the cognitive domain that has been most extensively investigated in TBI using functional neuroimaging.

One of the most commonly used tests to assess WM is a visual or auditory "*n*-back" task. The *n*-back is a WM task requiring continual monitoring and maintenance of individually presented items (e.g., letters) that are to be recalled when prompted. The first examination using fMRI to examine cognitive functioning in mTBI was performed by McAllister and colleagues (1999), who investigated a group of individuals within 1 mo of their injury. Using the *n*-back, these examiners, hypothesized that, compared with healthy adults, individuals with mTBI would show greater alterations in the neural networks associated with WM in response to changes in task load. Although reaction times were not measured, the authors noted that there were no between-group differences in task accuracy in any of the *n*-back conditions (e.g., 0, 1, or 2). Functional imaging results revealed increased right prefrontal activation in individuals with TBI in response to increasing the task load. This activation/ task load response was greater for individuals with TBI, compared with healthy controls, when the task load increased from 1-back to 2-back. The authors interpreted this increased activation as compensatory recruitment of additional cerebral resources that healthy adults do not require.

In a follow-up study, McAllister et al. (2001) again examined mTBI using the *n*-back (1-, 2-, and 3-back) to examine task load effects. The results revealed that in the moderate load condition (2-back), the mTBI group showed higher activation than healthy adults. In the highest working memory load (3-back), the mTBI group showed less activation than healthy controls. The authors interpreted this finding as a ceiling effect in the TBI sample; individuals with TBI reached a threshold where no additional resources were available for recruitment from the 2-back to the 3-back. What is important to consider regarding this interpretation is the method used to create these contrast images ("2-back" was 2-back minus 1-back, and "3-back" was 3-back minus 2-back). Because the mTBI sample showed a more elaborate neural network than did healthy adults during the 2-back task, a more extensive neural network was eliminated in order to create the 3-back contrast image. That is, in mTBI, the 3-back contrast eliminated much of the neural network responsible for responding to the increasing task load because, in the mTBI sample this network was already evident at 2-back. This is a basic problem with cognitive subtraction in functional imaging studies (see Gazzaley & D'Esposito, Chapter 4, this volume), and this issue is magnified in examining clinical samples in which there may be a fundamental difference between groups in the networks "removed" to create contrast effects.

Even considering the methodological shortcomings discussed here, the studies by McAllister and colleagues (1999, 2001) have provided reliable evidence that the neural networks representing WM in healthy adults and a mildly brain-injured TBI sample can be dissociated using fMRI. Moreover, regardless of the interpretation of the divergent activation patterns between groups, the work by McAllister and colleagues generally demonstrated that during tasks of WM, a disrupted neural network is associated with *increased* brain activation in the prefrontal, temporal, and parietal areas.

Christodoulou and colleagues (2001) later conducted the first examination of WM deficits using fMRI in a group of individuals with moderate and severe TBI. To examine the neural networks associated with working memory, these investigators used a modified version of the Paced Auditory Serial Addition Test (mPASAT) in the scanner. The mPASAT is a widely used and demanding WM task requiring rapid rehearsal and mental calculation of single digits. The mPASAT has been shown to be sensitive to WM and speeded the processing of impairments in TBI (Brooks et al., 1999). In this study, Christodoulou et al. hypothesized that the individuals with TBI would show increased activation in conjunction with diminished performance on this WM task. Although the healthy controls and individuals with TBI demonstrated overlapping regions of activation (i.e., middle frontal gyrus, superior and middle temporal gyrus, and inferior parietal gyrus), individuals with TBI consistently showed greater right-hemisphere activation, whereas healthy adults exhibited a neural network lateralized to the left hemisphere. Unfortunately, the design employed by these investigators did not allow for parametric manipulation of working memory load. Even so, the TBI sample performed significantly worse on the mPASAT task, so the observed increase in right-hemisphere activation was associated with poorer performance. These findings were consistent with work by McAllister and colleagues (1999, 2001) and again indicated that during WM tasks, individuals with TBI show a neural network requiring greater PFC involvement than do healthy adults. However, unlike those of McAllister et al., the findings by Christodoulou and colleagues (2001) revealed an important negative relationship between brain activation and task performance. Similar performance/activation relationships in TBI were more recently observed in a case study by Scheibel and colleagues (2003) and in the most recent study of working memory in moderate and severe TBI, in which investigators manipulated the WM load using the n-back (Perlstein et al., 2004). In fact, the work by Perlstein and colleagues (2004) revealed WM impairments both inside and outside the scanner, and, similar to the findings by Christodoulou and colleagues, individuals with TBI showed greater right dorsolateral–prefrontal cortex activation.

Although many WM tasks used in imaging studies have use verbally mediated materials, Chen and colleagues (2003) conducted a study of spatial working memory in mTBI. These investigators used PET to examine neural networks during a spatial working memory task in a group of individuals with mTBI. Interestingly, they found that in examining symptomatic patients as a group, individuals with mTBI had a smaller percentage change in regional CBF than controls in the right inferior frontal gyrus. Although the sample size in this study was quite small ($n = 5$ TBI, 5 controls), these data are consistent with prior work in humans and animals documenting reductions in CBF values.

In a more comprehensive investigation of mTBI, Chen et al. (2004) examined 16 athletes with concussion, using both a visual and a verbal working memory task during fMRI. It is important to note that the subjects did not differ significantly in their performance and displayed brain activation patterns similar to HCs. The athletes with concussion, however, showed less task-related activation in the right mid-dorsolateral prefrontal cortex and a negative relationship between the BOLD signal change and postconcussive symptom severity. Because of the negative relationship between the BOLD signal and the degree of symptomatology, these findings are inconsistent with prior work examining WM dysfunction in more severely injured populations. Although difficult to reconcile with the literature, the divergent findings in Chen et al. (2004) may be due to the type of task used or the mild nature of the injury in this sample.

Learning and Memory

Disturbed recognition memory for shapes following TBI was documented more than three decades ago (Levin et al., 1976) and "forgetfulness" has long been the most common deficit reported by patients with TBI (van Zomeren & van den Burg, 1985). Since that time, episodic memory deficits following TBI have been repeatedly observed, and examiners now maintain that most individuals with moderate and severe TBI experience some degree of memory disturbance (Levin, 1990; Rosenthal & Ricker, 2000). Surprisingly, the emphasis on examining new learning deficits in TBI has not transferred to the imaging literature, where much of the work thus far in TBI has focused on WM deficits.

In one study of episodic memory following TBI, Levine and colleagues (1998) used ^{15}O PET to examine an individual with severe TBI and isolated retrograde amnesia. The examiners hypothesized that, given the role of right prefrontal areas in episodic retrieval, the subject would show right frontal dysfunction, compared with healthy adults. The healthy controls showed activation patterns typical of encoding and retrieval: Greater left prefrontal activation was observed during encoding, whereas greater right prefrontal activation was observed during retrieval. However, in the patient with severe retrograde amnesia, decreased activation in right frontal regions was observed during retrieval, as well as increases in activation in posterior cortical areas during cued free recall. This case study illustrates trauma-induced alterations in traditionally well-established networks representing episodic memory.

Separately, Ricker et al. (2001b) were the first to use ^{15}O PET to examine regional cerebral blood flow (rCBF) changes during verbal recall and recognition in TBI. Using a small TBI sample size ($n = 5$), this study examined word recognition following a list-learning trial. The data revealed that during word recall, frontal lobe rCBF was reduced in individuals with TBI, as compared with HCs; however, there were increases in CBF in several posterior brain regions in cases of TBI. During recognition trials, both groups demonstrated bifrontal increases in activation. These findings corroborate what has been observed in behavioral studies examining episodic memory deficits following TBI; acquisition of novel material is often slowed or reduced, but individuals with TBI often show relatively spared recognition for recently presented material (DeLuca et al., 2000).

More recently, Levine et al. (2002) once again examined the functional organization of memory in six subjects with moderate to severe TBI using ^{15}O PET. The goal of the study was to document activation differences in individuals with TBI relative to controls, using a previously studied learning and retrieval paradigm. The investigators predicted that when compared with healthy adults, participants with TBI would show additional activation due to functional reorganization of function following the injury. Behaviorally, the subjects with TBI performed worse, but not significantly worse, than the healthy controls. In regard to functional imaging data, healthy adults and subjects with TBI showed a right-lateralized frontotemporal network; however, participants with TBI also exhibited a neural network that extended to areas contralateral and homologous to those regions active in the baseline neural network. In order to examine the influence of localized lesions on the findings, the investigators removed three subjects with focal sites of injury, and, after reanalysis, the results remained largely the same. These findings were important because they illustrated that individuals with TBI, regardless of lesion size or location, tend to show patterns of activation dissimilar to those of healthy individuals, which may imply that diffuse axonal injury may cause the altered activation patterns in this population. The consistency in these findings across individuals in what has classically been considered a heterogeneous sample is an important contribution provided by imaging, which discussed in greater detail in a following section, "Integrating the Findings."

Summary of Functional Imaging Studies to Date

This chapter has provided an overview of the current functional imaging studies examining cognitive dysfunction following TBI. It is important to remember that the neuroimaging studies discussed here are designed to establish a basic pattern of brain activation in HCs, which become the standard for comparison for individuals with TBI. These "normal" activation patterns are used to determine abnormality in the TBI sample, and any differences in the basic neural network are commonly attributed to the trauma. However, the nature of these basic brain activation patterns may vary from study to study, from group to group, and, in some cases, even within groups of healthy adults. This variability in basic neural networks (especially when occurring during roughly equivalent levels of behavioral performance) is important to consider and has implications for interpreting the "aberrant" activation observed in any single case of TBI. Moreover, conclusions, to date, are limited by the very small sample sizes; only the work by McAllister and colleagues (1999, 2001) have had a sample size of at least 20. The studies conducted thus far have focused largely on the neural networks of cognitive domains known to be impaired in TBI (see Table 9.1 for descriptions of important baseline and functional studies in TBI). Although various cognitive domains have been assessed, there are some commonalities across findings, and these are discussed below.

Integrating the Findings

A review of the current literature indicates that, very generally speaking, functional neuroimaging is sensitive to the basic brain alterations evident following TBI. This sensitivity has been consistently documented across studies, and, critically, the basic brain differences observed via functional imaging have typically been linked to specific performance decrements. The directionality of these activation/performance relationships is the basis for understanding how distinct brain structures, and even entire neural networks, contribute to the cognitive deficits observed in TBI.

Altered brain activation in TBI samples as compared with HCs has been occasionally interpreted as *compensatory* or indicative of *brain reorganization*. The term "compensation," as it has been used in the functional imaging literature to date, implies that brain activation observed in individuals with TBI operates to bolster the subject's performance. However, without directly examining the relationship between performance and activation (specifically using reaction time), it is difficult to determine if altered brain activation facilitates performance or is an indicator of an inefficient neural system. In several studies reviewed above, a negative relationship between performance and activation was observed (see Christodoulou et al., 2001; Perlstein et al., 2004). This negative relationship between neural activity and task performance indicates that either the observed neural networks are directly contributing to poor performance (e.g., neural disinhibition) or they represent a network that

TABLE 9.1. Influential Studies Examining Neurometabolism in TBI

Study	Imaging modality	Regions of interest	Sample size	Control sample size	Summary of findings
			MR spectroscopy		
Ashwal et al. (2004)	pMRS	Occipital grey and parietal white matter	38 children with TBI	10 matched controls	Elevated Glx levels, Glx did not correlate with outcome.
Brooks et al. (2000)	pMRS	Occipitoparietal grey and white matter	19 TBI, longitudinally over 6 mo	28 controls	Neuropsychological deficits correlated with decreased NAA and increased Cho; NAA at 1.5 mo correlated with outcome at 6 mo.
Carpentier et al. (2006)	pMRS	Brain stems	40 severe TBI 17.5 ± 6.4 d after injury	None	pMRS sensitive to otherwise undetected brain stem injury.
Friedman et al. (1998)	pMRS	Normal-appearing occipitoparietal white and occipital grey matter	12 TBI	14 controls	Reduced NAA in white matter and increased Cho in grey matter; NAA and Cr correlated with neuropsychological performance.
Friedman et al. (1999)	pMRS	Occipitoparietal white and grey matter	14 TBI at 1.5 and 6 mo postinjury	14 matched controls	NAA levels correlated with neuropsychological testing performance and GOS.
Garnett et al. (2000)	pMRS	Lesioned areas	19 TBI 3–38 d postinjury	None	NAA decreased and Cho increased postinjury; the severity of the injury correlated with the decline of the NAA/Cr ratio.
Ross et al. (1998)	pMRS	Lesioned areas	12 children, 13 adults with acute TBI	None	Reductions in NAA after injury in lesioned areas; in children, detectable lipid/lactate levels and decreased NAA/Cr level correlated negatively with outcome.

(continued)

263

TABLE 9.1. *(continued)*

Study	Imaging modality	Regions of interest	Sample size	Control sample size	Summary of findings
			MR spectroscopy *(continued)*		
Shutter et al. (2004)	pMRS	Normal-appearing brain tissue	42 TBI 7 days out from injury	None	Glx and Cho were elevated in occipital grey and parietal white matter in participants with poor outcomes. MRS was more accurate in predicting outcome than somatosensory evoked potentials.
Uzan et al. (2003)	pMRS	Thalamus	14 TBI: 8 in PVS, 6 who emerged from PVS	5 controls	MRS showed severe brain damage in the thalamus by detecting NAA/Cr ratios where conventional MRI did not. NAA/Cr ratios were correlated with group prediction on persistent vegetative or emergent status.
			Baseline PET		
Bergsneider et al. (1997)	[18]FDG PET	Whole brain, focus on lesioned areas	28 TBI with severe injures	None	First study to document hyperglycolysis after TBI using imaging; hyperglycolysis shown in lesioned areas, perilesioned areas, and globally.
Coles et al. (2002)	[15]O PET	Whole brain	33 TBI within 7 d of injury	14 controls	Hyperventilation led to increases in intracranial perfusion pressure, but also correlated with ischemic brain tissue.
Coles et al. (2004)	[15]O PET	Whole brain	12 TBI	10 matched controls	24 h after TBI, ischemic brain volume correlated with poor GOS at 6 mo; PET was more sensitive to ischemia than bedside monitoring procedures.
Diringer et al. (2002)	[15]O PET	Whole brain	13 severe TBI; 9 underwent moderate	None	Hyperventilation caused decreases in oxygen and CBF; these changes did not translate to energy

264

Study	PET method	Region	Sample	Control	Findings
			hyperventilation, 4 underwent severe hyperventilation		failure due to increased OEF and lower baseline metabolic rate.
Hutchinson et al. (2002)	Triple oxygen PET	Frontal areas defined by microdialysis	17 TBI with severe injuries	None	Significant relationship between lactate/pyruvate ratio and OEF. Combining PET and microdialysis effective and safe.
Jansen et al. (1996)	^{55}Co PET	Whole brain	5 TBI with moderate injuries	None	^{55}Co PET detected greater damage than did MRI or CT; detected damage in perilesional areas also detected by EEG.
Kraus et al. (2005)	^{18}FDG PET	Prefrontal cortex	22 total TBI; 6 underwent PET	None	NMDA agonist (amantidine), increased left prefrontal cortex glucose metabolism.
Langfitt et al. (1986)	^{133}Xe PET	Lesioned areas	3 TBI with elevated intracranial pressure	None	^{133}Xe PET detected greater cerebral damage than did MRI or CT, especially in the anterior temporal lobe.
Schroder et al. (1996)	^{15}O PET	Whole brain; ventricular size	33 severe TBI; 3 mo postinjury	None	Early CBF did not correlate with atrophy; did correlate with outcome; new thresholds for ischemia suggested.
Steiner et al. (2003)	^{15}O PET	Perilesional areas	18 TBI	18 nonlesioned areas in same TBI	Increased cerebral perfusion pressure and CBF in areas of lesion.
Wu et al. (2004)	^{15}O and ^{18}FDG PET	Grey and white matter in nonlesioned areas	10 TBI with moderate–severe injuries	16 controls	Decreases in the global white matter oxygen-to-glucose metabolism ratio indicated TBI has unrecognized diffuse effects.

(continued)

TABLE 9.1. (continued)

Study	Imaging modality	Regions of interest	Sample size	Control sample size	Summary of findings
				Functional imaging	
Chen et al. (2003)	^{15}O PET	Whole brain	5 TBI	5 controls	Mild TBI had a smaller % increase in regional CBF in the inferior frontal gyrus.
Chen et al. (2004)	fMRI	Whole brain	16 mild TBI	8 controls	TBI participants showed less activation in the right DLPFC; negative correlation between activation and post concussive symptoms.
Christodoulou et al. (2001)	fMRI	Whole brain	9 TBI	7 matched controls	TBI participants showed more right PFC, temporal activation during modified PASAT; greater "dispersion" of activation.
Humayun et al. (1989)	^{18}FDG PET	Whole brain	3 TBI	3 matched controls	Decreased glucose metabolism in medial temporal, posterior temporal, posterior frontal areas; increased metabolism in anterior temporal and frontal lobes.
Kirkby et al. (1996)	^{15}O PET	Whole brain	1 TBI; uninjured MZ twin	10 pairs of uninjured MZ twins	Injured MZ twin greater activation in the hippocampus and less activation in the left inferior frontal gyrus.
Levine et al. (1998)	^{15}O PET	Whole brain	1 amnesic participant	5 moderate to severe TBI w/o amnesia; 12 controls	Decreased right prefrontal activation during episodic memory retrieval compared to controls; increased activation in posterior cortical areas.
Levine et al. (2002)	^{15}O PET	Frontotemporal areas	6 moderate–severe TBI	11 matched controls	All participants showed right frontotemporal activation; TBIs also activated a contralateral homologue.

Study	Method	Region	TBI	Controls	Findings
Lombardi et al. (1999)	^{18}FDG PET	Whole brain	8 TBI	None	Negative correlation between perseverative responses and metabolism in the right but not left dorsolateral prefrontal cortex and caudate nucleus.
McAllister et al. (1999)	fMRI	Whole brain	12 TBI	11 matched controls	Mild TBI showed increased right PFC activation in working memory circuits with increasing task load compared with HCs.
McAllister et al. (2001)	fMRI	Whole brain	18 TBI (including the 12 from above)	12 matched controls	TBI showed greater right PFC activation and greater increase from 1–2 back and less from 2–3 back compared with the HCs.
Ricker et al. (2001a)	^{15}O PET	Whole brain	5 TBI	4 matched controls	TBI participants had decreased frontal activation during verbal memory recall, and increases in posterior cortical regions.
Ruff et al. (1994)	^{18}FDG PET	Various regions	9 TBI	24 controls	PET confirmed positive neuropsychological test results where conventional MRI and CT did not.
Scheibel et al. (2003)	fMRI	Prefrontal cortex	1 TBI	4 controls	Bilateral activation of PFC during a response inhibition task and a working memory task where HCs were unilateral.
Soeda et al. (2005)	fMRI	Whole brain	5 TBI	11 controls	TBI participants had less ACC activation during the Stroop task than did the HCs.

Note. HC, healthy control participant; CBF, cerebral blood flow; OEF, oxygen extraction fraction; PFC, prefrontal cortex; DLPFC, dorsolateral prefrontal cortex; ACC, anterior cingulate gyrus; MZ, monozygotic; FDG, fluorodeoxyglucose; Xe, xenon; Co, cobalt; PVS, persistent vegetative state; GOS, Glasgow Outcome Score; Glx, glutamate/glutamine; NAA, N-acetyl-aspartate; Cho, choline; Cr, creatine; PASAT, Paced Auditory Serial Addition Test is brought online owing to diminishing performance (e.g., cognitive control mechanisms). Thus, increases in brain activation that can be directly linked to performance decrements should not be interpreted as facilitative and certainly not indicative of "brain reorganization." Moreover, it is important to note that on tasks of WM, there is evidence that even healthy adults recruit prefrontal cortical networks during periods of increased task load (Braver et al., 1997; Culham et al., 2001; Manoach et al., 1997; Rypma & D'Esposito, 1999; Rypma et al., 1999). These findings indicate that increased neural activity during periods of poor performance may reflect basic mechanisms in place to tolerate fluctuating increases in task load and is not necessarily directly related to the injury. For this reason, the task–performance relationship has critical implications for interpreting activation in TBI. For a comprehensive review of this issue, see Hillary et al. (2006).

Whereas the findings from studies examining attention, WM, and episodic memory reveal negative task performance–activation relationships, studies examining other cognitive domains such as response inhibition and sustained attention have shown positive activation–task performance relationships. In the case of TBI, prefrontal areas have often shown increases in activation as performance diminishes; however, as noted by Scheibel et al. (2003), failure to integrate (or "activate") the ACC during a task of sustained attention was associated with poorer task performance. This positive relationship between performance and activation was also observed in investigations of more "hard-wired" functions, such as motor skills (Lotze et al., 2006; Prigatano et al., 2004), further indicating that activation–performance relationships may be dissociable across neural networks. Appropriate interpretation of imaging results thus requires performance (i.e., HC performance) and the directionality of activation–performance relationships in the TBI sample.

Future Directions for Functional Imaging and TBI

The application of functional imaging techniques to examine TBI thus far has been promising, yet there remain a great number of phenomena to be studied and methodological shortcomings to be addressed. First, at the most fundamental level, future work should continue to document the basic relationships between observable deficits and the neural substrate associated with those deficits. As noted repeatedly, the directionality of the activation–performance relationships is the basis for understanding how distinct brain structures, and even entire neural networks, contribute to the cognitive deficits observed in TBI. For this reason, future work should not aim simply to document the *existence* of altered patterns of activation in TBI, because for any between-group comparison, some differences likely exist. What is essential to characterize is the relationship between task performance and the specific neural network associated with that performance; such efforts allow for analysis of discrete cognitive deficits and their specific neurofunctional correlates.

The next generation of functional imaging studies in TBI should aim to examine a broader range of the basic trauma-induced deficits. Such examinations should include motor and sensory deficits, as well as a broader range of cognitive deficits commonly observed following TBI, including basic speed of information-processing deficits and the varied manifestations of frontal lobe dysfunction including perseveration, impulsivity, and planning/problem solving. Future work should focus less on ROI analysis and seek to examine basic cognitive deficits in the context of understanding how complete neural networks are altered following trauma. Approaches using whole-brain analyses also offer an opportunity to test models of connectivity to discern how neural networks operate in concert during any cognitive, sensory, or motor task (e.g., independent or principle components analysis). Connectivity analyses such as independent component analyses and principle components analysis provide information about how alterations at one area of a distributed neural network may influence functioning, not only in connected components, but in distant components of the same network (for a more complete review of connectivity methods, see McIntosh & Grady, Chapter 5, this volume). As noted, future work will require parametric manipulations in order to better characterize activation–performance relationships.

An important consideration in using functional imaging to examine brain injury and disease is the influence pathology may have directly on the imaging method. For example, although many of the current imaging techniques provide direct measurement of neural activity (e.g., MEG, EEG) or related neurophysiology (e.g., glucose uptake, oxygen utilization), because it is an indirect measure of neuronal firing, fMRI does not enjoy the same advantages. Thus, there remain important obstacles for investigators attempting to use fMRI to reliably examine the subtypes of TBI and the various stages of recovery. First, there has been no systematic examination of the effects of changes in cerebrovascular physiology on the fMRI signal over the course of recovery from TBI. As documented above, TBI results in widespread disruption of baseline cerebrovascular parameters, and recent work in humans has shown that the basic components of the fMRI signal (e.g., CBF, OEF, and blood flow transit time) are influenced in brain areas adjacent to a brain lesion (Hillary & Biswal, 2007; see Plate 9.2). To date, however, there has been no systematic examination of the influence of focal or diffuse brain lesions on the fMRI signal in humans. Moreover, the relationship between the fMRI signal and various clinical factors, such as time since injury, injury severity, and lesion presence, remains unknown. In order to more precisely examine the cognitive, motor, and emotional consequences of TBI using fMRI, it will be critical to determine the influence of these clinical factors on the fMRI signal.

Summary and Conclusions

Functional imaging has provided important insights into the basic brain changes commonly occurring following brain trauma. Through the use of multiple technologies, imaging now provides the opportunity to integrate information about the structural, metabolic, and functional brain changes associated with brain trauma. Findings have been instrumental in documenting baseline alterations in cerebrovascular reactivity in humans in areas adjacent to and distant from focal lesions. Examinations of neurometabolism via pMRS methods have been used to isolate important predictors of later cognitive and functional outcomes. Recent work using PET and fMRI methods have isolated localized and whole-brain alterations to the basic neural networks associated with attentional, memorial, and higher-order functioning. The next generation of studies should also work to examine other areas of deficit following TBI, including sensory and motor deficits, psychiatric problems, and common cognitive deficits not yet studied (e.g., speed of information processing, problem solving, impulsivity). Future work requires greater methodological precision by linking behavioral performance to brain activation through parametric manipulation of task load. Such methods allow examiners to directly examine the relationship between basic changes in the neural network and task performance as the task varies in demand. By including whole-brain and network analyses and continually refining current methods, functional imaging has the flexibility necessary for examining the various influences of brain trauma on human behavior.

REFERENCES

Ashwal, S., Holshouser, B., Tong, K., et al. (2004). Proton spectroscopy detected glutamate/glutamine is detected in children with traumatic brain injury. *Journal of Neurotrauma, 21*(11), 1539–1552.

Berg, E. (1948). A simple objective technique for measuring flexibility in thinking. *Journal of General Psychology, 39*, 15–22.

Bergsneider, M., Hovda, D. A., McArthurs, D. L., et al. (2001). Metabolic recovery following human traumatic brain injury based on fdg-pet: Time course and relationship to neurological disability. *Journal of Head Trauma Rehabilitation, 16*(2), 135–148.

Bouma, G. J., Muizelaar, J. P., Choi, S. C., et al. (1991). Cerebral circulation and metabolism after severe traumatic brain injury: The elusive role of ischemia. *Journal of Neurosurgery, 75*(5), 685–693.

Braver, T. S., Cohen, J. D., Nystrom, L. E., et al. (1997). A parametric study of prefrontal cortex involvement in human working memory. *NeuroImage, 5*(1), 49–62.

Brooks, D. N. (1976). Wechsler Memory Scale performance and its relationship to brain damage after severe closed head injury. *Journal of Neurology, Neurosurgery and Psychiatry, 39*(6), 593–601.

Brooks, J., Fos, L. A., Greve, K. W., et al. (1999). Assessment of executive function in patients with mild traumatic brain injury. *Journal of Trauma, 46*(1), 159–163.

Brooks, W. M., Friedman, S. D., & Gasparovic, C. (2001). Magnetic resonance spectroscopy in traumatic brain injury. *Journal of Head Trauma Rehabilitation, 16*(2), 149–164.

Brooks, W. M., Stidley, C. A., Petropoulos, H., et al. (2000). Metabolic and cognitive response to human traumatic brain injury: A quantitative proton magnetic resonance study. *Journal of Neurotrauma*, 17(8), 629–640.

Carpentier, A., Galanaud, D., Puybasset, L., et al. (2006). Early morphologic and spectroscopic magnetic resonance in severe traumatic brain injuries can detect "invisible brain stem damage" and predict "vegetative states." *Journal of Neurotrauma*, 23(5), 674–685.

Chen, J. K., Johnston, K. M., Frey, S., et al. (2004). Functional abnormalities in symptomatic concussed athletes: An fMRI study. *NeuroImage*, 22(1), 68–82.

Chen, S. H., Kareken, D. A., Fastenau, P. S., et al. (2003). A study of persistent postconcussion symptoms in mild head trauma using positron emission tomography. *Journal of Neurology, Neurosurgery and Psychiatry*, 74(3), 326–332.

Christodoulou, C., DeLuca, J., Ricker, J. H., et al. (2001). Functional magnetic resonance imaging of working memory impairment after traumatic brain injury. *Journal of Neurology, Neurosurgery and Psychiatry*, 71, 161–168.

Cicerone, K., & Giacino, J. (1992). Remediation of executive function deficits after traumatic brain injury. *Neurorehabilitation*, 2, 12–22.

Coles, J. P., Fryer, T. D., Smielewski, P., et al. (2004). Defining ischemic burden after traumatic brain injury using ^{15}O PET imaging of cerebral physiology. *Journal of Cerebral Blood Flow and Metabolism*, 24(2), 191–201.

Coles, J. P., Minhas, P. S., Fryer, T. D., et al. (2002). Effect of hyperventilation on cerebral blood flow in traumatic head injury: Clinical relevance and monitoring correlates. *Critical Care Medicine*, 30(9), 1950–1959.

Courtney, S. M. (2004). Attention and cognitive control as emergent properties of information representation in working memory. *Cognitive, Affective, and Behavioral Neuroscience*, 4(4), 501–516.

Culham, J. C., Cavanagh, P., & Kanwisher, N. G. (2001). Attention response functions: Characterizing brain areas using fMRI activation during parametric variations of attentional load. *Neuron*, 32(4), 737–745.

Cummings, J. L. (1993). Frontal-subcortical circuits and human behavior. *Archives of Neurology*, 50(8), 873–880.

Cunningham, A. S., Salvador, R., Coles, J. P., et al. (2005). Physiological thresholds for irreversible tissue damage in contusional regions following traumatic brain injury. *Brain*, 128(Pt. 8), 1931–1942.

DeLuca, J., Schultheis, M. T., Madigan, N. K., et al. (2000). Acquisition versus retrieval deficits in traumatic brain injury: Implications for memory rehabilitation. *Archives of Physical Medicine and Rehabilitation*, 81(10), 1327–1333.

Demaree, H. A., DeLuca, J., Gaudino, E. A., et al. (1999). Speed of information processing as a key deficit in multiple sclerosis: Implications for rehabilitation. *Journal of Neurology, Neurosurgery and Psychiatry*, 67(5), 661–663.

Diringer, M. N., Videen, T. O., Yundt, K., et al. (2002). Regional cerebrovascular and metabolic effects of hyperventilation after severe traumatic brain injury. *Journal of Neurosurgery*, 96(1), 103–108.

Faden, A. I., O'Leary, D. M., Fan, L., et al. (2001). Selective blockade of the mGluR1 receptor reduces traumatic neuronal injury in vitro and improves outcome after brain trauma. *Experimental Neurology*, 167(2), 435–444.

Fontaine, Azouvi, Remy, et al. (1996). Functional anatomy of neuropsychological deficits after severe traumatic brain injury. *Neurology*, 53(9), 1963–1968.

Friedman, S. D., Brooks, W. M., Jung, R. E., et al. (1999). Quantitative 1H-MRS predicts outcome following traumatic brain injury. *Neurology, 52,* 1384–1391.

Friedman, S. D., Brooks, W. M., Jung, R. E., et al. (1998). Proton MR spectroscopic findings correspond to neuropsychological function in traumatic brain injury. *American Journal of Neuroradiology, 19,* 1879–1885.

Garnett, M. R., Blamire, A. M., Rajagopalan, B., et al. (2000). Evidence for cellular damage in normal-appearing white matter correlates with injury severity in patient following TBI: A magnetic resonance spectroscopy study. *Brain, 123,* 1403–1409.

Gennarelli, T. A., Thibault, L. E., Adams, J. H., et al. (1982). Diffuse axonal injury and traumatic coma in the primate. *Annals of Neurology, 12*(6), 564–574.

Gentilini, M., Nichelli, P., Schoenhuber, R., et al. (1985). Neuropsychological evaluation of mild head injury. *Journal of Neurology, Neurosurgery, and Psychiatry, 48*(2), 137–140.

Golding, E. M. (2002). Sequelae following traumatic brain injury. The cerebrovascular perspective. *Brain Research Reviews, 38*(3), 377–388.

Grant, D. A., & Berg, E. A. (1948). A behavioral analysis of degree of reinforcement and ease of shifting to new responses in a Weigl-type card sorting problem. *Journal of Experimental Psychology, 50,* 237–244.

Gross, H., Kling, A., Henry, G., et al. (1996). Local cerebral glucose metabolism in patients with long-term behavioral and cognitive deficits following mild traumatic brain injury. *Journal of Neuropsychiatry and Clinical Neurosciences, 8*(3), 324–334.

Guerrero, J. L., Thurman, D. J., & Sniezek, J. E. (2000). Emergency department visits associated with traumatic brain injury: United States, 1995–1996. *Brain Injury, 14*(2), 181–186.

Gutentag, S. S., Naglieri, J. A., & Yeates, K. O. (1998). Performance of children with traumatic brain injury on the Cognitive Assessment System. *Assessment, 5*(3), 263–272.

Hamm, R. J., Temple, M. D., Pike, B. R., et al. (1996).Working memory deficits following traumatic brain injury in the rat. *Journal of Neurotrauma, 13*(6), 317–323.

Hillary, F. G., Genova, H. M., Chiaravalloti, N. D., et al. (2006). Prefrontal modulation of working memory performance in brain injury and disease. *Human Brain Mapping, 27*(11), 837–847.

Hillary, F. G., & Biswal, B. (2007). The influence of neuropathology on the fMRI signal: A measurement of brain or vein? *Clinical Neuropsychologist, 21*(1), 58–72.

Hovda, D. A., Becker, D. P., & Katayama, Y. (1992). Secondary injury and acidosis. *Journal of Neurotrauma, 9*(Suppl. 1), S47–S60.

Humayun, M. S., Presty, S. K., Lafrance, N. D., et al. (1989). Local cerebral glucose abnormalities in mild closed head injured patients with cognitive impairments. *Nuclear Medicine Communications, 10*(5), 335–344.

Hutchinson, P. J., Gupta, A. K., Fryer, T. F., et al. (2002). Correlation between cerebral blood flow, substrate delivery, and metabolism in head injury: A combined microdialysis and triple oxygen positron emission tomography study. *Journal of Cerebral Blood Flow Metabolism, 22*(6), 735–745.

Inglis, F., Kuroda, Y., & Bullock, R. (1992). Glucose hypermetabolism after acute subdural hematoma is ameliorated by a competitive NMDA antagonist. *Journal of Neurotrauma, 9*(2), 75–84.

Jager, T. E., Weiss, H. B., Coben, J. H., et al. (2000). Traumatic brain injuries evaluated in U.S. emergency departments, 1992–1994. *Academic Emergency Medicine*, 7(2), 134–140.

Jang, S. H., Ahn, S. H., Yang, D. S., et al. (2005). Cortical reorganization of hand motor function to primary sensory cortex in hemiparetic patients with a primary motor cortex infarct. *Archives of Physical Medicine and Rehabilitation*, 86(8), 1706–1708.

Jansen, H. M., van der Naalt, J., van Zomeren, A. H., et al. (1996). Cobalt-55 positron emission tomography in traumatic brain injury: A pilot study. *Journal of Neurology, Neurosurgery and Psychiatry*, 60(2), 221–224.

Johnston, A. J., Steiner, L. A., Coles, J. P., et al. (2005). Effect of cerebral perfusion pressure augmentation on regional oxygenation and metabolism after head injury. *Critical Care Medicine*, 33(1), 189–195.

Katayama, Y., Becker, D. P., Tamura, T., et al. (1990). Massive increases in extracellular potassium and the indiscriminate release of glutamate following concussive brain injury. *Journal of Neurosurgery*, 73(6), 889–900.

Kirkby, B. S., Van Horn, J. D., Ostrem, J. L., et al. (1996). Cognitive activation during PET: A case study of monozygotic twins discordant for closed head injury. *Neuropsychologia*, 34(7), 689–697.

Kochanek, P. M., Hendrich, K. S., Dixon, C. E., et al. (2002). Cerebral blood flow at one year after controlled cortical impact in rats: Assessment by magnetic resonance imaging. *Journal of Neurotrauma*, 19(9), 1029–1037.

Kraus, M. F., Smith, G. S., Butters, M., et al. (2005). Effects of the dopaminergic agent and NMDA receptor antagonist amantadine on cognitive function, cerebral glucose metabolism and D2 receptor availability in chronic traumatic brain injury: A study using positron emission tomography (PET). *Brain Injury*, 19(7), 471–479.

Langfitt, T. W., Obrist, W. D., Alavi, A., et al. (1986). Computerized tomography, magnetic resonance imaging, and positron emission tomography in the study of brain trauma: Preliminary observations. *Journal of Neurosurgery*, 64(5), 760–767.

Leon-Carrion, J., Alarcon, J. C., Revuelta, M., et al. (1998). Executive functioning as outcome in patients after traumatic brain injury. *International Journal of Neuroscience*, 94(1–2), 75–83.

Levin, H. S. (1990). Memory deficit after closed head injury. *Journal of Clinical and Experimental Neuropsychology*, 12(1), 129–153.

Levin, H. S. (1992). Neurobehavioral recovery. *Journal of Neurotrauma*, 9(Suppl. 1), S359–S373.

Levin, H. S., Gary, H. E., Jr., Eisenberg, H. M., et al. (1990). Neurobehavioral outcome 1 year after severe head injury. *Journal of Neurosurgery*, 73, 699–709.

Levin, H. S., Grossman, R. G., & Kelly, P. J. (1976). Short-term recognition memory in relation to severity of head injury. *Cortex*, 12(2), 175–182.

Levin, H. S., Grossman, R. G., Rose, J. E., et al. (1979). Long-term neuropsychological outcome of closed head injury. *Journal of Neurosurgery*, 50(4), 412–422.

Levine, B., Black, S. E., Cabeza, R., et al. (1998). Episodic memory and the self in a case of isolated retrograde amnesia. *Brain*, 121(Pt. 10), 1951–1973.

Levine, B., Cabeza, R., McIntosh, A. R., et al. (2002). Functional reorganisation of memory after traumatic brain injury: A study with $H_2^{15}O$ positron emission tomography. *Journal of Neurology, Neurosurgery and Psychiatry*, 73(2), 173–181.

Lewine, J. D., Davis, J. T., Sloan, J. H., et al. (1999). Neuromagnetic assessment of pathophysiologic brain activity induced by minor head trauma. *American Journal of Neuroradiology, 20*(5), 857–866.

Lombardi, W. J., Andreason, P. J., Sirocco, K. Y., et al. (1999). Wisconsin Card Sorting Test performance following head injury: Dorsolateral fronto-striatal circuit activity predicts perseveration. *Journal of Clinical and Experimental Neuropsychology, 21*(1), 2–16.

Lotze, M., Grodd, W., Rodden, F. A., et al. (2006). Neuroimaging patterns associated with motor control in traumatic brain injury. *Neurorehabilitation and Neural Repair, 20*(1), 14–23.

Manoach, D. S., Schlaug, G., Siewert, B., et al. (1997). Prefrontal cortex fMRI signal changes are correlated with working memory load. *Neuroreport, 8*(2), 545–549.

McAllister, T. W., Saykin, A. J., Flashman, L. A., et al. (1999). Brain activation during working memory 1 month after mild traumatic brain injury: A functional MRI study. *Neurology, 53*(6), 1300–1308.

McAllister, T. W., Sparling, M. B., Flashman, L. A., et al. (2001). Differential working memory load effects after mild traumatic brain injury. *NeuroImage, 14*(5), 1004–1012.

McDonald, B. C., Flashman, L. A., & Saykin, A. J. (2002). Executive dysfunction following traumatic brain injury: Neural substrates and treatment strategies. *Neurorehabilitation, 17*, 333–344.

McDowell, S., Whyte, J., & D'Esposito, M. (1997). Working memory impairments in traumatic brain injury: Evidence from a dual-task paradigm. *Neuropsychologia, 35*(10), 1341–1353.

McIntosh, T. K., Smith, D. H., Meaney, D. F., et al. (1996). Neuropathological sequelae of traumatic brain injury: Relationship to neurochemical and biomechanical mechanisms. *Laboratory Investigation, 74*(2), 315–342.

Munson, S., Schroth, E., & Ernst, M. (2006). The role of functional neuroimaging in pediatric brain injury. *Pediatrics, 117*(4), 1372–1381.

Oddy, M., Coughlan, T., Tyerman, A., et al. (1985). Social adjustment after closed head injury: A further follow-up seven years after injury. *Journal of Neurology, Neurosurgery and Psychiatry, 48*(6), 564–568.

Ommaya, A. K., & Hirsch, A. E. (1971). Tolerances for cerebral concussion from head impact and whiplash in primates. *Journal of Biomechanics, 4*, 13–20.

Perlstein, W. M., Cole, M. A., Demery, J. A., et al. (2004). Parametric manipulation of working memory load in traumatic brain injury: Behavioral and neural correlates. *Journal of the International Neuropsychological Society, 10*(5), 724–741.

Ponsford, J., & Kinsella, G. (1992). Attentional deficits following closed-head injury. *Journal of Clinical and Experimental Neuropsychology, 14*(5), 822–838.

Prigatano, G. P., Johnson, S. C., & Gale, S. D. (2004). Neuroimaging correlates of the Halstead Finger Tapping Test several years post-traumatic brain injury. *Brain Injury, 18*(7), 661–669.

Richards, H. K., Simac, S., Piechnik, S., et al. (2001). Uncoupling of cerebral blood flow and metabolism after cerebral contusion in the rat. *Journal of Cerebral Blood Flow and Metabolism, 21*(7), 779–781.

Ricker, J. H., Hillary, F. G., & DeLuca, J. (2001a). Functionally activated brain imaging (^{15}O PET and fMRI) in the study of learning and memory after traumatic brain injury. *Journal of Head Trauma Rehabilitation, 16*(2), 191–205.

Ricker, J. H., Muller, R. A., Zafonte, R. D., et al. (2001b). Verbal recall and recognition following traumatic brain injury: A ^{15}0-water positron emission tomography study. *Journal of Clinical and Experimental Neuropsychology, 23*(2), 196–206.

Rieger, M., & Gauggel, S. (2002). Inhibition of ongoing responses in patients with traumatic brain injury. *Neuropsychologia, 40,* 76–85.

Rosenthal, M., & Ricker, J. H. (2000). In R. G. Frank & T. R. Elliot (Eds.), *Handbook of rehabilitation psychology* (pp. 56–57). Washington, DC: American Psychological Association.

Ross, B. D., Ernst, T., Kreis, R., et al. (1998). 1H MRS in acute traumatic brain injury. *Journal of Magnetic Resonance Imaging, 8*(4), 829–840.

Ruff, R. M., Crouch, J. A., Troster, A. I., et al. (1994). *Brain Injury, 8*(4), 297–308.

Rypma, B., & D'Esposito, M. (1999). The roles of prefrontal brain regions in components of working memory: Effects of memory load and individual differences. *Proceedings of the National Academy of Sciences, 96*(11), 6558–6563.

Rypma, B., Prabhakaran, V., Desmond, J. E., et al. (1999). Load-dependent roles of frontal brain regions in the maintenance of working memory. *NeuroImage, 9*(2), 216–226.

Salthouse, T. A. (1996). The processing-speed theory of adult age differences in cognition. *Psychological Review, 103*(3), 403–428.

Salthouse, T. A., & Coon, V. E. (1993). Influence of task-specific processing speed on age differences in memory. *Journal of Gerontology, 48*(5), 245–255.

Scheibel, R. S., Pearson, D. A., Faria, L. P., et al. (2003). An fMRI study of executive functioning after severe diffuse TBI. *Brain Injury, 17*(11), 919–930.

Schiff, N. D., Ribary, U., Moreno, D. R., et al. (2002). Residual cerebral activity and behavioural fragments can remain in the persistently vegetative brain. *Brain, 125*(Pt. 6), 1210–1234.

Schroder, M. L., Muizelaar, J. P., Kuta, A. J., et al. (1996). Thresholds for cerebral ischemia after severe head injury: Relationship with late CT findings and outcome. *Journal of Neurotrauma, 13*(1), 17–23.

Shallice, T., & Burgess, P. W. (1991). Deficits in strategy application following frontal lobe damage in man. *Brain, 114*(Pt. 2), 727–741.

Shutter, L., Tong, K. A., & Holshouser, B. A. (2004). Proton MRS in acute traumatic brain injury: Role for glutamate/glutamine and choline for outcome prediction. *Journal of Neurotrauma, 21*(12), 1693–1705.

Smith, D. H., Cecil, K. M., Meaney, D. F., et al. (1998). Magnetic resonance spectroscopy of diffuse brain trauma in the pig. *Journal of Neurotrauma, 15,* 665–674.

Soeda, A., Nakashima, T., Okumura, A., et al. (2005). Cognitive impairment after traumatic brain injury: A functional magnetic resonance imaging study using the Stroop task. *Neuroradiology, 47*(7), 501–506.

Sosin, D. M., Sacks, J. J., & Smith, S. M. (1989). Head injury-associated deaths in the United States from 1979 to 1986. *Journal of the American Medical Association, 262*(16), 2251–2255.

Sosin, D. M., Sniezek, J. E., & Waxweiler, R. J. (1995). Trends in death associated with traumatic brain injury, 1979 through 1992: Success and failure. *Journal of the American Medical Association, 273*(22), 1778–1780.

Steiner, L. A., Coles, J. P., Johnston, A. J., et al. (2003). Responses of posttraumatic pericontusional cerebral blood flow and blood volume to an increase in cerebral perfusion pressure. *Journal of Cerebral Blood Flow and Metabolism, 23*(11), 1371–1377.

Stroop, J. R. (1935). Studies of interference in serial verbal reactions. *Journal of Experimental Psychology, 18*, 643–662.

Stuss, D. T., Ely, P., Hugenholtz, H., et al. (1985). Subtle neuropsychological deficits in patients with good recovery after closed head injury. *Neurosurgery, 17*(1), 41–47.

Stuss, D. T., Stethem, L. L., Hugenholtz, H., et al. (1989). Reaction time after head injury: Fatigue, divided and focused attention, and consistency of performance. *Journal of Neurology, Neurosurgery and Psychiatry, 52*(6), 742–748.

Sunami, K., Nakamura, T., Ozawa, Y., et al. (1989). Hypermetabolic state following experimental head injury. *Neurosurgical Review, 12*(Suppl. 1), 400–411.

Thurman, D. J., Alverson, C., Dunn, K. A., et al. (1999). Traumatic brain injury in the United States: A public health perspective. *Journal of Head Trauma Rehabilitation, 14*(6), 602–615.

Unterberg, A. W., Stover, J., Kress, B., et al. (2004). Edema and brain trauma. *Neuroscience, 129*(4), 1021–1029.

Uzan, M., Albayram, S., Dashti, S. G., et al. (2003). Thalamic proton magnetic resonance spectroscopy in vegetative state induced by traumatic brain injury. *Journal of Neurology, Neurosurgery, and Psychiatry, 74*(1), 33–38.

van Zomeren, A. H., & van den Burg, W. (1985). Residual complaints of patients two years after severe head injury. *Journal of Neurology, Neurosurgery, and Psychiatry, 48*(1), 21–28.

Vespa, P., Bergsneider, M., Hattori, N., et al. (2005). Metabolic crisis without brain ischemia is common after traumatic brain injury: A combined microdialysis and positron emission tomography study. *Journal of Cerebral Blood Flow and Metabolism, 25*(6), 763–774.

Vespa, P. M., McArthur, D., O'Phelan, K., et al. (2003). Persistently low extracellular glucose correlates with poor outcome 6 months after human traumatic brain injury despite a lack of increased lactate: A microdialysis study. *Journal of Cerebral Blood Flow and Metabolism, 23*(7), 865–877.

Vespa, P., Prins, M., Ronne-Engstrom, E., et al. (1998). Increase in extracellular glutamate caused by reduced cerebral perfusion pressure and seizures after human traumatic brain injury: A microdialysis study. *Journal of Neurosurgery, 89*(6), 971–982.

Wiese, H., Stude, P., Nebel, K., et al. (2004). Impaired movement-related potentials in acute frontal traumatic brain injury. *Clinical Neurophysiology, 115*(2), 289–298.

Wu, H. M., Huang, S. C., Hattori, N., et al. (2004). Subcortical white matter metabolic changes remote from focal hemorrhagic lesions suggest diffuse injury after human traumatic brain injury. *Neurosurgery, 55*(6), 1306–1315.

Yamaki, T., Imahori, Y., Ohmori, Y., et al. (1996a). Cerebral hemodynamics and metabolism of severe diffuse brain injury measured by PET. *Journal of Nuclear Medicine, 37*(7), 1166–1170.

Yamaki, T., Yoshino, E., Fujimoto, M., et al. (1996b). Chronological positron emission tomographic study of severe diffuse brain injury in the chronic stage. *Journal of Trauma, 40*(1), 50–56.

CHAPTER 10

Functional Neuroimaging in Multiple Sclerosis

Gerald T. Voelbel
Nancy D. Chiaravalloti
John DeLuca

Although structural neuroimaging (i.e., magnetic resonance imaging; MRI) has become a key element of diagnosis and care for persons with multiple sclerosis (MS), the application of functional imaging to the study of brain function is a relatively new area of research in MS. Initial studies applying functional imaging to MS utilized positron emission tomography (PET) and single photon emission computed tomography (SPECT). More recently, functional magnetic resonance imaging (fMRI), which has numerous advantages over PET and SPECT, has begun to be used in persons with MS. fMRI examines changes in cortical activation during motor and cognitive processes, and it has been applied to MS only since the late 1990s. The increased utilization of functional imaging techniques to study clinical issues in MS over the past 10 years has provided a wealth of new knowledge about brain–behavior relationships in MS. However, this rapidly increasing body of new knowledge must be met with the appropriate scientific scrutiny regarding its interpretation and application.

The primary aim of this chapter is to provide an overview of the functional imaging studies of MS, focusing primarily on studies using fMRI. Following a brief background of MS itself, this chapter reviews and discusses the implications of functional imaging studies focusing on the physical and cognitive symptoms associated with the disease, as well as the current findings of this functional imaging research. Finally, we discuss the possible limitations of this work.

Description of MS

MS is a chronic neurological disease that is characterized by white matter plaques and lesions in the brain and spinal cord. The lesions and plaques affect the myelin sheath, which in turn inhibits the nerve transmission of the axons (Skoff, 2003). New evidence suggests that direct involvement of axonal loss is a major cause of neurological disabilities (Peterson & Trapp, 2005). Four clinical courses have been used to describe MS. Each of the disease courses is based on the rate of progression of the disease: relapsing–remitting, secondary progressive, progressive relapsing, and primary progressive (Lublin & Reingold, 1996). Relapsing–remitting MS is characterized by periods in which symptoms are exacerbated and full recovery is noted between attacks. Approximately 80% of individuals with relapsing–remitting MS later develop secondary progressive MS (Herndon, 2003). In secondary progressive MS, the symptoms gradually worsen with or without occasional relapses or minor remissions. Progressive–relapsing MS is characterized by a progressive decline from the onset of the disease, punctuated by acute periods of symptom relapse. There may or may not be recovery from these acute periods. Finally, primary progressive MS is a continuous and gradual worsening of the symptoms with no distinct symptom exacerbation or remission.

MS is diagnosed after observation of two clinical attacks and objective evidence (e.g., MRI) of two lesions separated in space and time (McDonald et al., 2001). The primary method to assess the lesions is the use of two T2 or gadolinium-enhanced MRI scans at least 3 mo apart from each other (McDonald et al., 2001). The lesions detected by MRI are areas of inflamed tissue, demyelinated axons, plaques, and scarring of the axon's myelin sheath (Herndon, 2003). The plaques and scarring can be found throughout the central nervous system, but they are primarily detected in the periventricular regions, optic nerves, juxtacortical areas, corpus callosum, cerebellum, and brain stem (Calabresi, 2004; Herndon, 2003).

Symptoms of MS

The symptomatic sequelae of MS are highly unpredictable and heterogeneous. Symptoms can include fatigue, cognitive difficulties, depression, bladder and bowel difficulties, vertigo, visual impairment, weakness and numbness in limbs, spasticity and tremors, speech and swallowing difficulties, sexual dysfunction, and heat sensitivity (Calabresi, 2004; Kesselring, 2004). The most commonly reported symptom of MS is fatigue, which can be subjectively reported as either physical or mental, is often unrelated to physical disability, and is worsened by heat (Freal et al., 1984; Krupp et al., 2005; Schwartz et al., 1993). Several hypotheses have been proposed to identify the mechanisms of MS-related fatigue, including immune system dysregulation, impaired nerve conduction, neuroendocrine/neurotransmitter dysregulation, autonomic nervous system involvement, and energy depletion (Krupp et al., 2005). However, no single mechanism has been successfully invoked to explain the fatigue observed in individuals with MS.

Cognitive deficits are observed in up to 65% of persons with MS (Peyser et al., 1990; Rao et al., 1991; Ron et al., 1991), at both the earlier and later stages of the disease (Pelosi et al., 1997; Piras et al., 2003), and are generally unrelated to degree of physical disability (Archibald & Fisk, 2000; Foong et al., 1997). The most common cognitive problems in MS are in episodic and working memory (Bobholz & Rao, 2003; Grafman et al., 1990; Kenealy et al., 2002). Although early studies of episodic memory in MS suggested difficulties in retrieval from long-term storage (Caine et al., 1986; Rao, 1986; Rao et al., 1989), more recent studies have shown that the primary memory problem in MS is in the initial acquisition (or learning) of information (DeLuca et al., 1994, 1998; Demaree et al., 2000; Gaudino et al., 2001; Thornton et al., 2002; see Thornton & Raz, 1997, for a review). Another very common cognitive deficit that is characteristic of MS is slowed information processing (DeLuca et al., 2004; Janculjak et al., 2002). Such deficits in information-processing speed are often observed concurrently with other cognitive deficits commonly seen in MS (DeLuca et al., 2004). These include deficits in working memory and episodic memory (Gaudino et al., 2001; Janculjak et al., 2002; Lengenfelder et al., 2003), with some studies linking deficits in speed of information processing to these memory impairments seen in MS (Archibald & Fisk, 2000; DeLuca et al., 1994; Gaudino et al., 2001). Other significant cognitive impairments observed in MS are found in executive functions (i.e., abstract reasoning, fluency, planning, and organization) (Foong et al., 1997; Lazeron et al., 2004; Denney et al., 2005), perceptual skills (Vleugels et al., 2000), and sustained attention (Janculjak et al., 2002; Olivares et al., 2005).

In addition to impairing cognitive functioning, the central nervous system damage in MS also affects sensory and motor functions. One of the more prominent sensory symptoms associated with MS is vision difficulties, such as optic neuritis, diplopia, and internuclear ophthalmoplegia (Frohman et al., 2005). Other sensory dysfunctions noted in patients with MS include numbness, tingling, vertigo, proprioceptive dysfunction, and neuralgia (De Simone et al., 2005). MS symptoms affecting the motor system are also common, including paresis, spasticity, dysarthria, myoclonus, and restless leg syndrome (Merson & Rolnick, 1998; Pantano et al., 2002; Rizzo et al., 2004; Yokota et al., 1991).

The fatigue and the cognitive, sensory, and motor deficits resulting from MS can severely reduce the patient's quality of life. Because the onset of MS typically occurs between the ages of 20 and 40, when individuals are most active and productive in many aspects of their lives (Reingold, 1995), the disease often leads to the loss of gainful employment for a large number of patients (Beatty et al., 1995). Between 50 and 80% of patients with MS are unemployed within 10 years of the onset of the disease (Gronning et al., 1990; Kornblith et al., 1986; LaRocca et al., 1985). Although a number of factors have been shown to be related to employment status in MS, including the presence of a working spouse (Genevie et al., 1987), age (Rozin et al., 1975), duration and course of the disease (Bauer et al., 1965), physical symptom severity, fatigue, and visual impairment (LaRocca et al., 1985), individuals with MS have identified cognitive problems such as information processing and memory deficits as presenting significant obstacles to maintaining meaningful employment (Roessler & Rumrill, 1995). Not only were information-processing and memory problems identified subjectively to affect employment status, but objective evidence of poor information-processing and memory performance predicted unemployment status as well (Beatty et al., 1995).

Taken together, the symptoms of MS affect a wide range of intra- and interindividual systems. Although MS symptoms are heterogeneous in nature, the impact of the disease on the central nervous system has led to the investigation of the neural mechanisms affected by MS through neuroimaging techniques.

Functional Neuroimaging Studies in MS

Although neuropsychological and behavioral studies are essential to increasing our understanding of the heterogeneous symptoms characteristic of MS, neuroimaging techniques provide valuable information about the integrity of brain structure and function. Such techniques are essential to achieve a complete understanding of the impact of MS on brain functioning. Functional neuroimaging studies have been conducted in MS, examining symptoms in various realms of functioning, including motor skills, fatigue, and cognitive abilities, each of which is reviewed below. Studies that identified possible confounds that affect the observed patterns of cortical activation are also discussed. Numerous studies have been conducted relating structural imaging studies to cognitive, motor, and other (e.g., fatigue) aspects of MS (see Marrie et al., 2005; Miller & Frank, 1998; Rao, 1990, for a review). This chapter focuses on functional neuroimaging studies.

Motor System

Functional MRI studies of the motor system in MS have primarily involved the upper extremities, focusing mainly on fine movements of the digits. Such studies have shown significant differences in patterns of cortical activation, or blood-oxygen-level-dependent (BOLD) responses, during motor tasks as compared with healthy control adults (Lee et al., 2000; Filippi et al., 2002, 2004; Morgen et al., 2004; Pantano et al., 2002; Reddy et al., 2000, 2002; Rocca et al., 2002, 2003). Relative to controls, increased cortical activation during simple fine motor movements has been observed in relapsing–remitting, secondary progressive, and primary progressive MS, and probable subjects with MS who experienced a single event resulting in hemiparesis (Filippi et al., 2002;

Pantano et al., 2002; Reddy et al., 2000; Rocca et al., 2003). The pattern of activation in individuals with MS shows both increased contralateral and ipsilateral cerebral activation of the sensorimotor cortex as compared with healthy control participants (Filippi at al., 2002; Pantano et al., 2002; Rocca et al., 2003). The relative increase in contralateral cortical activation that has been demonstrated by the MS groups suggests that the motor tasks are recruiting additional cortical resources from the motor areas that are used to perform these tasks. The increase of ipsilateral–cortical activation during motor tasks in individuals with MS, as compared with healthy controls, has been interpreted as evidence that the motor areas in individuals with MS undergo a functional reorganization (Filippi et al., 2002; Pantano et al., 2002). However, there may be confounding factors affecting the observed patterns of cortical activation that need to be investigated before definitely drawing such conclusions.

Three main factors have been identified as potentially confounding the observation of cortical activation patterns in a population of individuals with MS: task difficulty, repetitive use, and lesion load. Recent research has begun to examine these factors, specifically in regard to their impact on patterns of cortical activation in MS. *Task difficulty* is the first factor potentially affecting patterns of cerebral activation in the MS sample. It has been suggested that the complexity of motor tasks may affect the differences in observed patterns of cortical activation between participants with MS and healthy control groups. One study compared the patterns of cortical activation between a group of participants with MS and a healthy control group on a "simple task" (i.e., repetitive flexion–extension of the last four fingers) and a "complex task" (i.e., manipulation of a pen, glass, and toothbrush; Filippi et al., 2004). When the pattern of activation was compared between the simple task and the complex task, both groups showed increased contralateral frontal cortical activation during the complex task, which suggests that the increase in the complexity of the task recruited additional cortical resources. However, in examining differences in cortical activation between the two groups on the simple task, the group with MS demonstrated additional activation in regions associated only with performance of the complex task in healthy samples. These results validate that the group with MS required additional resources, usually associated with more complex pathways, to complete fine motor tasks. Such studies suggest that the level of complexity or difficulty of the motor task affects the pattern of observed results and how one interprets cerebral reorganization.

Repetitive use is a second possible confounding factor in examining cortical activation patterns in MS. A recent study examined whether patterns of cerebral activation associated with motor functions changed after motor training that consisted of repetitive flexion and extensions of the thumb in participants with MS (Morgen et al., 2004). The observed level of activation of the contralateral primary somatosensory and parietal associative cortices decreased with training in the control group. However, the observed level of activation of the same cortical regions did not decrease in the MS group with training. The authors concluded that the participants with MS did not have task-specific cortical reorganization, inasmuch as the control group demonstrated a reduction in cortical activation after thumb extension training, which was not observed in the MS group. The authors proposed two possible explanations for this finding. One possible reason was that the thumb movement was more effortful for the MS group than for the control group, evidenced by the MS group requiring more training to learn the movements. Another possible explanation is that the axonal damage and lesions that occur in MS may prevent task-specific plasticity. Additional research is necessary to determine which explanation is more accurate and appropriate.

The role of *lesion load* in patterns of cerebral activation is a third possible confounding factor in examining patterns of cerebral activation in MS during motor movements. That is, how do the cortical and subcortical lesions that are characteristic of MS affect patterns of cortical activation during fMRI? The influence of such lesions on fMRI activation remains unclear. Two fMRI studies of motor functions in participants with MS have reported that the extent of the lesion load affects the patterns of cortical activation observed (Filippi et al., 2002; Lee et al., 2000). Both studies reported that increased lesion load was associated with activation of the ipsilateral hemisphere in the MS group. In addition, Lee and colleagues (2000) reported that the center of the cortical activation site shifted posteriorly as the lesion volume increased. These studies suggest that as the lesion load increases, alternative cortical areas are recruited, even for simple motor tasks. It has been proposed that the shift in areas of cortical activation serves as an adaptive function to compensate for damaged areas (Filippi et al., 2002). In contrast, at least one study (Pantano et al., 2002) found that the cerebral lesions have little effect on the pattern of cortical activation and that lesions on the corticospinal tract play a larger role in cortical reorganization in the motor areas. Given the paucity of research examining this question, the influence of lesion load on patterns of cerebral activation of the sensorimotor system remains unclear and more studies in MS should address this very important issue.

Fatigue

Although motor system dysfunction is the most objectively observable symptom of MS, fatigue is perhaps the least objective symptom. Nonetheless, fatigue results in significant disruption in the lives of individuals with MS. There have been few functional imaging studies that have addressed the effect of fatigue on brain activity in MS. MS-related fatigue has been associated with neuropathology in a number of neuroimaging studies that have compared the structural integrity of individuals diagnosed with MS with and without fatigue (Colombo et al., 2000; Tartaglia et al., 2004). The vast majority of these studies find little to no relationship between structural neuroimaging and self-reported fatigue (Krupp et al., 2005). However, a study that examined neuronal integrity by using magnetic resonance spectroscopy (MRS) reported that the N-acetylaspartate/creatine ratio (NAA/Cr), which is an indicator of neuronal integrity, was significantly lower in an MS group with fatigue than an MS group without fatigue (Tartaglia et al., 2004). Other neuroimaging studies have also reported differences between persons with MS and fatigue as compared with persons with MS, but without reported fatigue. Thus, one study demonstrated that reduced glucose metabolism was associated with self-reported fatigue in MS, using PET (Roelcke et al., 1997). Specifically, reduced glucose metabolism was revealed bilaterally in the lateral and medial pre-frontal cortex, premotor cortex, posterior parietal cortex, and right supple-mentary motor area, and subcortically in the internal capsule and ventral putamen in an MS group with fatigue, as compared with an MS group with-out fatigue. More recently, Filippi and colleagues (2002) compared the pat-tern of the BOLD response during a simple motor task between MS groups with and without fatigue and found that patients with MS with fatigue showed a distinct pattern of activation as compared with a group with MS without fatigue. Specifically, the MS group without fatigue showed greater activation than the MS group with fatigue in the ipsilateral cerebellar hemisphere, inferior frontal region (rolandic operculum), parietal cortex (precuneus), contralateral middle frontal gyrus, and thalamus; whereas the MS group with fatigue showed increased activation in the cingulate motor area. Examination of the extent of the lesion load between these MS groups revealed no significant difference, and no relationship was found between the lesion load and the BOLD response. The subjective level of fatigue was, how-ever, related to the level of activation found in the contralateral intraparietal sulcus, thalamus, and ipsilateral operculum. There is also preliminary evi-dence that persons with MS require more cerebral resources to maintain the same level of cognitive performance as do healthy adults (DeLuca et al., 2006), which has been suggested as a measure of cognitive fatigue (DeLuca, 2005).

Although the pathophysiology of fatigue in MS is still unclear, the afore-mentioned neuroimaging studies demonstrate that there are clear differences between persons with MS who suffer from fatigue and those with MS and do not suffer from fatigue at the level of NAA/Cr, glucose utilization, and pat-terns of cerebral activation during fine motor tasks. It is possible that persons with MS who report greater fatigue have greater neuropathology at the neuronal level, which may not be detected by the examination of structural lesions. Clearly, more studies are needed to elucidate the cause of fatigue in MS and to explain why such neuroimaging differences exist between those with fatigue and without fatigue.

Cognition

Although limited in number, existing studies examining cognition in MS uti-lizing functional neuroimaging have already yielded an increased understand-ing of how the cognitive changes that accompany MS are related to functional cerebral activity. Thus far, functional imaging studies that have investigated cognitive processes in MS have concentrated on three main domains: working memory (WM), attention, and executive functions.

Working Memory

WM can be defined as a system for temporarily storing and manipulating information for performance on cognitive tasks (Baddeley, 1992). WM deficits have been detected in the earliest stage of MS (Audoin et al., 2005) as well as across the disease course (i.e., relapsing–remitting and progressive MS; Grigsby et al., 1994). Most of the functional imaging studies examining cognition in groups with MS have been in the area of WM. fMRI studies of participants with MS have predominantly used three different verbal working memory cognitive tasks: the Paced Auditory Serial Addition Test (PASAT; Audoin et al., 2005) or a modification of the PASAT referred to as the mPASAT (Chiaravalloti et al., 2005), the *n*-back test (Sweet et al., 2004), and the Sternberg paradigm (Hillary et al., 2003).

In general, two patterns of performance have been observed in MS using the PASAT and mPASAT. First, in contrast to healthy controls who tend to show more focal left frontal activation (i.e., left dorsolateral prefrontal cortex and the left frontopolar) on fMRI studies with the PASAT and mPASAT, participants with MS show bilateral frontal cortical activation (Audoin et al., 2003, 2005; Chiaravalloti et al., 2005; Mainero et al., 2004; Staffen et al., 2002). Second, as compared with healthy control groups, the groups with MS show significantly greater activation dispersed throughout other brain regions, such as bilateral parietal lobe (Chiaravalloti et al., 2005; Mainero et al., 2004; Staffen et al., 2002), bilateral temporal lobe (Mainero et al., 2004), and the right cerebellum (Audoin et al., 2003). Therefore, not only is there bilateral frontal lobe activation in the participants with MS relative to healthy controls, but participants with MS recruit additional cortical areas throughout the brain while performing the PASAT or mPASAT.

As a way to investigate whether the observed patterns of cerebral activation of WM during the PASAT are associated with MS in general or associated with the presence of cognitive impairment, participants with MS with impaired WM and participants with MS without impaired WM have been compared with healthy controls (Audoin et al., 2005; Chiaravalloti et al., 2005; Mainero et al., 2004). Chiaravalloti and colleagues (2005) reported that while performing the mPASAT, the group with impaired WM had a more diffuse pattern of activation than the group with intact WM and the healthy control group. In fact, when compared with the control group, the group with impaired WM showed significantly greater activation in the right frontal and right parietal lobes, whereas the group with intact WM demonstrated patterns of activation similar to those of the control group (Chiaravalloti et al., 2005). In contrast, the distinct pattern of cerebral activation between groups with impaired WM and those with intact WM was not found by Audoin and colleagues (2005). Both groups with MS in the Audoin et al. (2005) study showed increased activation in the right frontal region as compared with the control group, and the group with intact WM showed increased activation over the control group in the left frontal region. However, the pattern of activation was not significantly different between the MS group with intact WM and the MS group with impaired WM. In another WM study that used the PASAT, Mainero and colleagues (2004) also examined patterns of activation between a group with impaired WM and a group with intact WM during the mPASAT. In contrast to the Chiaravalloti et al. (2005) and Audoin et al. (2005) studies, the group with intact WM in the Mainero et al. (2004) study had an increased level of activation as compared with the group with impaired WM.

There are several methodological differences between the Chiaravalloti et al. (2005), Audoin et al. (2005), and Mainero et al. (2004) WM studies that could account for the divergent results. Whereas the Chiaravalloti et al. (2005) and Mainero et al. (2004) studies used a modified version of the PASAT, in which the participants were required to respond with a button press when the serially present numbers summed to 10 (Figure 10.1), the Audoin et al. (2005) study used the a standard PASAT paradigm, which requires a verbal response of the sum of two previously presented numbers. Although both tasks tap into verbal WM, the difference in response requirements (verbal vs. simple motor) may contribute to the disparate patterns of cortical activation between the studies. Two additional differences in the studies may have affected the pattern of cortical activation observed. First, the Chiaravalloti et al. (2005) study used an auditory monitoring control task, which was subtracted from the mPASAT activation during the analyses for the purpose of narrowing the observed pattern of activation to working memory specifically (rather than attention, auditory processing, etc.). In contrast, the

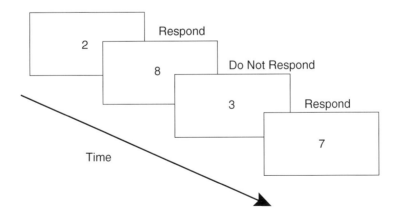

FIGURE 10.1. Schematic representation of the modified PASAT paradigm. "Press the button only when two consecutive numbers add up to 10."

Mainero et al. (2004) study did not have a control task to narrow the pattern of activation to WM processes. Second, the Mainero et al. study presented the stimuli to participants every 3 s, whereas the Chiaravalloti et al. study presented the stimuli to participants every 2 s. The increased demand in processing speed required of the 2-s version may have put a greater demand on the working memory system in the WM-impaired individuals but not in the WM-intact group, which may be associated with increased cortical areas required for processing (Lengenfelder et al., 2006; Wishart et al., 2004). Overall, future studies need to address the disparate WM results observed in the currently reviewed studies examining WM in MS using the PASAT or mPASAT.

As mentioned previously, the *n*-back is another task that has been experimentally used to assess WM functioning in groups with MS (Sweet et al., 2004; Wishart et al., 2004). The *n*-back requires the participants to respond after a consonant is repeated at a designated interval during a string of consonants; for example, a 2-back task requires the participant to respond when the current letter that is presented matches the letter that was presented two letters prior (Figure 10.2). fMRI studies of the 2-back WM task suggest that the *pattern* of activation between the participants with MS and healthy controls is similar when performance is similar between groups (Sweet et al., 2004; Wishart et al., 2004). Therefore, the same cortical regions (frontal and parietal areas) in healthy controls that were activated during the 2-back task were also activated in the groups with MS. However, the *level* of activation within these frontal and parietal regions was found to be significantly different between the healthy control groups and the groups with MS. That is, the MS group in the Sweet and colleagues (2004) study showed greater activation than the control group in the left dorsolateral prefrontal cortex, primary motor cortex, somatosensory cortex, premotor cortex, dorsolateral cortex, anterior cingulate, and bilateral supplementary motor area, whereas the MS groups in

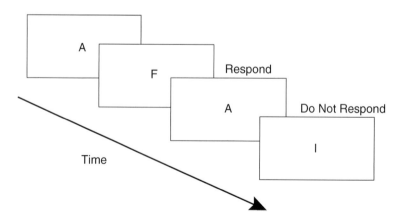

FIGURE 10.2. *n*-back, 2-back condition. When the letter presented matches the one presented 2-back, the subject responds by pressing the response key.

the Wishart and colleagues (2004) study showed greater activation than the control group in the bilateral medial frontal gyrus and middle temporal gyrus, right cingulate gyrus, right parietal cortex, and right occipital lobe. The results of these studies demonstrate that the MS groups have greater hemodynamic responses in similarly activated regions as the healthy control groups, but neither study demonstrated increased levels of activation in areas that are not generally associated with the n-back task.

The third task used to study WM in fMRI studies with participants who have MS is the Sternberg paradigm, which consists of presenting a string of letters to the participants, followed by a delay, after which a single target letter is presented. The participants are required to respond if the target letter was included in the string of letters presented prior to the delay (Figure 10.3). Using the Sternberg paradigm, Hillary and colleagues (2003) reported that both groups activated the left frontal cortex and left temporal lobe, with no significant differences noted in level of activation between the groups. In contrast, the MS group had significantly greater activation in the right frontal cortex and right temporal lobe than the healthy control group. Interestingly, when participants were grouped together, an inverse relationship between behavioral performance on the Sternberg and level of activation within the right temporal lobe and right frontal cortex activation was revealed. That is, the participants with poorer Sternberg performance demonstrated increased activation in the right frontal cortex and right temporal lobe. A similar inverse relationship was reported by Chiaravalloti (2005) between performance on the PASAT and the level of activation of the right frontal and parietal regions.

Although the cerebellum has historically been thought to strictly serve motor functions, recent studies have identified the cerebellum as an active contributor to WM functions as well (Desmond et al., 1997; Harris et al.,

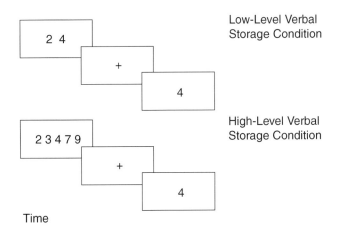

FIGURE 10.3. Modified Sternberg paradigm.

2001). Li and colleagues (2004) utilized the Sternberg paradigm to investigate patterns of activation within the cerebellum in an MS group as compared with an HC group. Results showed a significant decrease in the number of voxels activated in the right and left cerebellar hemispheres in the MS group compared with the HC group. Results of the Li et al. (2004) study suggest that the cognitive processes of the cerebellum are disrupted in MS, which is possibly caused by a disruption in the pathways between the cerebellum and the cerebrum.

Functional neuroimaging studies of WM have reported significant differences in the patterns of cortical activation between MS groups and healthy control groups. The preponderance of findings reveals that most MS groups investigated show altered patterns of activation than the healthy control groups. The altered pattern of activation during tasks of WM involve increased levels of activation in the same loci as shown in healthy control groups, as well as areas of activation in the right frontal and parietal lobes, which are not significantly activated in the healthy control groups. Interestingly, when individuals with MS and intact WM are compared with healthy control groups, the patterns of activation are similar. However, those with impaired WM are most likely to have the altered pattern of cerebral activation as compared with healthy control groups.

Attention

Cognitive studies of attention are difficult to conduct because of the difficulty in isolating attention from other cognitive processes involved in the same task (Sarter et al., 2001). For example, tasks of WM in which behavioral responses are required when stimuli are presented repeatedly, involve sustained attention, divided attention, visual or auditory attention, simple motor movements, and auditory processing (i.e., PASAT). It is difficult for any given study to distinguish between these varied cognitive processes, in that there is considerable overlap between the involved cognitive constructs. However, two studies have attempted to circumvent this problem by using a visual attention task (Penner et al., 2003) and an auditory attention task (Santa Maria et al., 2004). Both studies have shown significant differences in patterns of cortical activation during the attention tasks between groups with MS and healthy control groups. Penner and colleagues (2003) divided the participants with MS into groups, based on their performance levels on an attention task that was administered during an fMRI scan. The task required participants to press a button as quickly as possible when a cross appeared on the screen. Both MS groups showed a diffuse pattern of activation relative to the control group, but the pattern was even more diffuse in the group of mildly impaired patients with MS (Penner et al., 2003). Specifically, the mildly impaired group had significantly greater activation in the right dorsolateral prefrontal cortex, right superior temporal gyrus, right lateral cerebellum, left angular gyrus, and bilateral inferior parietal cortex, whereas the severely impaired group had significantly greater activation than the control group in the left inferior parietal lobe.

Significantly altered patterns of cerebral activation in MS have also been shown utilizing positron emission tomography (PET) during a selective auditory attention task (Santa Maria et al., 2004). As compared with the control group, the group with MS had significantly less glucose utilization in the right anterior cingulate gyrus and increased activation in the left superior temporal gyrus (Santa Maria et al., 2004), which represents the level of cerebral activity. However, when Santa Maria and colleagues (2004) compared high and low cognitively performing participants with MS with each other, no differences in glucose utilization was observed. The decreased activity in the anterior cingulate gyrus, which plays a major role in attention, suggests that either neural transmission within the cingulate is disrupted or the pathway to the cingulate may be disrupted in individuals with MS.

The two functional neuroimaging studies of attention (Penner, 2003; Santa Maria, 2004) investigated separate aspects of attention: sustained attention and auditory selective attention. The differences in the attention modalities examined in these functional imaging studies make it difficult to make direct comparisons of the results between these two studies; however, both studies support prior cognitive functional neuroimaging studies by providing evidence that there are differences in the level of activation between groups with MS and control groups in the loci of the neural substrates that subserve these cognitive processes.

Executive Functions

Although it is known that persons with MS show evidence of difficulties on tasks of planning and problem solving, an area of executive function (Arnett et al., 1997; Foong et al., 1997; Stablum et al., 2004), there is only one known fMRI study that investigated planning abilities in participants with MS (Lazeron et al., 2004). Lazeron and colleagues administered a modified version of the Tower of London (TOL), with varying levels of difficulty based on the number of moves to complete the task. The group with MS and the control group showed comparable activation of the bilateral frontal and parietal lobes during the TOL, even though the MS group performed significantly worse than the control group on the task. The behavioral data from the group with MS and the control group suggest that the task was very difficult for both groups. In an attempt to explore whether the pattern of activation noted was due to the level of difficulty of the task, the difficult trials of TOL (six to eight moves) were compared with the easy trials of TOL (two to four moves). However, no significant group difference in the pattern of cortical activation was observed. Clearly, there is a paucity of evidence to make any conclusions about the functional cerebral activity involved in executive functions in MS, and more studies are needed to investigate the pattern of cerebral activity during other measures of planning and problem solving.

Neural Plasticity and Reorganization

Many of the functional neuroimaging studies of fine motor ability, fatigue, and cognition report significantly different patterns of cortical activation in groups with MS as compared with the healthy control groups. The nature of these differences vary across the three domains. Nonetheless, two main patterns of differences can be identified. First, the BOLD responses are often observed in MS groups in regions where no activation was reported in healthy control groups. Second, the regions of cortical activation are largely similar between groups with MS and healthy control groups, but the level of activation may be increased and the area demonstrating activation may be more diffuse in the MS groups. Despite the fact that these general patterns can be identified, there is a lack of consistency in the extent to which a given set of results conforms to the pattern. Researchers often look to methodology to explain these inconsistencies. Yet a definitive explanation for differing patterns and levels of cerebral activation in MS remains elusive.

Multiple theories have been proposed to explain the differing patterns of cerebral activation noted in MS. The explanation most commonly articulated is one of cerebral reorganization (Mainero et al., 2004; Filippi & Rocca, 2004). The most clear-cut support for such cerebral reorganization is derived from the functional neuroimaging studies of fine motor performance. As previously stated, BOLD responses are observed primarily in the contralateral–sensorimotor cortex during fine motor movements in healthy control groups. However, in samples of patients with MS, significant ipsilateral activation in the sensorimotor cortex is observed relative to healthy controls (Filippi et al., 2002; Pantano et al., 2002). Cerebral reorganization in MS is thought to recruit additional cortical regions as a compensatory mechanism to decrease the effects of MS-related motor and cognitive impairments (Rocca et al., 2002; Wishart et al., 2004). Such a theory suggests that axons develop new connections and synapses with other neurons at a remote region away from a site of lesion in order to limit the effects of the lesioned area. This model is consistent with what is typically observed in the animal literature. Specifically, animal models of ischemic injuries to the primary motor regions that represent the hand have shown cortical reorganization with postmortem histological analyses, in which the axons near the site of lesion create new connections with neurons at a substantial distance away from the site of lesion (Dancause et al., 2005).

It remains unclear as to whether the altered activation patterns seen in MS are permanent (Buckle, 2005). One longitudinal study addressed that question by having groups with MS and healthy controls undergo two fMRI scans between 15 and 26 mo apart. The motor tasks during both fMRI studies consisted of touching the thumb to the four fingers sequentially (Pantano et al., 2005). Results showed that the group with MS had greater bilateral activation, as compared with the healthy control group, during both fMRI studies. However, during the second scan the group with MS demonstrated reduced activation of the ipsilateral sensorimotor cortex and contralateral cerebellum as compared with the baseline study. No changes were detected in the healthy control group from the first to the second scan. Age, lesion load, and new relapses were reported as identified factors that affected the level of change of activation of the ipsilateral sensorimotor cortex of the MS group. Specifically, those who were younger and had a better clinical course between baseline and follow-up had the greatest change in level of activation in the ipsilateral sensorimotor cortex. Although it is still unclear whether the cerebral reorganization is permanent in motor regions, the Pantano et al. (2005) study does suggest that the pattern of activation during fine motor tasks may be affected by age and clinical course.

Although cerebral reorganization is certainly a feasible explanation for the altered patterns of cerebral activation in motor and cognitive functional imaging studies, viable alternative theories have certainly been proposed. A second theory that needs to be explored further emphasizes a threshold at which a task becomes very difficult for an individual. It stipulates that the patterns of activation seen in MS may be due to additional cerebral resources being recruited when the task demand reaches a certain threshold (Hillary et al., 2006). The "threshold" may be based on the individual's experience of task difficulty. This theory of cortical recruitment is based on a hypothesis that the pathways and sites of cortical activation are more transitory and not permanent. Therefore, at a certain level of task difficulty, the level of cortical recruitment may increase, providing additional cortical resources from the surrounding focal regions and the homologous region in the other hemisphere. Specifically, the level of task demand in WM studies has been shown to be positively correlated with level of activation. The positive relationship between level of activation and demand in WM has been shown in both healthy controls (Rypma & D'Esposito, 1999; Rypma et al., 2002) and individuals with MS (Wishart et al., 2004). It would follow from the threshold theory that the altered pattern of cerebral activation in patients with MS, as compared with healthy controls, is due to individuals with MS having a lower threshold level of task difficulty than healthy controls. In other words, do groups with MS recruit additional cortical resources for cognitive functions at one level of cognitive difficulty, whereas the recruitment of the same additional cortical areas occurs at a more difficult cognitive task level in healthy controls?

The threshold theory is helpful in explaining differences in the patterns of activation between cognitively intact and cognitively impaired groups with MS. As previously reported, in general, cognitively intact MS groups show similar patterns of cortical activation to the healthy controls, but the cognitively impaired groups with MS show altered patterns of activation as compared with the healthy control groups. Thus, it is suggested that the cognitively impaired groups with MS have a lowered threshold as compared with the cognitively intact groups, which requires additional cortical resources to perform at similar cognitive levels.

The presence of lesions in the brains of patients with MS creates an additional challenge in the interpretation of neuroimaging findings in MS. Neuronal integrity may in fact affect the patterns of activation observed in functional neuroimaging studies, either directly or indirectly. Specifically, it has been hypothesized that the lesions in the periventricular region and white matter tracts to the frontal lobe affect blood flow to regions near and connected to the sites of lesions (Feeney & Baron, 1986; Pozzilli et al., 1991; Rao et al., 1989). It is important to note that the BOLD fMRI procedure assumes that "an increase in neuronal activity within the brain region results in an increase in local blood flow" (Hillary et al., 2002). Therefore, the presence of lesions in the brain characteristic of MS that may affect blood flow could also potentially affect the patterns of activation in MS. However, because functional imaging studies have shown more diffuse regions of activation in individuals with MS as compared with healthy controls, it may be hypothesized that the extent of the lesions cause increased blood flow broadly to regions surrounding the cortical areas that subserve functional behaviors.

In a more indirect manner, it has been hypothesized that neuronal integrity affects behavioral performance on motor and cognitive tasks, which in turn causes an increase in recruited cortical resources. To support this relationship, studies have shown that measures of lesion load, which is one method of identifying neuronal integrity, are inversely correlated with behavioral performance on cognitive tasks (Christodoulou et al., 2003; Foong et al., 1997; Huber et al., 1992; Sperling et al., 2001). However, the investigation of the relationship between lesion load and level of functional cerebral activation during cognitive performance has resulted in mixed findings. Once again, differences in methodological techniques may be able to explain such mixed findings. Specifically, the technique utilized to quantify lesion load may significantly alter one's results. Some studies utilizing gross measures of lesions report no relationship between lesion load and level of cerebral activation (Audoin et al., 2003; Chiaravalloti et al., 2005; Hillary et al., 2003), whereas more sensitive measures of lesion load, including quantification in terms of volumetric techniques, have demonstrated a positive correlation between increased regions of activation on fMRI and lesion load volume (Filippi et al., 2002; Lee et al., 2000; Mainero et al., 2004). Such findings suggest that neuronal integrity can affect the patterns of cerebral activation observed in clinical populations.

Neuronal integrity may also have an effect at a microscopic level, which can be measured through a number of neuroimaging techniques. Specifically, magnetic resonance spectroscopy (MRS) studies of MS have reported reduced ratios of NAA/Cr in patients with MS, as compared with healthy control groups (Foong et al., 1999; Tartaglia et al., 2004). NAA/Cr ratios have been positively correlated with behavioral performance on cognitive tasks, subjective levels of fatigue, the Expanded Disability Status Scale, duration of the disease, and lesion load (Christodoulou et al., 2003; Gadea et al., 2004; Pan et al., 2001; Tartaglia et al., 2004.

Magnetization transfer ratio (MTR), a measure of diffuse disease activity in normal-appearing white matter (NAWM), has also been used to examine neuronal integrity at a microscopic level. Decreased MTR is suggestive of demyelination and axonal loss. Decreased MTR of NAWM is reportedly related to cognitive impairment (Audoin et al., 2004; Ranjeva et al., 2005). Audoin et al. (2004) noted an inverse correlation between the level of activation in the right frontal lobe during a WM task and the level of MTR. In a study that examined the functional connectivity between neuroanatomical regions activated during the PASAT, the reduced level of MTR was correlated with the reduced level of functional connectivity between the left prefrontal lobe and anterior cingulate cortex (Au Duong et al., 2005).

Neuroimaging studies have reported altered cerebral activation patterns in groups with MS, as compared with healthy control groups, which is widely accepted as evidence that in MS the brain undergoes cerebral reorganization to compensate for reduced or lost cerebral functions. Although this is a valid theory, in this section we have postulated that there are other interpretations of these findings and that more careful studies are needed to examine how levels of effort, lesions, and neuronal integrity affect the patterns of cerebral activation before definitive conclusions can be made about the altered patterns of cerebral activation.

Conclusions and Future Directions

The current review of functional imaging studies in MS demonstrates that there are clear differences in the patterns of cerebral activation between those with MS and healthy adults in functional neuroimaging studies of motor functions, fatigue, and cognition. However, the patterns of activation are not consistent across studies, which is likely due to the types of tasks utilized, neuronal integrity, and level of effort needed to perform the tasks. The current interpretation of the altered patterns of activation is that in MS, the brain undergoes cerebral reorganization to compensate for the loss of functions. Although this is a reasonable explanation, there are alternative explanations, specifically in regard to individualized threshold levels for the recruitment of additional cortical resources. Although we are still at the beginning of investigating the changes that occur functionally in the central nervous system of people with MS, the functional neuroimaging studies reviewed above have demonstrated that the disease exerts a significant impact on motor functions, cognitive skills, and fatigue at a very basic level of brain function.

Further longitudinal research is needed to understand the impact of physical and cognitive interventions on the central nervous system in MS. Two studies have demonstrated changes in the WM circuit in healthy adults after WM training using fMRI (Hempel et al., 2004; Olesen et al., 2004). Because deficits in WM is one of the predominant complaints of patients with MS, such WM intervention techniques could be applied in MS. The impact of cognitive interventions can help lead the way to elucidate the nature of neuroplasticity and training-induced cortical rewiring in the MS neural system and whether axons can be redirected and maintained. In addition to the Pantano et al. (2005) study previously described, other longitudinal studies are needed to explore the relationship of age, clinical course, neuronal integrity, and level of effort on the changes that occur in cerebral activation patterns and cerebral reorganization in MS over time.

REFERENCES

Archibald, C. J., & Fisk, J. D. (2000). Information processing efficiency in patients with multiple sclerosis. *Journal of Clinical and Experimental Neuropsychology*, 22(5), 686–701.

Arnett, P. A., Rao, S. M., Grafman, J., et al. (1997). Executive functions in multiple sclerosis: An analysis of temporal ordering, semantic encoding, and planning abilities. *Neuropsychology*, 11(4), 535–544.

Audoin, B., Au Duong, M. V., Ranjeva, J. P., et al. (2005). Magnetic resonance study of the influence of tissue damage and cortical reorganization on PASAT performance at the earliest stage of multiple sclerosis. *Human Brain Mapping*, 24(3), 216–228.

Audoin, B., Ibarrola, D., Ranjeva, J. P., et al. (2003). Compensatory cortical activation observed by fMRI during a cognitive task at the earliest stage of MS. *Human Brain Mapping*, 20(2), 51–58.

Audoin, B., Ranjeva, J. P., Au Duong, M. V., et al. (2004). Voxel-based analysis of MTR images: A method to locate gray matter abnormalities in patients at the earliest stage of multiple sclerosis. *Journal of Magnetic Resonance Imaging*, 20(5), 765–71.

Au Duong, M. V., Audoin, B., Boulanouar, K., et al. (2005). Altered functional connectivity related to white matter changes inside the working memory network at the very early stage of MS. *Journal of Cerebral Blood Flow and Metabolism*, 25(10), 1245–1253.

Baddeley, A. (1992). Working memory. *Science*, 255(5044), 556–559.

Bauer, H. J., Firnhaber, W., & Winkler, W. (1965). Prognostic criteria in multiple sclerosis. *Annals of the New York Academy of Sciences*, 122, 542–551.

Beatty, W. W., Paul, R. H., Wilbanks, S. L., et al. (1995). Identifying multiple sclerosis patients with mild or global cognitive impairment using the Screening Examination for Cognitive Impairment (SEFCI). *Neurology*, 45(4), 718–723.

Bobholz, J. A., & Rao, S. M. (2003). Cognitive dysfunction in multiple sclerosis: A review of recent developments. *Current Opinions in Neurology*, 16(3), 283–288.

Buckle, G. J. (2005). Functional magnetic resonance imaging and multiple sclerosis: The evidence for neuronal plasticity. *Journal of Neuroimaging*, 15(Suppl. 4), 82S–93S.

Caine, E. D., Bamford, K. A., Schiffer, R. B., et al. (1986). A controlled neuropsychological comparison of Huntington's disease and multiple sclerosis. *Archives of Neurology*, 43(3), 249–254.

Calabresi, P. A. (2004). Diagnosis and management of multiple sclerosis. *American Family Physician*, 70(10), 1935–1944.

Chiaravalloti, N., Hillary, F., Ricker, J., et al. (2005). Cerebral activation patterns during working memory performance in multiple sclerosis using fMRI. *Journal of Clinical and Experimental Neuropsychology, 27*(1), 33–54.

Christodoulou, C., Krupp, L. B., Liang, Z., et al. (2003). Cognitive performance and MR markers of cerebral injury in cognitively impaired MS patients. *Neurology, 60*(11), 1793–1798.

Colombo, B., Martinelli Boneschi, F., Rossi, P., et al. (2000). MRI and motor evoked potential findings in nondisabled multiple sclerosis patients with and without symptoms of fatigue. *Journal of Neurology, 247*(7), 506–509.

Dancause, N., Barbay, S., Frost, S. B., et al. (2005). Extensive cortical rewiring after brain injury. *Journal of Neuroscience, 25*(44), 10167–10179.

DeLuca, J. (2005). Fatigue, cognition and mental effort. In J. DeLuca (Ed.), *Fatigue as a window to the brain* (pp. 37–57). Cambridge, MA: MIT Press.

DeLuca, J., Barbieri-Berger, S., & Johnson, S. K. (1994). The nature of memory impairments in multiple sclerosis: Acquisition versus retrieval. *Journal of Clinical and Experimental Neuropsychology, 16*(2), 183–189.

DeLuca, J., Chelune, G. J., Tulsky, D. S., et al. (2004). Is speed of processing or working memory the primary information processing deficit in multiple sclerosis? *Journal of Clinical and Experimental Neuropsychology, 26*(4), 550–562.

DeLuca, J., Gaudino, E. A., Diamond, B. J., et al. (1998). Acquisition and storage deficits in multiple sclerosis. *Journal of Clinical and Experimental Neuropsychology, 20*(3), 376–390.

DeLuca, J., Genova, H., & Wylie, G. R. (2006). *Cerebral mechanisms of cognitive fatigue in multiple sclerosis using fMRI.* Paper presented at the 20th annual meeting of Human Brain Mapping, Florence, Italy.

Demaree, H. A., Gaudino, E. A., DeLuca, J., et al. (2000). Learning impairment is associated with recall ability in multiple sclerosis. *Journal of Clinical and Experimental Neuropsychology, 22*(6), 865–873.

Denney, D. R., Sworowski, L. A., & Lynch, S. G. (2005). Cognitive impairment in three subtypes of multiple sclerosis. *Archives of Clinical Neuropsychology, 20*(8), 967–981.

De Simone, R., Marano, E., Brescia Morra, V., et al. (2005). A clinical comparison of trigeminal neuralgic pain in patients with and without underlying multiple sclerosis. *Neurological Sciences, 26*(Suppl. 2), S150–S151.

Desmond, J. E., Gabrieli, J. D., Wagner, A. D., et al. (1997). Lobular patterns of cerebellar activation in verbal working-memory and finger-tapping tasks as revealed by functional MRI. *Journal of Neuroscience, 17*(24), 9675–9685.

Feeney, D. M., & Baron, J. C. (1986). Diaschisis. *Stroke, 17*(5), 817–830.

Filippi, M., & Rocca, M. A. (2004). Cortical reorganisation in patients with MS. *Journal of Neurology, Neurosurgery and Psychiatry, 75,* 1087–1089.

Filippi, M., Rocca, M. A., Falini, A., et al. (2002). Correlations between structural CNS damage and functional MRI changes in primary progressive MS. *NeuroImage, 15*(3), 537–546.

Filippi, M., Rocca, M. A., Mezzapesa, D. M., et al. (2004). A functional MRI study of cortical activations associated with object manipulation in patients with MS. *NeuroImage, 21*(3), 1147–1154.

Foong, J., Rozewicz, L., Davie, C. A., et al. (1999). Correlates of executive function in multiple sclerosis: The use of magnetic resonance spectroscopy as an index of focal pathology. *Journal of Neuropsychiatry and Clinical Neurosciences, 11*(1), 45–50.

Foong, J., Rozewicz, L., Quaghebeur, G., et al. (1997). Executive function in multiple sclerosis: The role of frontal lobe pathology. *Brain, 120*(Pt. 1), 15–26.

Freal, J. E., Kraft, G. H., & Coryell, J. K. (1984). Symptomatic fatigue in multiple sclerosis. *Archives of Physical Medicine and Rehabilitation, 65*(3), 135–138.

Frohman, E. M., Frohman, T. C., Zee, D. S., et al. (2005). The neuro-ophthalmology of multiple sclerosis. *Lancet Neurology, 4*(2), 111–121.

Gadea, M., Martinez-Bisbal, M. C., Marti-Bonmati, L., et al. (2004). Spectroscopic axonal damage of the right locus coeruleus relates to selective attention impairment in early stage relapsing-remitting multiple sclerosis. *Brain, 127*(Pt. 1), 89–98.

Gaudino, E. A., Chiaravalloti, N. D., DeLuca, J., et al. (2001). A comparison of memory performance in relapsing-remitting, primary progressive and secondary progressive, multiple sclerosis. *Neuropsychiatry, Neuropsychology, and Behavioral Neurology, 14*(1), 32–44.

Genevie, L., Kallos, J. E., & Struenig, E. L. (1987). Job retention among people with multiple sclerosis. *Journal of Neurologic Rehabilitation, 1*, 131–155.

Grafman, J., Rao, S. M., & Litvan, I. (1990). Disorders of memory. In S. M. Rao (Ed.), *Neurobehavioral aspects of multiple sclerosis* (pp. 102–117). New York: Oxford University Press.

Grigsby, J., Ayarbe, S. D., Kravcisin, N., et al. (1994). Working memory impairment among persons with chronic progressive multiple sclerosis. *Journal of Neurology, 241*(3), 125–131.

Gronning, M., Hannisdal, E., & Mellgren, S. I. (1990). Multivariate analyses of factors associated with unemployment in people with multiple sclerosis. *Journal of Neurology, Neurosurgery, and Psychiatry, 53*(5), 388–390.

Harris, I. M., Fulham, M. J., & Miller, L. A. (2001). The effects of mesial temporal and cerebellar hypometabolism on learning and memory. *Journal of the International Neuropsychological Society, 7*(3), 353–362.

Hempel, A., Giesel, F. L., Garcia Caraballo, N. M., et al. (2004). Plasticity of cortical activation related to working memory during training. *American Journal of Psychiatry, 161*(4), 745–747.

Herndon, R. M. (2003). The pathology of multiple sclerosis and its variants. In R. M. Herndon (Ed.), *Multiple sclerosis: Immunology, pathology, and pathophysiology* (pp. 185–198). New York: Demos.

Hillary, F. G., Chiaravalloti, N. D., Ricker, J. H., et al. (2003). An investigation of working memory rehearsal in multiple sclerosis using fMRI. *Journal of Clinical and Experimental Neuropsychology, 25*(7), 965–978.

Hillary, F. G., Genova, H. M., Chiaravalloti, N. D., et al. (2006). Prefrontal modulation of working memory performance in brain injury and disease. *Human Brain Mapping, 27*(11), 837–847.

Hillary, F. G., Steffener, J., Biswal, B. B., et al. (2002). Functional magnetic resonance imaging technology and traumatic brain injury rehabilitation: Guidelines for methodological and conceptual pitfalls. *Journal of Head Trauma Rehabilitation, 17*(5), 411–430.

Huber, S. J., Bornstein, R. A., Rammohan, K. W., et al. (1992). Magnetic resonance imaging correlates of neuropsychological impairment in multiple sclerosis. *Journal of Neuropsychiatry and Clinical Neuroscience, 4*(2), 152–158.

Janculjak, D., Mubrin, Z., Brinar, V., et al. (2002). Changes of attention and memory in a group of patients with multiple sclerosis. *Clinical Neurology and Neurosurgery, 104*(3), 221–227.

Kenealy, P. M., Beaumont, J. G., Lintern, T. C., et al. (2002). Autobiographical memory in advanced multiple sclerosis: Assessment of episodic and personal semantic memory across three time spans. *Journal of the International Neuropsychological Society, 8*(6), 855–860.

Kesselring, J. (2004). Neurorehabilitation in multiple sclerosis—what is the evidence-base? *Journal of Neurology, 251*(Suppl. 4), IV25–IV29.

Kornblith, A. B., La Rocca, N. G., & Baum, H. M. (1986). Employment in individuals with multiple sclerosis. *International Journal of Rehabilitation Research, 9*(2), 155–165.

Krupp, L. B., Christodoulou, C., & Schombert H. (2005). Multiple sclerosis and fatigue. In J. DeLuca (Ed.), *Fatigue as a window to the brain* (pp. 61–71). Cambridge, MA: MIT Press.

LaRocca, N., Kalb, R., Scheinberg, L., et al. (1985). Factors associated with unemployment of patients with multiple sclerosis. *Journal of Chronic Diseases, 38*(2), 203–210.

Lazeron, R. H., Rombouts, S. A., Scheltens, P., et al. (2004). An fMRI study of planning-related brain activity in patients with moderately advanced multiple sclerosis. *Multiple Sclerosis, 10*(5), 549–555.

Lee, M., Reddy, H., Johansen-Berg, H., et al. (2000). The motor cortex shows adaptive functional changes to brain injury from multiple sclerosis. *Annals of Neurology, 47*(5), 606–613.

Lengenfelder, J., Bryant, D., Diamond, B. J., et al. (2006). Processing speed interacts with working memory efficiency in multiple sclerosis. *Archives of Clinical Neuropsychology, 21*(3), 229–238.

Lengenfelder, J., Chiaravalloti, N. D., Ricker, J. H., et al. (2003). Deciphering components of impaired working memory in multiple sclerosis. *Cognitive and Behavioral Neurology, 16*(1), 28–39.

Li, Y., Chiaravalloti, N. D., Hillary, F. G., et al. (2004). Differential cerebellar activation on functional magnetic resonance imaging during working memory performance in persons with multiple sclerosis. *Archives of Physical and Medical Rehabilitation, 85*(4), 635–639.

Lublin, F. D., & Reingold, S. C. (1996). Defining the clinical course of multiple sclerosis: Results of an international survey. National Multiple Sclerosis Society (USA) Advisory Committee on Clinical Trials of New Agents in Multiple Sclerosis. *Neurology, 46* (4), 907–911.

Mainero, C., Caramia, F., Pozzilli, C., et al. (2004). fMRI evidence of brain reorganization during attention and memory tasks in multiple sclerosis. *NeuroImage, 21*(3), 858–867.

Marrie, R. A., Fisher, E., Miller, D. M., et al. (2005). Association of fatigue and brain atrophy in multiple sclerosis. *Journal of the Neurological Sciences, 228*(2), 161–166.

McDonald, W. I., Compston, A., Edan, G., et al. (2001). Recommended diagnostic criteria for multiple sclerosis: Guidelines from the International Panel on the Diagnosis of Multiple Sclerosis. *Annals of Neurology, 50*(1), 121–127.

Merson, R. M., & Rolnick, M. I. (1998). Speech-language pathology and dysphagia in multiple sclerosis. *Physical and Medical Rehabilitation Clinics of North America*, *9*(3), 631–641.

Miller, D. H., & Frank, J. A. (1998). Magnetic resonance imaging techniques to monitor short term evolution of multiple sclerosis and to use in preliminary trials. *Journal of Neurology, Neurosurgery, and Psychiatry*, *64*(Suppl. 1), S44–S46.

Morgen, K., Kadom, N., Sawaki, L., et al. (2004). Training-dependent plasticity in patients with multiple sclerosis. *Brain*, *127*(Pt. 11), 2506–2517.

Olesen, P. J., Westerberg, H., & Klingberg, T. (2004). Increased prefrontal and parietal activity after training of working memory. *Nature Neuroscience*, *7*(1), 75–79.

Olivares, T., Nieto, A., Sanchez, M. P., et al. (2005). Pattern of neuropsychological impairment in the early phase of relapsing-remitting multiple sclerosis. *Multiple Sclerosis*, *11*(2), 191–197.

Pan, J. W., Krupp, L. B., Elkins, L. E., et al. (2001). Cognitive dysfunction lateralizes with NAA in multiple sclerosis. *Applied Neuropsychology*, *8*(3), 155–160.

Pantano, P., Mainero, C., Iannetti, G. D., et al. (2002). Contribution of corticospinal tract damage to cortical motor reorganization after a single clinical attack of multiple sclerosis. *NeuroImage*, *17*(4), 1837–1843.

Pantano, P., Mainero, C., Lenzi, D., et al. (2005). A longitudinal fMRI study on motor activity in patients with multiple sclerosis. *Brain*, *128*(Pt. 9), 2146–2153.

Pelosi, L., Geesken, J. M., Holly, M., et al. (1997). Working memory impairment in early multiple sclerosis: Evidence from an event-related potential study of patients with clinically isolated myelopathy. *Brain*, *120*(Pt. 11), 2039–2058.

Penner, I. K., Rausch, M., Kappos, L., et al. (2003). Analysis of impairment related functional architecture in MS patients during performance of different attention tasks. *Journal of Neurology*, *250*(4), 461–472.

Peterson, J. W., & Trapp, B. D. (2005). Neuropathobiology of multiple sclerosis. *Neurological Clinics*, *23*(1), 107–129, vi–vii.

Peyser, J. M., Rao, S. M., LaRocca, N. G., et al. (1990). Guidelines for neuropsychological research in multiple sclerosis. *Archives of Neurology*, *47*(1), 94–97.

Piras, M. R., Magnano, I., Canu, E. D., et al. (2003). Longitudinal study of cognitive dysfunction in multiple sclerosis: Neuropsychological, neuroradiological, and neurophysiological findings. *Journal of Neurology, Neurosurgery and Psychiatry*, *74*(7), 878–885.

Pozzilli, C., Passafiume, D., Bernardi, S., et al. (1991). SPECT, MRI and cognitive functions in multiple sclerosis. *Journal of Neurology, Neurosurgery and Psychiatry*, *54*(2), 110–115.

Ranjeva, J. P., Audoin, B., Au Duong, M. V., et al. (2005). Local tissue damage assessed with statistical mapping analysis of brain magnetization transfer ratio: Relationship with functional status of patients in the earliest stage of multiple sclerosis. *American Journal of Neuroradiology*, *26*(1), 119–127.

Rao, S. M. (1990). *Neurobehavioural aspects of multiple sclerosis*. New York: Oxford University Press.

Rao, S. M. (1986). Neuropsychology of multiple sclerosis: A critical review. *Journal of Clinical and Experimental Neuropsychology*, *8*(5), 503–542.

Rao, S. M., Leo, G. J., Bernardin, L., et al. (1991). Cognitive dysfunction in multiple sclerosis. I. Frequency, patterns, and prediction. *Neurology*, *41*(5), 685–891.

Rao, S. M., Leo, G. J., & St Aubin-Faubert, P. (1989). On the nature of memory disturbance in multiple sclerosis. *Journal of Clinical and Experimental Neuropsychology, 11*(5), 699–712.

Reddy, H., Narayanan, S., Arnoutelis, R., et al. (2000). Evidence for adaptive functional changes in the cerebral cortex with axonal injury from multiple sclerosis. *Brain, 123*(Pt. 11), 2314–2320.

Reddy, H., Narayanan, S., Woolrich, M., et al. (2002). Functional brain reorganization for hand movement in patients with multiple sclerosis: Defining distinct effects of injury and disability. *Brain, 125*(Pt. 12), 2646–2657.

Reingold, S. C. (1995). The new partnership in multiple sclerosis: Relations with industry. *Multiple Sclerosis, 1*(3), 141–142.

Rizzo, M. A., Hadjimichael, O. C., Preiningerova, J., et al. (2004). Prevalence and treatment of spasticity reported by multiple sclerosis patients. *Multiple Sclerosis, 10*(5), 589–595.

Rocca, M. A., Falini, A., Colombo, B., et al. (2002). Adaptive functional changes in the cerebral cortex of patients with nondisabling multiple sclerosis correlate with the extent of brain structural damage. *Annals of Neurology, 51*(3), 330–339.

Rocca, M. A., Mezzapesa, D. M., Falini, A., et al. (2003). Evidence for axonal pathology and adaptive cortical reorganization in patients at presentation with clinically isolated syndromes suggestive of multiple sclerosis. *NeuroImage, 18*(4), 847–855.

Roelcke, U., Kappos, L., Lechner-Scott, J., et al. (1997). Reduced glucose metabolism in the frontal cortex and basal ganglia of multiple sclerosis patients with fatigue: A 18F-fluorodeoxyglucose positron emission tomography study. *Neurology, 48*(6), 1566–1571.

Roessler, R. T., & Rumrill, P. D., Jr. (1995). The relationship of perceived worksite barriers to job mastery and job satisfaction for employed people with multiple sclerosis. *Rehabilitation Counseling Bulletin, 39*, 2–14.

Ron, M. A., Callanan, M. M., & Warrington, E. K. (1991). Cognitive abnormalities in multiple sclerosis: A psychometric and MRI study. *Psychological Medicine, 21*(1), 59–68.

Rozin, R., Schiff, Y., Kahana, E., et al. (1975). Vocational status of multiple sclerosis patients in Israel. *Archives of Physical Medicine and Rehabilitation, 56*(7), 300–304.

Rypma, B., Berger, J. S., & D'Esposito, M. (2002). The influence of working-memory demand and subject performance on prefrontal cortical activity. *Journal of Cognitive Neuroscience, 14*(5), 721–731.

Rypma, B., & D'Esposito, M. (1999). The roles of prefrontal brain regions in components of working memory: Effects of memory load and individual differences. *Proceedings of the National Academy of Sciences of the United States of America, 96*(11), 6558–6563.

Santa Maria, M. P., Benedict, R. H., Bakshi, R., et al. (2004). Functional imaging during covert auditory attention in multiple sclerosis. *Journal of the Neurological Sciences, 218*(1–2), 9–15.

Sarter, M., Givens, B., & Bruno, J. P. (2001). The cognitive neuroscience of sustained attention: Where top-down meets bottom-up. *Brain Research: Brain Research Reviews, 35*(2), 146–160.

Schwartz, J. E., Jandorf, L., & Krupp, L. B. (1993). The measurement of fatigue: A new instrument. *Journal of Psychosomatic Research, 37*(7), 753–762.

Skoff, R. (2003). Morphology of ologodendrocytes and myelin. In R. M. Herndon

(Ed.), *Multiple sclerosis: Immunology, pathology, and pathophysiology* (pp. 7–24). New York: Demos.

Sperling, R. A., Guttmann, C. R., Hohol, M. J., et al. (2001). Regional magnetic resonance imaging lesion burden and cognitive function in multiple sclerosis: A longitudinal study. *Archives of Neurology, 58*(1), 115–121.

Stablum, F., Meligrana, L., Sgaramella, T., et al. (2004). Endogenous task shift processes in relapsing-remitting multiple sclerosis. *Brain and Cognition, 56*(3), 328–331.

Staffen, W., Mair, A., Zauner, J., et al. (2002). Cognitive function and fMRI in patients with multiple sclerosis: Evidence for compensatory cortical activation during an attention task. *Brain, 125*, 1275–1282.

Sweet, L. H., Rao, S. M., Primeau, M., et al. (2004). Functional magnetic resonance imaging of working memory among multiple sclerosis patients. *Journal of Neuroimaging, 14*(2), 150–157.

Tartaglia, M. C., Narayanan, S., Francis, S. J., et al. (2004). The relationship between diffuse axonal damage and fatigue in multiple sclerosis. *Archives of Neurology, 61*(2), 201–207.

Thornton, A. E., & Raz, N. (1997). Memory impairment in multiple sclerosis: A quantitative review. *Neuropsychology, 11*(3), 357–366.

Thornton, A. E., Raz, N., & Tucke, K. A. (2002). Memory in multiple sclerosis: Contextual encoding deficits. *Journal of the International Neuropsychological Society, 8*(3), 395–409.

Vleugels, L., Lafosse, C., van Nunen, A., et al. (2000). Visuoperceptual impairment in multiple sclerosis patients diagnosed with neuropsychological tasks. *Multiple Sclerosis, 6*(4), 241–254.

Wishart, H. A., Saykin, A. J., McDonald, B. C., et al. (2004). Brain activation patterns associated with working memory in relapsing–remitting MS. *Neurology, 62*(2), 234–238.

Yokota, T., Hirose, K., Tanabe, H., et al. (1991). Sleep-related periodic leg movements (nocturnal myoclonus) due to spinal cord lesion. *Journal of the Neurological Sciences, 104*(1), 13–18.

CHAPTER 11

Alcohol Intoxication and Brain Imaging

CHALLENGES AND FINDINGS

Vince D. Calhoun
Godfrey D. Pearlson

The behavioral effects of alcohol intoxication are well known. In contrast to the effects of many other drugs of abuse, it is widely believed that multiple extracellular signaling pathways are involved in the cognitive and behavioral effects of acute alcohol consumption. Much less is known about how brain function and specific brain circuits are affected by alcohol. There is relatively little imaging evidence examining how exposure to alcohol might transiently modulate brain function. Current brain-imaging tools enable us to examine the impact of alcohol intoxication on the brain noninvasively. In this chapter, we provide a brief review of previous work using functional magnetic resonance imaging (fMRI) to study the neural correlates of acute alcohol intoxication. We also discuss some of the challenges involved in using fMRI as a tool to study alcohol intoxication. Finally, we describe in detail two studies from our own work, the first involving a visual perception paradigm, and the second involving a naturalistic behavior, simulated driving. In both studies we found specific circuits that were modulated by alcohol, both global and local effects of alcohol were revealed, and relationships between behavior, brain function, and alcohol blood levels were examined.

Basic Alcohol Effects on Physiology

For such a simple substance, alcohol has complex effects on brain transmitter systems, including glutamate, the brain's major excitatory neurotransmitter. Alcohol has profound inhibitory effects at low concentrations at a particular subtype of glutamate receptor, the N-methyl-D-aspartate (NMDA) ionotropic receptor, a receptor-gated ion channel (see review of Krystal & Tabakoff, 2004). In turn, these NMDA effects likely influence the regulation and release of a series of other neurotransmitters. Alcohol also has dose-dependent sedative-hypnotic effects that are mediated via potentiation of gamma-aminobutyric acid (GABA) receptors. The wide range of ethanol effects in humans depend in part on dose, blood level, whether levels are rising or falling, and their speed of alteration, plus psychological factors related to expectation and social setting.

The behavioral effects of alcohol intoxication are well known. For example, alcohol depresses neural activity, with an immediate effect "on all cognitive–motor processing . . . from decreased sensory acuity, delayed and aberrant judgment and decision making" to slowed motor responses (Mongrain & Standing, 1989). Even blood alcohol levels within legal limits significantly impair multiple attentional abilities; larger doses produce major impairments (Neill et al., 1991). Brewer and Sandow (1980) examined real accidents and found that the drivers with blood alcohol concentrations (BACs) ≥ 0.05 were more likely to have been engaged in secondary activities at the time of the accident (Brewer & Sandow, 1980). Consistent with this finding, sustained and divided attentional tasks are most impaired by alcohol (Moskowitz & Sharma, 1974). Thus, accidents are caused less by deficits in basic vehicle handling, simple perception, or reaction time than by interference with higher-order cognitive aspects such as working memory (WM) and divided visual attention. Comprehensive reviews such as those of Perrine (1976) and Mitchell (1985) conclude that information processing, decision making, and judgment are most consistently affected by alcohol.

Acute alcohol administration interferes with performance on neuropsychological tasks assessing a wide variety of cognitive processes, including immediate memory span (Tarter & Jones, 1971; Jones, 1973; Parker et al., 1974), short-term memory (Rosen & Lee, 1976; Tarter et al., 1991), conceptual and abstracting processes, and motor speed and coordination (Tarter & Jones, 1971), which may relate to prefrontal cortex moderation of complex motor skills (Peterson et al., 1990b). Although some evidence suggests no alcohol-induced differences on attention tests (Tarter & Jones, 1971), other findings indicate detrimental effects on attention allocation (Lamb & Robertson, 1987). Learning and memory are also negatively affected by alcohol (Ryback, 1971; Mungas et al., 1994). There is no single, simple alcohol-related effect on cognition that subsumes the multiple, differently dose-related consequences summarized in Table 11.1.

TABLE 11.1. Effects of Alcohol on Cognitive Tasks

Cognitive/psychomotor task	Alcohol-related impairment
Pursuit motor and tracking accuracy	Manno et al. (1970), Hansteen et al. (1976), Kvalseth (1977), Belgrave et al. (1979), Landauer & Howat (1983), Fagan et al. (1987), Peterson et al. (1990a)
Simple perception	Mitchell (1985) (least affected)
Hand and body steadiness, coordination	Manno et al. (1971),[a] Hansteen et al. (1976), Belgrave et al. (1979), Tagawa et al. (2000)
Increased choice reaction time	Tagawa et al. (2000),[a] Pickworth et al. (1997),[b] Perrine (1976),[c] Sugarman et al. (1973),[c] Landauer & Howat (1983),[c] Maylor & Rabbitt (1987) (not at lower doses), Eadson & Vogel-Sprott (2000)
Visual search	Moskowitz et al. (1976)[c]
Divided visual attention/useful field of view	Linnoila (1974), Moskowitz et al. (1985), Niaura et al. (1987), Mills et al. (1996), Kerr & Hindmarch (1998), Wesnes et al. (2000)
Sustained attention (continuous performance task)	Rohrbaugh et al. (1988), Mongrain & Standing (1989)
Perception of danger/risk taking, hazard perception latency	Allen (1972), Klonoff (1974), Hansteen et al. (1976), Rimm et al. (1982), McMillen & Wells-Parker (1987), McMillen et al. (1989), West et al. (1993), Deery & Love (1996)
Working memory	Petros et al. (1985), Minocha et al. (1985), Baker et al. (1986), Haut et al. (1989), Peterson et al. (1990a), Pickworth et al. (1997), Finn et al. (1999), Wesnes et al. (2000)
Go/no-go/response inhibition	Finn et al. (1999), Eadson & Vogel-Sprott (2000)
Planning/executive function	Peterson et al. (1990a), Giancola & Moss (1998), Cherek (2000)
Judgment of own driving performance	Flanagan et al. (1983)
Time estimation	Tinklenberg et al. (1976),[a,b] Bech et al. (1973),[c] Lapp et al. (1994)
Distance estimation	Bech et al. (1973)[c]
Digit symbol substitution task	Pickworth et al. (1997)
Serial addition/subtraction	Pickworth et al. (1997)

[a] Dose-dependent effect.
[b] Negative study.
[c] Actually driving in automobiles or driving simulators.

In addition, psychophysical measures (Wegner et al., 2001), including event-related potential (ERP) measures (Ahveninen et al., 2000), are impaired by intoxication. An analysis of literature examining the P300 ERP response (a positive peak appearing approximately 300 ms poststimulus) to alcohol challenge suggests slower information processing (Colrain et al., 1993; Krull et al., 1993). Both neuropsychological and neurological deficits in executive function, visuospatial performance, and functions of gait and balance are detectable as the result of *chronic* use in alcoholic men even after a month of sobriety (Sullivan et al., 2002b). Functions most severely affected in alcoholic women involve visuospatial and verbal and nonverbal WM processes, as well as gait and balance (Sullivan et al., 2002a). In general, these acute and chronic studies support a deleterious effect of alcohol on cognitive functioning.

The Use of Imaging to Examine Alcohol Effects

There has been relatively little imaging evidence in examining how exposure to alcohol may transiently modulate brain function in the context of cognitive task performance (Mathew & Wilson, 1986; Volkow et al., 1988; Volkow et al., 1990; Schwartz et al., 1993; Tiihonen et al., 1994). Alcohol's action on brain blood flow and metabolism are summarized in Table 11.2. Even

TABLE 11.2. Effects of Alcohol on Cerebral Blood Flow and Metabolism

Brain region	Alcohol effect
Generalized effects	↓ Overall cortical rCGM after alcohol (and at baseline in chronic alcoholic subjects) (Volkow et al., 1990)
	↑ Overall cortical rCBF (Mathew & Wilson, 1986; Schwartz et al., 1993)
	Mixed effects (DeWitt et al., 1990)
	↑ Overall cortical rCGM with alcohol *withdrawal* in alcoholic subjects (Volkow et al., 1994)
Cerebellum	↓ rCGM (Volkow et al., 1990)
	↓ rCBF (Volkow et al., 1988)
Prefrontal cortex	↑ rCBF (Mathew & Wilson, 1986; Volkow et al., 1988; Tiihonen et al., 1994)
Basal ganglia	Spared (Volkow et al., 1990)
Corpus callosum	Spared (Volkow et al., 1990)
Right temporal lobe	↑ rCBF (Mathew & Wilson, 1986; Volkow et al., 1988)
Parietal lobe	↑ rCBF (Mathew & Wilson, 1986)

Note. rCBF, regional cerebral blood flow; rCGM, regional cerebral glucose metabolism.

these results are partly contradictory and methodologically problematic (e.g., Schlaepfer & Pearlson, 1995). Alcohol may depress cerebellar activity, but increase prefrontal cortical activity. However, the prefrontal cortex (PFC) is a large heterogeneous anatomic area, and more discrete local changes remain to be defined. Only one study (Haier et al., 1999) has examined alcohol-induced changes in cerebral activation during performance of a cognitive (divided attention) task. Task performance differences between conditions were significantly correlated with metabolic rates in the parietal lobe and inversely with rates in the putamen and anterior cingulate. Within individuals, alcohol-induced parietal metabolic rate changes significantly correlated with attention performance changes.

Significant work needs to be done to map acute alcohol effects on brain function, including specific cognitive impairment, dose–response relationships, and effects of acute versus acute-on-chronic dosing. For example, Melgaard et al. (1990) and Volkow et al. (1992) assessed chronic effects on regional cerebral blood flow (rCBF) and showed metabolic reversible decreases after detoxification (Volkow et al., 1994). There may be continuing effects on executive and visuospatial abilities (Bates et al., 1997), suggesting prefrontal and parietal damage, which are stable over 21 days of treatment.

There has been some work examining differences in brain activation between chronic alcoholic individuals and healthy controls (Pfefferbaum et al., 2001). In general, it is reported that frontal activity is modified in chronic alcohol users. On a WM task, after controlling for baseline vigilance response, Tapert et al. (2001) found decreases in the right superior and inferior parietal, right middle frontal, right postcentral, and left superior frontal cortex. Another fMRI study suggested a reorganization of brain function resulting from long-term alcohol exposure and reported changes in WM, decreases in Brodmann's areas (BAs) 9, 10, and 45 and increases in BA 47 (Pfefferbaum et al., 2001). Neural correlates of alcohol craving have been reported in subcortical basal ganglia, amygdala, hippocampus (Schneider et al., 2001), prefrontal (George et al., 2001), and orbitofrontal regions (Wrase et al., 2002). From the Wrase et al. study, it is not clear that brain regions showing changes due to chronic alcohol use are the same as regions that demonstrate transient functional changes in response to acute alcohol use. Although some of alcohol's acute and chronic effects on the brain are beginning to be understood (see review by Krystal & Tabakoff, 2002), and its cognitive effects are reasonably well documented, there is a paucity of publications using brain-imaging techniques to probe the cerebral basis of specific alcohol effects on cognition. This is especially so in regard to dose–response relationships and compensatory brain strategies, such as input from regions ordinarily not concerned with mediating a particular task that become active under conditions of intoxication. Brain-imaging explorations of alcohol-induced task impairment under conditions of distraction or sleep deprivation are also under-explored, as are interactions with other commonly coabused substances, such as marijuana.

Challenges to the Use of Imaging in Alcohol Studies

The results just mentioned are suggestive of a widespread impact of alcohol intoxication on neuronal activity. Tools for measuring brain activity, including fMRI and positron emission tomography (PET) have been in use for a decade or more. However, there have been relatively few imaging studies addressing the impact of alcohol intoxication on brain activity. This is because of specific challenges related to the invasiveness of a radioactive tracer injection (in the case of PET) or, for fMRI, the hardware (e.g., any in-scanner equipment must be nonmagnetic and not generate radio frequency signals that interfere with the fMRI scan) or the environment (e.g., typical MRI scanners require participants to lie on their backs). Additional challenges are present for fMRI data because of the impact of alcohol on the blood vasculature, presenting a potential confound, or in the case of virtual reality, the analysis of the data provides additional complexities.

Alcohol is known to have vasoactive properties, confounding fMRI studies relying on phenomenological hemodynamic changes. Global changes (more specifically, decreases) in fMRI signal changes are likely confounded by such changes. A previous fMRI study reported that alcohol resulted in a significant activation decrease in visual areas, with slightly more right-sided decreases (Levin et al., 1998). There have been few studies addressing the effect of alcohol on brain activity, and to our knowledge, no cognitive imaging studies were conducted at two or more alcohol doses.

Recent Examples Using Functional Imaging and Alcohol

We now describe two studies from our own work, part of a larger study of simulated driving, both of which used fMRI to study the impact of two blood alcohol concentrations on brain activity. The first study serves as an example of an examination of the influences of alcohol on cognition using a visual perception task (Calhoun et al., 2001a, 2004a). Visual perception has been investigated in skills such as object recognition (Sugio et al., 1999), visual attention (Nakamura et al., 2000), and examination of the visual properties of letters (Raij, 1999). The Motor-Free Visual Perception Test—Revised (MVPT-R; Colarusso & Hammill, 1995) was designed to provide a reliable and valid measure of overall visual perceptual processing ability. It has been employed previously as a predictor of driving ability according to the following characteristics: (1) relevance to highway safety; (2) relation to on-the-road driving behavior or crashes; (3) capability of assessment on a driving simulator; and (4) sensitivity to alcohol effects (Sivak et al., 1981; Stokx & Gaillard, 1986; Kaszniak et al., 1991; Keyl et al., 1997).

The second study provides an example of an advanced approach; participants were administered placebo or two amounts of alcohol immediately prior to performing an in-scanner simulated driving paradigm (Calhoun et al.,

2002, 2004b). Such a task involves multiple interacting cognitive domains and was analyzed using independent component analysis. Driving while intoxicated (DWI) remains a persistent public health risk in the United States, resulting in more than 17,000 fatalities and an estimated 250,000 injuries related to intoxicated driving in 2002 (National Highway Traffic Safety Administration, 2002). One of the most common experimental tools in intoxicated driving research is the driving simulator, and many studies to date have employed driving simulators to assess the effects of various abused substances and prescribed medications, as well as the effects of normal aging, sleep deprivation, and other adverse conditions on driving and driving-related skills (Linnoila & Mattila, 1973; Rimm et al., 1982; Deery & Fildes, 1999; Arnedt et al., 2001; Verster et al., 2002). We have previously demonstrated the validity of a similar simulated driving environment to evaluate performance measures in sober and alcohol-intoxicated subjects as compared directly with real on-road driving (McGintyet al., 2001). Acute alcohol effects on behavioral and cognitive functions necessary for driving were summarized above (see also the review in Mitchell, 1985).

Summary of Study Design

An outline of the study design is presented in Figure 11.1. Participants were scanned in two sessions on two different days. Sessions were held at the same time of day (midmorning). For the first scan session, participants received a placebo, after which they were removed from the scanner and received a dose of beverage alcohol individualized to participant body weight, age, and sex, calculated using a published algorithm (Kapur, 1989) and designed to produce a BAC of 0.04 or 0.08% (the dose was counterbalanced between day 1 and day 2). The alcohol beverage was administered orally in single-blind fashion as 190 pf (95% v/v) ethanol diluted in chilled fruit juice to a constant volume, consumed over 10 m. Placebo drinks were of the same total volume, including 15 cc of alcohol floating on the surface. All beverages were served in identical glass containers, wrapped in an alcohol-soaked cloth to help disguise the contents (Hammersley et al., 1992). BACs were determined immediately before and after the scan session, using a handheld breath meter (Intoximeters, Inc.), and subjects were blind to BACs. No subject in either study reported here experienced nausea or was unable to complete the study.

The experimental paradigms are presented in Figure 11.2. Fifteen MVPT-R figures (approximately half the test battery) were presented an average of 17 s apart. A white asterisk on a black background was visible during the interstimulus intervals. For each item, a central test stimulus was presented above four other figures (one target and three distracters). Simulated driving involved a 10-min task consisting of 1-min epochs of (1) an asterisk fixation task, (2) active simulated driving, and (3) watching a simulated driving scene (while randomly moving fingers over the controller). Subjects were instructed to stay in the right lane except in order to pass, to avoid collisions, to stay

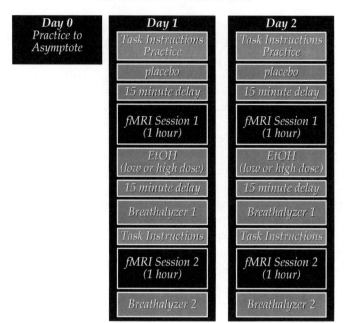

Day 0	Day 1	Day 2
Practice to Asymptote	Task Instructions Practice	Task Instructions Practice
	placebo	placebo
	15 minute delay	15 minute delay
	fMRI Session 1 (1 hour)	fMRI Session 1 (1 hour)
	EtOH (low or high dose)	EtOH (low or high dose)
	15 minute delay	15 minute delay
	Breathalyzer 1	Breathalyzer 1
	Task Instructions	Task Instructions
	fMRI Session 2 (1 hour)	fMRI Session 2 (1 hour)
	Breathalyzer 2	Breathalyzer 2

FIGURE 11.1. Study design. Outline of study design consisting of 2 days with two scan sessions on each day. Boxes are not proportional to the amount of time spent on each task.

within a speed range of 100–140 (the units were not specified), and to drive normally. Additional details on scanning and fMRI preprocessing may be found in a number of journal articles (Calhoun et al., 2001a, 2002, 2004a, 2004b).

At the lower BAC (mean 0.041 ± 0.016) on the 5-point analog scale (where 5 indicated maximal intoxication), participants indicated subjective intoxication of mean 1.0 ± 0.7, and at the higher BAC (mean 0.096 ± 0.040), participants self-rated intoxication of mean 3.1 ± 0.8. The difference on the subjective intoxication scores was highly significant ($p < .000001$).

Global versus Local Dose Response Effects in a Visual Perception Task

All participants performed well on the MVPT-R task, having an 85% average correct response (within 5% of the norm). Participants receiving the low dose of alcohol tended ($p < .07$) toward slightly decreased reaction time, whereas participants receiving the high dose of alcohol slightly ($p < .08$) increased in reaction time. No significant differences in accuracy were found ($p > .47$; low dose; $p > .11$; high dose). fMRI data from each participant were entered into a general linear model group analysis framework using the software package

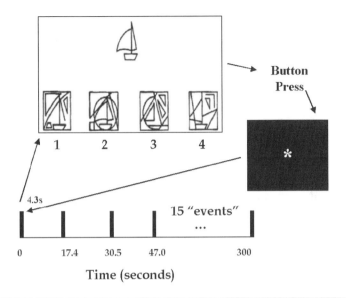

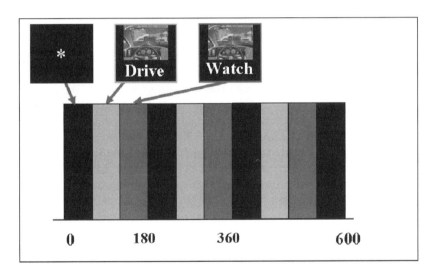

FIGURE 11.2. Time line of the MVPT-R and simulated driving paradigm. For the MVPT-R paradigm (top), figures were presented with an interstimulus interval of approximately 17 s. The participants were asked to indicate which of the four lower figures contained the upper figure by pressing 1, 2, 3, or 4, after which an asterisk was presented until the next figure appeared. The correct answer for this figure is 2. The driving paradigm (bottom) consisted of ten 1-min epochs of (a) a fixation target, (b) driving the simulator, and (c) watching a simulation while randomly moving fingers over the controller. The paradigm was presented twice, changing the order of the (b) and (c) epochs and counterbalancing the first order across subjects.

SPM (Statistical Parametric Mapping; *www.fil.ion.ucl.uk/spm*). The resultant statistics were height corrected for multiple comparisons to $p < .05$, using a method derived from Gaussian random field theory (Friston et al., 1996). The main effect group analysis for (1) (mean) sober (colored red/orange), (2) low dose (colored blue/cyan), and (3) high dose (colored green/yellow) is displayed in Plate 11.1. The SPM analysis revealed activation in visual and visual association areas as well as frontal eye fields (FEF)/dorsolateral–prefrontal cortex (DLPFC), and the supplementary motor area (SMA). At the highest dose, some regions (FEF/DLPFC/SMA) became more diffusely activated, that is, at the given threshold, the cluster size in each of these regions was greater.

We observed both global and local hemodynamic effects of alcohol. There was a global decrease evident both by visual inspection of the left side of Plate 11.1 and by examination of the maximum t-value (sober = 13.64, low dose = 11.49, high dose = 7.56) located in the lingual gyrus for all doses. In addition to the global effects, there were also localized increases and decreases. In particular, the contrast-to-noise (as measure by the t-value) in frontal regions increased (relative to sober) at the low dose and decreased (relative to sober) at the high dose (see Figure 11.3).

For the correlation analysis, a small, but detectable, effect was observed at a threshold of $p < .05$ (uncorrected) controlled for false positives with a contiguity filter of $k = 50$ voxels. The largest dose-dependent decreases were observed in bilateral parietal visual areas such as the precuneus and in the bilateral visual area middle temporal (MT) (although this was not independently verified with visual cortical mapping). The largest cluster demonstrating a dose-dependent increase was observed in the precentral gyrus. Corresponding images are presented on the right side of Plate 11.1.

We hypothesized that frontal and cerebellar regions would exhibit a dose-dependent decrease (Sullivan et al., 2000b). Consistent with our hypothesis, bilateral negative correlations were observed in frontal regions just anterior and superior to the frontal eye fields. In particular, the CNR in frontal regions increased (relative to sober) at the low dose and decreased (relative to sober) at the high dose. From Figure 11.3, it can thus be seen that there is an inverted 'U' relationship between dose and activation for prefrontal regions. This may indicate more active (but the same) frontal regions at the low dose of alcohol as participants attempt to perform the task during mild intoxication, whereas at the high dose, additional frontal regions are recruited and are activated less efficiently. Contrary to our hypothesis, we observed no dose-dependent decreases in cerebellar activation. Occipital and parietal visual areas demonstrated the largest dose-dependent decreases (but the relationship was linear in this case). Though most of the primary visual cortex did not meet our significance criterion, there was a dose-dependent trend in many of these areas. This is evident upon visual inspection of Plate 11.1.

We observed a dose-dependent decrease in regions consistent with visual area MT (VMT). VMT additionally revealed robust activation for the main effect of the MVPT-R task (see Plate 11.1). It was recently shown that area MT, an area primarily responsive to motion, is also responsible for processing

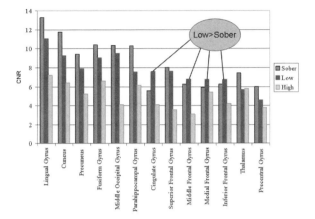

FIGURE 11.3. Graphic view of CNR differences detected in the main effects analysis. Bar graph comparison of CNR-by-area in the (mean) sober, low-dose, and high-dose studies. Visual areas demonstrate a clear dose-dependent decrease in CNR, whereas frontal regions appear to be higher in the low-dose condition and then lower in the high-dose condition.

shape (Kourtzi et al., 2002), and hence may reflect the task performance. The largest dose-dependent increases observed in medial prefrontal and precentral gyri were consistent with greater effort as the participants tried to overcome their impairment. Increases were also observed in the right insula, consistent with a PET study that found alcohol increases in right temporal and prefrontal regions (Volkow et al., 1988). The same study also demonstrated decreased cerebellar metabolism. A dose-dependent increase was observed in the right precentral gyrus. It has been shown that alcohol produces a psychomotor performance deficit in a dose-dependent manner (Hiltunen, 1997).

Virtual Reality and Alcohol Intoxication: Simulated Driving

We have also examined the impact of alcohol intoxication on fMRI activity during a simulated driving experiment that employed an off-the-shelf driving skill videogame software program. While in the scanner, participants held a Nintendo-like controller, shielded in copper foil, with all ferromagnetic components removed. In-scanner subject movement was not a problem, even at the higher alcohol dose. Driving performance was rated on eight different measures; vehicle collisions, near vehicle collisions, number of lane deviations, duration of lane deviations, number of instances over maximum speed limit, total time over maximum speed limit, number of instances below minimum speed limit, and total time below minimum speed limit. As compared with sober baseline, at the lower BAC, performance slightly improved and participants reduced average speed. At the higher BAC, subjects drove more at higher speeds ($p < .008$, corrected), and there was a trend toward increased collisions with other cars ($p < .15$, corrected).

For the fMRI analysis, we used a group ICA (independent component analysis) approach (Calhoun et al., 2001b), available in a toolbox implemented in Matlab (*icatb.sourceforge.com*). We calculated the average sober-condition ICA maps for each of the 25 components, and, using these 25 images, we generated single-subject component time courses for *all* datasets using spatial multiple regression of the component images onto the fMRI data for each time point (that is, we flattened each fMRI volume/time point into a row vector and computed the regressor of the spatial component with the fMRI volume and a spatial intercept regressor). We were thus computing a multiple regression of all components (and all voxels) onto the data at once, as a way to generate ICA time courses from component images. This approach is distinct from a regions-of-interest approach such as that which may be utilized in a typical general linear model (GLM) analysis. Rather, given a set of (fixed) independent component images, we were essentially generating their companion time courses. Finally, we selected the components that were highly correlated with the paradigm for further analysis.

ICA imaging results from the fixed-average-spatial (FAS) analysis are summarized in Plate 11.2, with different colors coding for each component. The average time courses for each scan session are presented in the middle and right panels of Plate 11.2, respectively. For visualization, the three epoch cycles were averaged together and presented as "fixation," "drive," and "watch." The 25 time courses were sorted according to their correlation with the driving paradigm and then visually inspected for task-related or transiently task-related activity (based on their periodicity with the paradigm). Of the 25 components, 7 demonstrated such a relationship. This is consistent with previous results (Calhoun et al., 2002), with the exception that the primary/supplemental motor and cerebellar networks were divided into two separate components (albeit with similar temporal patterns on average).

The left panel of Plate 11.2 displays the thresholded average components of interest [i.e., "weighted regions of interest (networks)"] determined from the sober-condition data. Cerebellar networks are depicted in the same color as the motor and supplementary motor regions, except with a turquoise border surrounding the region. The middle panel displays the average calibrated time courses (computed via spatial regression of the component maps onto the raw data for each subject) from the sober condition and low-dose condition, with color used as in the spatial component maps (the alcohol condition is indicated with the color gray). The right panel display is the same for the fMRI session consisting of the sober condition and corresponding (same day) high-dose condition (also indicated with the color gray).

Analysis 1: Behavior/fMRI/Alcohol

A direct comparison of significant behavioral measures (vehicular collisions and speed over 140), alcohol dose, and fMRI signal, was performed by computing the dose-related correlation of the behavior results with these parameterized results. All *p* values were greater than .2 except for two results:

The cerebellar component (D_40 – FW_40) exhibited a highly significant dose-related effect with driving greater than 140 ($p < .001$, corrected) and the frontoparietocingulate component (D_40 – FW_40) showed a weak dose-related correlation with vehicular collisions ($p < .15$, corrected). This may be due to less efficient processing of the complex motor coordination required at higher speeds. At BACs approaching 0.10%, there is a significant increase in collisions or near-collisions (Voas & Tippetts, 1999; Weiler et al., 2000). The dose-related cerebellar involvement is also consistent with previous studies implicating a detrimental effect of alcohol on complex motor control (Peterson et al., 1990c) and alcohol-associated decreases in cerebellar blood flow (Volkow et al., 1988). Because visual and attentional fields narrow, inebriated drivers are less responsive to peripheral events and often exhibit depressed perceptual and motor functioning (Mascord et al., 1995). We did not find significant differences in the frontoparietal region, contrary to hypotheses. The lack of significant findings in these regions, coupled with findings for the other regions discussed, suggests that decreased motor functioning during intoxication may be due less to attentional differences than to the impact of alcohol on cerebellar/motor and orbitofrontal regions.

Analysis 2: Disruption Score/Alcohol

The change in the fMRI disruption score with respect to dose is shown in Plate 11.3 (coloring is identical to that used in Plate 11.2). All components were found to be temporally less correlated for the high-dose experiment than for the low-dose experiment. Significant differences were found for the orbitofrontal component and the primary motor/SMA component ($p < .001$). Because of a significant speed-related relationship to both the orbitofrontal rate parameter and the D_40 – FW_40 activity in the orbitofrontal component in a previous study (Calhoun et al., 2002), we suggested that both the vigilance network and the error-monitoring network could be interpreted as a "switching" influence of the vigilance network on the error-monitoring network. In this context, awareness of driving (vigilance) is initiated once the driving condition begins (manifesting as an exponential decrease in fMRI signal). Error correction and disinhibition are revealed as a gradual decline of this component at a rate determined in part by the vigilance network. When subjects drive faster, the vigilance component changes more; thus, the error correction and disinhibition component decreases at a faster rate. In the present study, the speed was not modulated to a large degree (although a small but significant increase in the high-dose condition was observed). However, the orbitofrontal (OF) network was modulated by alcohol, but the frontoparietal (FP) network was not. Thus, the current results are consistent with a dissociation of the OF and FP networks (the latter network is modulated by alcohol, whereas the former network is not), manifesting as a problem in the OF network primarily (whereas the FP network does not appear to be affected).

The components identified by our analysis lend themselves naturally to interpretation in terms of well-known neurophysiological networks as discussed in Calhoun et al. (2002). In Plate 11.4 the seven components are divided into four patterns, with alcohol- and speed-related effects (Calhoun et al., 2002) indicated. Hypothesized functions of these networks are (1) vigilance, (2) error monitoring and inhibition, (3) motor, (4) higher-order motor (cerebellar), (5) visual, (6) higher-order visual, and (7) visual monitoring. We delineated the networks affected by driving speed in the previous study, as well as the networks affected by alcohol dose in the current study. We have discussed the involvement of these circuits in the context of simulated driving in detail previously, and the reader is referred to this work for further discussion (Groeger, 2000; Calhoun et al., 2002).

Future Work

Future work should include additional types of imaging information (such as perfusion) in order to quantify the global effects of alcohol on resting cerebral blood flow. In addition, because we did not collect physiological information such as cardiac rate, respiratory rate, skin conductivity, or eye movements, it is not possible to rule out whether these may have been associated with dose-related changes.

The behavioral and physiological effects of alcohol are complicated and can differ even at the same BAC within an individual, depending on whether the person is on the ascending or descending limb of the BAC curve (Conrod et al., 1997). It was for this reason that we measured BAC before and after the scan session and attempted to scan participants as close to their peak BACs as possible. However, more frequent measurement of BAC would have been useful. It would have also been useful to have a third, higher dose of alcohol, inasmuch as a trend toward behavioral decrements were observed only at the high dose. We would expect, in this case, to see greater dose-related decreases in frontal regions and increased amplitude changes in regions associated with the visual perception task.

The use of simulation and virtual reality paradigms or movies in order to provide an etiologically valid and more robust stimulation of the brain is an important area, which should be further studied. As virtual reality hardware becomes more "scanner-friendly," we predict that such approaches will become more widely used. Moreover, the study of alcohol intoxication can potentially be augmented through the combining of multiple tasks and multimodal data (Calhoun et al. 2005a, 2005b).

REFERENCES

Ahveninen, J., Jaaskelainen, I. P., Pekkonen, E., et al. (2000). Global field power of auditory N1 correlates with impaired verbal-memory performance in human alcoholics. *Neuroscience Letters*, *285*, 131–134.

Allen, J. E. (1972). Pilot study of marijuana effects is conducted. *Accident Reports*.

Arnedt, J. T., Wilde, G. J., Munt, P. W., et al. (2001). How do prolonged wakefulness and alcohol compare in the decrements they produce on a simulated driving task? *Accident Analysis and Prevention, 33,* 337–344.

Baker, S. J., Chrzan, G. J., Park, C. N., et al. (1986). Behavioral effects of 0 and 0.05% blood alcohol in male volunteers. *Neurobehavioral Toxicology and Teratology, 8,* 77–81.

Bates, M. E., Haier, R. J., Schandler, S. L., et al. (1997). Stability of neuropsychological assessments early in alcoholism treatment. Journal of Studies on Alcohol 58, 617–621.

Bech, P., Rafaelsen, L., & Rafaelsen, O. J. (1973). Cannabis and alcohol: Effects on estimation of time and distance. *Psychopharmacologia, 32,* 373–381.

Belgrave, B. E., Bird, K. D., Chesher, G. B., et al. (1979). The effect of (–) trans-delta9-tetrahydrocannabinol, alone and in combination with ethanol, on human performance. *Psychopharmacology, 62,* 53–60.

Brewer, N., & Sandow, B. (1980). Alcohol effects on driver performance under conditions of divided attention. *Ergonomics, 23,* 185–190.

Calhoun, V. D., Adali, T., Giuliani, N., et al. (2005a). A method for multimodal analysis of independent source differences in schizophrenia: Combining gray matter structural and auditory oddball functional data. *Human Brain Mapping, 27*(1), 47–62.

Calhoun, V. D., Adali, T., McGinty, V., et al. (2001a). fMRI activation in a visual-perception task: Network of areas detected using the general linear model and independent components analysis. *NeuroImage, 14,* 1080–1088.

Calhoun, V. D., Adali, T., Pearlson, G. D., et al. (2001b). A method for making group inferences from functional MRI data using independent component analysis. *Human Brain Mapping, 14,* 140–151.

Calhoun, V. D., Altschul, D., McGinty, V., et al. (2004a). Alcohol intoxication effects on visual perception: An fMRI study. *NeuroImage, 21,* 15–26.

Calhoun, V. D., Keihl, K. A., & Pearlson, G. D. (2005b). A method for multi-task fMRI data fusion applied to schizophrenia. *Human Brain Mapping, 27*(7), 598–610.

Calhoun, V. D., Pekar, J. J., McGinty, V. B., et al. (2002). Different activation dynamics in multiple neural systems during simulated driving. *Human Brain Mapping, 16,* 158–167.

Calhoun, V. D., Pekar, J. J., & Pearlson, G. D. (2004b). Alcohol intoxication effects on simulated driving: Exploring alcohol-dose effects on brain activation using functional MRI. *Neuropsychopharmacology, 29,* 2097–2107.

Cherek, D. R. (2000). Executive cognitive functioning, alcohol, and aggression: Comment on Giancola (2000). *Experimental and Clinical Psychopharmacology, 8,* 604–606.

Colarusso, R. P., & Hammill, D. D. (1995). *Motor-free visual perception test— Revised.* Novato, CA: Academic Therapy Publications.

Colrain, I. M., Taylor, J., McLean, S., et al. (1993). Dose dependent effects of alcohol on visual evoked potentials. *Psychopharmacology, 112,* 383–388.

Conrod, P. J., Peterson, J. B., Pihl, R. O., et al. (1997). Biphasic effects of alcohol on heart rate are influenced by alcoholic family history and rate of alcohol ingestion. *Alcoholism: Clinical and Experimental Research, 21,* 140–149.

Deery, H. A., & Fildes, B. N. (1999). Young novice driver subtypes: Relationship to high-risk behavior, traffic accident record, and simulator driving performance. *Human Factors, 41,* 628–643.

Deery, H. A., & Love, A. W. (1996). The effect of a moderate dose of alcohol on the traffic hazard perception profile of young drink-drivers. *Addiction*, 91, 815–827.

DeWitt, H., Metz, J., Wagner, N., et al. (1990). Behavioral and subjective effects of ethanol: Relationship to cerebral metabolism using PET. *Alcoholism: Clinical and Experimental Research*, 14, 482–489.

Eadson, C., & Vogel-Sprott, M. (2000). Alcohol and behavioral control: Impaired response inhibition and flexibility in social drinkers. *Experimental and Clinical Psychopharmacology*, 8, 387–394.

Fagan, D., Tiplady, B., & Scott, D. B. (1987). Effects of ethanol on psychomotor performance. *British Journal of Anaesthesia*, 59, 961–965.

Finn, P. R., Justus, A., Mazas, C., et al. (1999). Working memory, executive processes and the effects of alcohol on go/no-go learning: Testing a model of behavioral regulation and impulsivity. *Psychopharmacology*, 146, 465–472.

Flanagan, N. G., Strike, P. W., Rigby, C. J., et al. (1983). The effects of low doses of alcohol on driving performance. *Medicine, Science and the Law*, 23, 203–208.

Friston, K. J., Holmes, A., Poline, J. B., et al. (1996). Detecting activations in PET and fMRI: Levels of inference and power. *NeuroImage*, 4, 223–235.

George, M. S., Anton, R. F., Bloomer, C., et al. (2001). Activation of prefrontal cortex and anterior thalamus in alcoholic subjects on exposure to alcohol-specific cues. *Archives of General Psychiatry*, 58, 345–352.

Giancola, P. R., & Moss, H. B. (1998). Executive cognitive functioning in alcohol use disorders. *Recent Developments in Alcoholism*, 14, 227–251.

Groeger, J. (2000). *Understanding driving: Applying cognitive psychology to a complex everyday task*. New York: Psychology Press.

Haier, R., Schandler, S., MacLachlan, A., et al. (1999). Alcohol induced changes in regional cerebral glucose metabolic rate during divided attention. *Personality and Individual Differences*, 26, 425–439.

Hammersley, R., Finnigan, F., & Millar, K. (1992). Alcohol placebos: You can only fool some of the people all of the time. *British Journal of Addiction*, 87, 1477–1480.

Hansteen, R. W., Miller, R. D., Lonero, L., et al. (1976). Effects of cannabis and alcohol on automobile driving and psychomotor tracking. *Annals of the New York Academy of Sciences*, 282, 240–256.

Haut, J. S., Beckwith, B. E., Petros, T. V., et al. (1989). Gender differences in retrieval from long-term memory following acute intoxication with ethanol. *Physiology and Behavior*, 45, 1161–1165.

Hiltunen, A. J. (1997). Acute alcohol tolerance in cognitive and psychomotor performance: Influence of the alcohol dose and prior alcohol experience. *Alcohol*, 14, 125–130.

Jones, B. M. (1973). Memory impairment on the ascending and descending limbs of the blood alcohol curve. *Journal of Abnormal Psychology*, 82, 24–32.

Kapur, B. M. (1989). *Computer blood alcohol calculator V1.20 ARF software*. Toronto: Addiction Research Foundation.

Kaszniak, A. W., Keyl, P. M., & Albert, M. S. (1991). Dementia and the older driver. *Human Factors*, 33, 527–537.

Kerr, J., & Hindmarch, I. (1998). The effects of alcohol alone or in combination with other drugs on information processing, task performance and subjective responses. *Human Psychopharmacology*, 13, 1–9.

Keyl, P. M., Rebok, G. W., & Gallo, J. J. (1997). *Screening elderly drivers in general medical setting: Toward the development of a valid and feasible assessment procedure.* Washington, DC: AARP Andrus Foundation.

Klonoff, H. (1974). Marijuana and driving in real-life situations. *Science, 186,* 317–324.

Kourtzi, Z., Bulthoff, H. H., Erb, M., et al. (2002). Object-selective responses in the human motion area MT/MST. *Nature Neuroscience, 5,* 17–18.

Krull, K. R., Smith, L. T., Sinha, R., et al. (1993). Simple reaction time event-related potentials: Effects of alcohol and sleep deprivation. *Alcoholism: Clinical and Experimental Research, 17,* 771–777.

Krystal, J. H., & Tabakoff, B. (2002). Ethanol abuse, dependence, and withdrawal: Neurobiology and clinical implications. In K. L. Davis, D. Charney, J. T. Coyle, et al. (Eds.), *Neuropsychopharmacology: The 5th generation of progress* (pp. 1425–1443). Philadelphia: Lippincott Williams & Wilkins.

Kvalseth, T. O. (1977). Effects of marijuana on human reaction time and motor control. *Perception and Motor Skills, 45,* 935–939.

Lamb, M. R., & Robertson, L. C. (1987). Effect of acute alcohol on attention and the processing of hierarchical patterns. *Alcoholism: Clinical and Experimental Research, 11,* 243–248.

Landauer, A. A., & Howat, P. (1983). Low and moderate alcohol doses, psychomotor performance and perceived drowsiness. *Ergonomics, 26,* 647–657.

Lapp, W. M., Collins, R. L., Zywiak, W. H., et al. (1994). Psychopharmacological effects of alcohol on time perception: The extended balanced placebo design. *Journal of Studies on Alcohol, 55,* 96–112.

Levin, J. M., Ross, M. H., Mendelson, J. H., et al. (1998). Reduction in BOLD fMRI response to primary visual stimulation following alcohol ingestion. *Psychiatry Research, 82,* 135–146.

Linnoila, M. (1974). Effect of drugs and alcohol on psychomotor skills related to driving. *Annals of Clinical Research, 6,* 7–18.

Linnoila, M., & Mattila, M. J. (1973). Interaction of alcohol and drugs on psychomotor skills as demonstrated by a driving simulator. *British Journal of Pharmacology, 47,* 671P–672P.

Manno, J. E., Kiplinger, G. F., Haine, S. E., et al. (1970). Comparative effects of smoking marihuana or placebo on human motor and mental performance. *Clinical Pharmacology and Therapeutics, 11,* 808–815.

Manno, J. E., Kiplinger, G. F., Scholz, N., et al. (1971). The influence of alcohol and marihuana on motor and mental performance. *Clinical Pharmacology and Therapeutics, 12,* 202–211.

Mascord, D., Walls, J., & Starmes, G. (1995). Fatigue and alcohol: Interactive effects on human performance in driving-related tasks. In L. Hartley (Eds.), *Fatigues and driving: Driver impairment, driver fatigue, and driving simulation* (pp. 189–205). London: Taylor & Francis.

Mathew, R. J., & Wilson, W. H. (1986). Regional cerebral blood flow changes associated with ethanol intoxication. *Stroke, 17,* 1156–1159.

Maylor, E. A., & Rabbitt, P. M. (1987). Effects of practice and alcohol on performance of a perceptual-motor task. *Quarterly Journal of Experimental Psychology, A 39,* 777–795.

McGinty, V. B., Shih, R. A., Garrett, E. S., et al. (2001). Assessment of intoxicated driving with a simulator: A validation study with on road driving. In *Proceedings on Human Centered Transportation Simulation Conference* (pp. 11–19). Iowa City, IA.

McMillen, D. L., Smith, S. M., & Wells-Parker, E. (1989). The effects of alcohol, expectancy, and sensation seeking on driving risk taking. *Addictive Behaviors, 14,* 477–483.

McMillen, D. L., & Wells-Parker, E. (1987). The effect of alcohol consumption on risk-taking while driving. *Addictive Behaviors, 12,* 241–247.

Melgaard, B., Henriksen, L., Ahlgren, P., et al. (1990). Regional cerebral blood flow in chronic alcoholics measured by single photon emission computerized tomography. *Acta Neurologica Scandinavia, 82,* 87–93.

Mills, K. C., Parkman, K. M., & Spruill, S. E. (1996). A PC-based software test for measuring alcohol and drug effects in human subjects. *Alcoholism: Clinical and Experimental Research, 20,* 1582–1591.

Minocha, A., Barth, J. T., Roberson, D. G., et al. (1985). Impairment of cognitive and psychomotor function by ethanol in social drinkers. *Veterinary and Human Toxicology, 27,* 533–536.

Mitchell, M. C. (1985). Alcohol-induced impairment of central nervous system function: Behavioral skills involved in driving. *Journal of Studies on Alcohol, 10*(Suppl.), 109–116.

Mongrain, S., & Standing, L. (1989). Impairment of cognition, risk-taking, and self-perception by alcohol. *Perception and Motor Skills, 69,* 199–210.

Moskowitz, H., Burns, M. M., & Williams, A. F. (1985). Skills performance at low blood alcohol levels. *Journal of Studies on Alcohol, 46,* 482–485.

Moskowitz, H., Hulbert, S., & McGlothin, W. H. (1976). Marijuana: Effects on simulated driving performance. *Accident Analysis and Prevention, 8,* 45–50.

Moskowitz, H., & Sharma, S. (1974). Effects of alcohol on peripheral vision as a function of attention. *Human Factors, 16,* 174–180.

Mungas, D., Ehlers, C. L., & Wall, T. L. (1994). Effects of acute alcohol administration on verbal and spatial learning. *Alcohol and Alcoholism, 29,* 163–169.

Nakamura, K., Honda, M., Okada, T., et al. (2000). Attentional modulation of parieto-occipital cortical responses: Implications for hemispatial neglect. *Journal of the Neurological Sciences, 176,* 136–143.

National Highway Traffic Safety Administration. (2002). *Traffic safety facts* (Report #DOT HS 809 606). Washington, DC: Author.

Neill, R. A., Delahunty, A. M., & Fenelon, B. (1991). Discrimination of motion in depth trajectory following acute alcohol ingestion. *Biological Psychology, 31,* 1–22.

Niaura, R. S., Nathan, P. E., Frankenstein, W., et al. (1987). Gender differences in acute psychomotor, cognitive, and pharmacokinetic response to alcohol. *Addictive Behaviors, 12,* 345–356.

Parker, E. S., Alkana, R. L., Birnbaum, I. M., et al. (1974). Alcohol and the disruption of cognitive processes. *Archives of General Psychiatry, 31,* 824–828.

Perrine, M. W. (1976). Alcohol and highway crashes: Closing the gap between epidemiology and experimentation. *Modern Problems of Pharmacopsychiatry, 11,* 22–41.

Peterson, J. B., Rothfleisch, J., Zelazo, P. D., et al. (1990). Acute alcohol intoxication and cognitive functioning. *Journal of Studies on Alcohol, 51,* 114–122.

Petros, T. V., Kerbel, N., Beckwith, B. E., et al. (1985). The effects of alcohol on prose memory. *Physiology and Behavior, 35,* 43–46.

Pfefferbaum, A., Desmond, J. E., Galloway, C., et al. (2001). Reorganization of frontal systems used by Alcoholics for Spatial Working Memory: An fMRI study. *NeuroImage, 14*, 7–20.

Pickworth, W. B., Rohrer, M. S., & Fant, R. V. (1997). Effects of abused drugs on psychomotor performance. *Experimental and Clinical Psychopharmacology, 5*, 235–241.

Raij, T. (1999). Patterns of brain activity during visual imagery of letters. *Journal of Cognitive Neuroscience, 11*, 282–299.

Rimm, D. C., Sininger, R. A., Faherty, J. D., et al. (1982). A balanced placebo investigation of the effects of alcohol vs. alcohol expectancy on simulated driving behavior. *Addictive Behavior, 7*, 27–32.

Rohrbaugh, J. W., Stapleton, J. M., Parasuraman, R., et al. (1988). Alcohol intoxication reduces visual sustained attention. *Psychopharmacology, 96*, 442–446.

Rosen, L. J., & Lee, C. L. (1976). Acute and chronic effects of alcohol use on organizational processes in memory. *Journal of Abnormal Psychology, 85*, 309–317.

Ryback, R. S. (1971). The continuum and specificity of the effects of alcohol on memory: A review. *Quarterly Journal of Studies on Alcohol, 32*, 995–1016.

Schlaepfer, T. E., & Pearlson, G. D. (1995). Pitfalls of SPECT studies of acute ethanol-induced changes in cerebral blood flow. *American Journal of Psychiatry, 152*, 1695–1696.

Schneider, F., Habel, U., Wagner, M., et al. (2001). Subcortical correlates of craving in recently abstinent alcoholic patients. *American Journal of Psychiatry, 158*, 1075–1083.

Schwartz, J. A., Speed, N. M., Gross, M. D., et al. (1993). Acute effects of alcohol administration on regional cerebral blood flow: The role of acetate. *Alcoholism: Clinical and Experimental Research, 17*, 1119–1123.

Sivak, M., Olson, P. L., Kewman, D. G., et al. (1981). Driving and perceptual/cognitive skills: Behavioral consequences of brain damage. *Archives of Physical Medicine and Rehabilitation, 62*, 476–483.

Stokx, L. C., & Gaillard, A. W. (1986). Task and driving performance of patients with a severe concussion of the brain. *Journal of Clinical and Experimental Neuropsychology, 8*, 421–436.

Sugarman, R. C., Cozad, C. P., & Zavala, A. (1973). *Alcohol-induced degradation of performance on simulated driving tasks* (Paper No. 730099). Detroit: Society of Automotive Engineers.

Sugio, T., Inui, T., Matsuo, K., et al. (1999). The role of the posterior parietal cortex in human object recognition: A functional magnetic resonance imaging study. *Neuroscience Letters, 276*, 45–48.

Sullivan, E. V., Fama, R., Rosenbloom, M. J., et al. (2002a). A profile of neuropsychological deficits in alcoholic women. *Neuropsychology, 16*, 74–83.

Sullivan, E. V., Rosenbloom, M. J., & Pfefferbaum, A. (2000b). pattern of motor and cognitive deficits in detoxified alcoholic men. *Alcoholism: Clinical and Experimental Research, 24*, 611–621.

Tagawa, M., Kano, M., Okamura, N., et al. (2000). Relationship between effects of alcohol on psychomotor performances and blood alcohol concentrations. *Japanese Journal of Pharmacology, 83*, 253–260.

Tapert, S. F., Brown, G. G., Kindermann, S. S., et al. (2001). fMRI measurement of brain dysfunction in alcohol-dependent young women. *Alcoholism: Clinical and Experimental Research, 25*, 236–245.

Tarter, R. E., Arria, A. M., & Van Thiel, D. H. (1991). Hepatic encephalopathy coexistent with alcoholism. *Recent Dev. Alcohol*, *9*, 205–224.

Tarter, R. E., & Jones, B. M. (1971). Absence of intellectual deterioration in chronic alcoholics. *Journal of Clinical Psychology*, *27*, 453–455.

Tiihonen, J., Kuikka, J., Hakola, P., et al. (1994). Acute ethanol-induced changes in cerebral blood flow. *American Journal of Psychiatry*, *151*, 1505–1508.

Tinklenberg, J. R., Roth, W. T., & Kopell, B. S. (1976). Marijuana and ethanol: Differential effects on time perception, heart rate, and subjective response. *Psychopharmacology*, *49*, 275–279.

Verster, J. C., Volkerts, E. R., & Verbaten, M. N. (2002). Effects of alprazolam on driving ability, memory functioning and psychomotor performance: A randomized, placebo-controlled study. *Neuropsychopharmacology*, *27*, 260–269.

Voas, R. B., & Tippetts, A. S. (1999). *The relationship of alcohol safety laws to drinking drivers in fatal crashes* (Report No. DOT HS 808 980). Washington, DC: National Highway Traffic Safety Administration.

Volkow, N. D., Hitzemann, R., Wang, G. J., et al. (1992). Decreased brain metabolism in neurologically intact healthy alcoholics. *American Journal of Psychiatry*, *149*, 1016–1022.

Volkow, N. D., Hitzemann, R., Wolf, A. P., et al. (1990). Acute effects of ethanol on regional brain glucose metabolism and transport. *Psychiatry Research*, *35*, 39–48.

Volkow, N. D., Mullani, N., Gould, L., et al. (1988). Effects of acute alcohol intoxication on cerebral blood flow measured with PET. *Psychiatry Research*, *24*, 201–209.

Volkow, N. D., Wang, G. J., Hitzemann, R., et al. (1994). Recovery of brain glucose metabolism in detoxified alcoholics. *American Journal of Psychiatry*, *151*, 178–183.

Wegner, A. J., Gunthner, A., & Fahle, M. (2001). Visual performance and recovery in recently detoxified alcoholics. *Alcohol and Alcoholism*, *36*, 171–179.

Weiler, J. M., Bloomfield, J. R., Woodworth, G. G., et al. (2000). Effects of fexofenadine, diphenhydramine, and alcohol on driving performance: A randomized, placebo-controlled trial in the Iowa Driving Simulator. *Annals of Internal Medicine*, *132*, 354–363.

Wesnes, K. A., Garratt, C., Wickens, M., et al. (2000). Effects of sibutramine alone and with alcohol on cognitive function in healthy volunteers. *British Journal of Clinical Pharmacology*, *49*, 110–117.

West, R., Wilding, J., French, D., et al. (1993). Effect of low and moderate doses of alcohol on driving hazard perception latency and driving speed. *Addiction*, *88*, 527–532.

Wrase, J., Grusser, S., Klein, S., et al. (2002). Development of alcohol-associated cues and cue-induced brain activation in alcoholics. *European Psychiatry*, *17*, 287.

CHAPTER 12

Functional Neuroimaging in Schizophrenia

J. Daniel Ragland

Schizophrenia is usually first diagnosed during late adolescence or early adulthood, when individuals are reaching their prime and preparing to take on adult responsibilities of career and family. As the individual's thinking becomes increasingly disorganized, with the presence of delusions and auditory hallucinations, and as his or her social functioning becomes constricted by negative symptoms such as anergia and anhedonia, the individual is no longer able to manage these responsibilities, experiences a psychotic break, and receives a diagnosis of schizophrenia after a period of sustained illness. Although this first psychotic break is usually unexpected, it reflects a lifelong neurodevelopmental abnormality in how the brain of that individual perceives, understands, and interprets the environment.

In the late 19th and early 20th century leading psychiatrists and neurologists, including Alzheimer, Kraepelin, and Bleuler, began investigating this disorder. In 1896, Emil Kraepelin coined the term *dementia praecox* to connote the devastating impact of the illness on brain function. The term was later changed to "schizophrenia" by Eugene Bleuler to emphasize that it is not truly a dementia but a "splitting" of mental capacities. In the past 100 years it has become clear that schizophrenia is not a classic neurodegenerative disorder like Alzheimer's disease but rather a progressive neurodevelopmental disorder resulting from problems in early and late brain development and neurotoxic effects of environmental stressors and untreated illness (Keshavan, 1999). During the past century neurobiological research of schizophrenia has grown exponentially from early postmortem studies of brain pathology to experiments using structural and functional neuroimaging methods, to recent molecular studies designed to identify the genes responsible for abnormal brain development and neural function.

The focus of this chapter is on how functional neuroimaging methods have improved our understanding of where and how things are going wrong in the brains of individuals with schizophrenia. The chapter discusses imaging methods designed to reveal functional changes in regional blood flow and metabolism, including ^{133}Xenon clearance, positron emission tomography (PET), and blood-oxygen-level-dependent (BOLD) functional magnetic resonance (fMRI) imaging. These techniques provide the primary means for studying *in vivo* changes in brain function and have assumed a central role in the neuroscientific investigation of schizophrenia and other major psychiatric illnesses. Although this chapter does not review results from neuropathological and structural imaging studies, those methods continue to play a central role in the study of schizophrenia and the reader is encouraged to explore several excellent reviews of research in these areas (Harrison & Roberts, 2000; Pearlson & Marsh, 1999; Shenton et al., 2001). Likewise, a comprehensive review of electrophysiological methods, including evoked response potential studies, and PET and single-photon emission tomography (SPECT) studies of receptor activity are beyond the scope of this chapter and can be explored further in several excellent review articles (Frankle & Laruelle, 2002; Light & Braff, 1999; McCarley et al., 1991).

Within the context of functional neuroimaging, this chapter introduces the reader to two prominent theories on the pathophysiology of schizophrenia and shows how these once competing theories have been reconciled over time. The discussion begins with a consideration of the "hypofrontality" theory of schizophrenia, followed by the presentation of data supporting a left-hemisphere temporal lobe model of brain dysfunction, and concluding with evidence supporting a combined model of distributed frontotemporal network dysfunction in schizophrenia. The chapter closes with several recent theories suggesting diffuse dysfunction throughout the brains of individuals with schizophrenia and emphasizing the importance of studying early information processing.

Frontal Lobe Model

The prefrontal cortex has been implicated in the pathophysiology of schizophrenia since the initial postmortem studies by Alzheimer in the late 19th century. The prefrontal cortex has rich reciprocal connections with the limbic system and the rest of the brain and is responsible for coordinating "the most elaborate and novel actions of the organism" (Fuster, 1999, p. 51). Dysfunction in this region could therefore help explain both generalized cognitive dysfunction (Blanchard & Neale, 1994) and more severe impairments in attention, problem solving, learning, and memory (Goldberg, 1985; Goldberg et al., 1987; Saykin et al., 1991) that are hallmarks of the disorder. On a phenomenological basis, patients with schizophrenia share many features of individuals with focal frontal lobe damage, including blunted affect, social withdrawal, poor insight, reduced motivation, distractibility, and poor impulse control (Strub & Black, 1985; Trimble, 1990; Weinberger, 1988). In the early 1970s the [133]Xenon clearance model was used to examine regional changes in cerebral metabolism and blood flow to test the hypothesis that patients had disrupted frontal lobe function.

Initial [133]Xenon clearance studies examined individuals when they were at rest and observed the distribution of blood flow across the cortex. In the first such study, Ingvar and Franzen (1974) compared the gradient of frontal to posterior cerebral blood flow in healthy volunteers and patients with schizophrenia. Although there was no group difference in whole-brain blood flow, patients showed a reduced gradient of frontal to posterior blood flow, leading to the conclusion that individuals with schizophrenia experience "hypofrontality" in their distribution of cerebral blood flow. A subsequent study by the same investigators observed that this pattern of hypofrontality was strongest in those patients with a restricted range of affect who were the most withdrawn and mute (Franzen & Ingvar, 1975). This pattern of resting hypofrontality was replicated by several subsequent imaging studies of cerebral blood flow and metabolism employing both [133]Xenon (Berman et al., 1986; Mathew et al., 1988) and PET functional imaging methods (Buchsbaum et al., 1982; Volkow et al., 1987). However, not all resting studies found evidence of hypofrontality (Catafau et al., 1994; Ebmeier et al., 1995), including a series of studies by Gur and colleagues (1983, 1985, 1987a, 1987b), who became increasingly critical of the hypofrontality model (Gur & Gur, 1995).

Although resting studies provide valuable and reproducible information on baseline cerebral perfusion and metabolism, lack of control over the individual's mental state makes it difficult to link regional patterns of activity to specific cognitive functions. Therefore, studies of hypofrontality in schizophrenia increasingly adopted "activation" paradigms in which changes in blood flow or metabolism were linked to specific neurobehavioral probes (Gur et al., 1992). The most widely studied neurobehavioral probe in these initial studies was the Wisconsin Card Sorting Task (WCST; Berg, 1948; Grant & Berg, 1948). The WCST is a measure of concept formation, cognitive flexibility, and working memory sensitive to frontal lobe lesions. It requires subjects to sort a deck of cards to one of four key cards that match the cards in the deck on several dimensions. The subject must use experimenter feedback ("correct" or "incorrect") to develop the correct sorting principle and switch to a new sorting principle when the rule changes.

In a series of studies Weinberger and colleagues (Weinberger et al., 1986, 1988; Berman et al., 1986, 1988) measured cerebral blood flow while patients and controls performed the WCST and a number-matching task designed to control for nonspecific activation (e.g., effects of attention, motor response, visual activation). These studies revealed that patients failed to show a normal increase in blood flow in the dorsolateral prefrontal cortex (DLPF) during

WCST performance. These results were specific to the WCST task, were replicated when patients were both on and off medication, and did not appear to be due to global cortical dysfunction. The consistency of these activation results and the inconsistency in the resting baseline results led to a reformulation of the hypofrontality hypothesis, stressing the importance of activation paradigms and clarifying that "hypofrontality appears to be dependent on the behavioral state of the patients during the brain imaging experiment" (Weinberger et al., 1991, p. 276). Andreasen and colleagues (1992) further clarified that hypofrontality may best be defined as "an inability for an individual to raise significantly his or her cerebral perfusion to the prefrontal region when given an experimental prefrontal cognitive challenge" (p. 955).

This revised form of the hypofrontality hypothesis was not immune to criticism. One concern raised was that of performance differences. Because patients performed worse on the WCST, it was not clear whether hypofrontality reflected inherent differences in prefrontal function or was a by-product of lower task performance (Ebmeier et al., 1995). This "chicken or the egg" criticism is notoriously difficult to address, because the tasks of greatest interest are often those that are most difficult for patients to perform. Efforts to address this criticism included studying other samples of patients who were also impaired but did not show hypofrontality, studying patients with schizophrenia on tasks on which they were impaired but showed normal prefrontal response, and studying low-performing controls and high-performing patients (Weinberger & Berman, 1996). Another concern about the hypofrontality hypothesis was that it might be limited to patients exhibiting prominent negative symptoms. This was suggested in a [133]Xenon-clearance study that found decreased activation during a frontal lobe task only in patients with high scores for negative symptoms (Andreasen et al., 1992). However, several subsequent studies found that the inverse correlation between negative symptoms and prefrontal cerebral blood flow did not occur during control task conditions (Vita et al., 1991; Lewis et al., 1992). Finally, a study of identical twins discordant for schizophrenia (Berman et al., 1992) found that prefrontal activation was lower in the affected twin than in the unaffected twin in all cases regardless of clinical symptomatology.

Left-Hemisphere Temporal Lobe Model

At the same time investigators were examining anterior-to-posterior gradients to test the frontal lobe model, efforts were being made to compare the gradient of left-to-right hemisphere blood flow and metabolism to establish laterality theories of schizophrenia. The left hemisphere is responsible for verbal, linguistic, and analytic functions, whereas the right hemisphere appears to be specialized for visuospatial and synthetic processes in healthy right-handed individuals. Features of thought disorder including analytic and language-processing deficits were suggestive of greater left-hemispheric dysfunction and motivated a search for laterality differences in schizophrenia.

The first studies were performed with the [133]Xenon clearance method and examined participants at rest and during performance of verbal analogy and spatial line orientation tasks. In the first such study (Gur et al., 1983) no group differences were found in anterior–posterior or left–right gradients of cerebral blood flow when patients and controls were at rest. However, during task performance patients failed to show the normal pattern of greater left-hemispheric increase for the verbal task and right-hemispheric increase for the spatial task. Patients did not produce any laterality effects for the verbal task; however, they showed greater left-hemispheric activation during the spatial task, providing initial support for a left-hemispheric overactivation model of the disorder. A subsequent study examined unmedicated patients with the same task paradigm (Gur et al., 1985). When not receiving medication, patients showed evidence of left-hemispheric overactivation both at rest and during task performance, leading to the conclusion that medication may serve to restore normal resting asymmetries in cerebral blood flow. Finally, a series of resting PET metabolism studies were performed to further test the laterality hypothesis. These studies found evidence of left-hemispheric overactivation in patients with severe versus mild clinical symptoms (Gur et al., 1987a) and that higher right- versus left-hemispheric metabolism was correlated with clinical improvement (Gur et al., 1987b). These studies also found evidence of a steeper subcortical-to-cortical gradient in schizophrenia, motivating a search for abnormalities in temporal and limbic brain regions.

In addition to helping explain analytic and language-processing deficits, a theory of left temporal lobe and hippocampal impairment could help account for clinical symptoms such hallucinations and delusions (Frith & Done, 1988) and for neuropsychological findings of differential impairments of verbal learning and memory (Saykin et al., 1991). Initial studies examined resting metabolism and blood flow and linked left temporal lobe hyperactivity with clinical symptoms. Increased activity in the left temporal lobe and underlying hippocampus and parahippocampal gyrus was associated with positive symptoms (Liddle et al., 1992), with auditory hallucinations (Anderson et al., 1991), and with overall symptom severity (DeLisi et al., 1989; Friston et al., 1992). In a resting glucose metabolism study using a high-resolution PET camera, Gur and colleagues (1995) found left-hemispheric overactivation of the midtemporal cortex in both first-episode and chronic patients with schizophrenia. This midtemporal activity also correlated with clinical features, including premorbid functioning and outcome. In a subsequent correlative study, Mozley and colleagues (1996) associated regional patterns of resting glucose metabolism with patient performance on a logical memory subtest of the Wechsler Memory Scale (WMS). Patients were divided between "good" and "poor" performers based on their recall scores, and regional glucose metabolism was contrasted between patient subgroups. The analysis revealed that patients who had worse memory performance also had higher left-hemispheric activation in inferior frontal, inferior temporal, midtemporal, and superior temporal brain regions. The study therefore provided a link between the left temporal overactivation model and memory performance in schizophrenia.

Evidence of resting abnormalities in temporal lobe metabolism and cerebral perfusion led to implementation of declarative memory (Squire, 1992) activation paradigms. The first memory activation study was performed by Wood and Flowers (1990). These investigators measured cerebral blood flow with [133]Xenon clearance in 24 healthy controls, 18 patients with schizophrenia, 22 patients with bipolar disorder, and 13 unipolar depressed subjects during two repeated word recognition memory tasks. Although hypofrontality occurred during both recognition tasks, it was not specific to diagnostic group and was associated with measures of anxiety, leading to the conclusion that hypofrontality was a state rather than trait variable. However, focal suppression of left-hemispheric perisylvian activation (in Broca's and Wernicke's areas) during task performance was specific to patients with schizophrenia, leading the investigators to conclude that the perisylvian finding represented a unique language-related focal deficit in schizophrenia. A subsequent [133]Xenon clearance study examined cerebral blood flow during both word and face recognition memory tasks (Gur et al., 1994). A sample of 18 unmedicated patients with schizophrenia and 18 demographically matched controls were examined. As in a previous study of healthy volunteers (Gur et al., 1993), controls showed appropriate laterality effects (left > right for verbal, and right > left for facial) restricted to the midtemporal cortex. The patients produced a much more diffuse pattern of findings. The patients had globally increased left-hemispheric cerebral blood flow changes and produced laterality effects in a distributed set of regions, including frontal pole, anterior temporal, and occipitotemporal regions. These abnormalities were related to poorer memory performance and greater symptom severity. Although the focus of the study was on the midtemporal lobe, frontal lobe abnormalities were also noted, making it increasingly problematic to discuss either frontal or temporal lobe models in isolation.

Distributed Network Model of Frontotemporal Dysfunction

Friston and colleagues (1992) were one of the first groups to suggest that frontal and temporal lobe findings may be related to an underlying frontotemporal network dysfunction in schizophrenia. Growing awareness of the reciprocal interconnectivity of prefrontal regions with the hippocampus (Goldman-Rakic et al., 1984) and the rest of the brain (Fuster, 1980; Nauta, 1971) made it increasingly difficult to isolate frontal and temporal lobe systems and argue that schizophrenia is either a focal frontal lobe or focal temporal lobe disorder. Evidence that impairment on frontal lobe tasks such as the WCST can result from temporal lobe pathology (Weinberger et al., 1992) provided further support for the conclusion that schizophrenia is best conceptualized as a disruption in the integration of widely distributed brain networks, rather than as a disorder of a single brain region (Andreasen et al., 1996).

In an effort to directly test this frontotemporal model, Ragland and colleagues developed the Paired Associate Recognition Test (PART; Ragland et al., 1995) as a measure of declarative memory, using WCST stimuli and response procedures to ensure compatibility of nonspecific aspects of perceptual and motor activation. The PART requires participants to learn and to retrieve paired associates (PAs), composed of two WCST cards, following a 2-min delay. During retrieval, participants indicate which of four WCST key cards were paired with previous targets. A normative study showed that the PART is a reliable and valid measure of declarative memory that correlates with Wechsler Memory Scale visual recall but does not correlate with WCST performance (Ragland et al., 1995). A neuropsychological study of 30 patients with schizophrenia and 30 healthy controls also found that patients were equally impaired on both tasks, and that impairment was not due to medication effects (Ragland et al., 1996). When the WCST and PART were administered during a PET study of cerebral blood flow in healthy volunteers (Ragland et al., 1997), there was bilateral activation over resting baseline in inferior frontal and occipitotemporal regions for both tasks, with more consistent dorsolateral–prefrontal activation for the WCST than for the PART. In addition, the best performers on the WCST activated only dorsolateral–prefrontal and inferior frontal regions, whereas the top PART performers activated only the occipitotemporal region. These combined results suggested the operation of an integrated frontotemporal network subserving both executive and declarative memory function that became more focal as performance increased. The next question was how the functioning of this network would be impacted by schizophrenia.

In a second PET cerebral blood flow study (Ragland et al., 1998) the PART and WCST were administered to 15 patients with schizophrenia and 15 healthy controls. As previously, controls activated inferior frontal, occipitotemporal, and temporal pole regions for both tasks, with better performance related to prefrontal activation during the WCST and occipitotemporal activation during the PART. In contrast, patients failed to activate any of these hypothesized regions during the WCST and produced dorsolateral prefrontal activation during the PART. Patients did not show any regional correlations with PART performance. Better patient performance on the WCST correlated with parahippocampal activation. These results provided evidence of both frontal and temporal lobe dysfunction and suggested that schizophrenia involves a breakdown in the integration of a distributed frontotemporal network. The finding that patients activated anterior (dorsolateral prefrontal) rather than posterior regions on the PART and showed performance correlations with temporal-limbic (parahippocampal gyrus) rather than anterior regions on the WCST also lent support to the hypothesis that schizophrenia

may produce a reversal in the normal reciprocal relationship between prefrontal and temporal-limbic brain regions (Volkow et al., 1986).

The notion that schizophrenia may cause a reversal in the normal inverse
relationship (Berman et al., 1986) between prefrontal and temporal-limbic
activity was also raised in one of the first fMRI studies of schizophrenia by
Yurgelun-Todd and colleagues (1996). In this verbal fluency study subjects
alternated between control (number counting) and phonemic fluency (generating words beginning with letter F, S, R, or T) blocks. Changes in the fMRI signal between the fluency and control conditions were measured in left
dorsolateral prefrontal and superior temporal regions of interest. Group comparisons revealed that controls showed greater prefrontal activation, whereas
patients had greater activation in the temporal lobe. Similar reversals (i.e.,
increased prefrontal and decreased temporal-limbic, or decreased prefrontal
and increased temporal-limbic activity) were documented in a series of more
recent fMRI studies of verbal learning and memory (see Weiss & Heckers,
2001, and Heckers, 2001, for reviews). These reversals led Weinberger (1987)
to suggest that mesocortical dopaminergic underactivity of the dorsolateral
prefrontal cortex may produce disinhibition of dopaminergic activity in
subcortical regions, leading to temporal-limbic overactivation.

Although this "top-down" model of reduced prefrontal inhibition of
temporal-limbic brain regions fits well with studies showing increased
temporal-limbic and decreased prefrontal activation, it is less successful at
explaining the reverse pattern of increased prefrontal and decreased hippocampal activation (e.g., Heckers et al., 1998; Weiss et al., 2003). In a recent
levels-of-processing word encoding and retrieval study (Ragland et al., 2005),
investigators found that prefrontal activation during word encoding could be
restored in patients with schizophrenia by providing them with semantic processing strategies (Plate 12.1). However, even when prefrontal activity was
restored, patients, continued to show evidence of temporal-limbic hyperactivity (Plate 12.2). These results suggest that when strategic memory demands
are reduced by providing patients with organizational strategies, they can successfully engage in semantic processing and activate their left prefrontal cortex. This contrasts with previous "hypofrontality" findings that were obtained
when patients had to generate strategies (e.g., during the WCST). However,
once the left prefrontal cortex is engaged, it appears that patients have difficulty modulating brain function and have a much less focal and task-specific
pattern of activity, with significant temporal-limbic overactivation.

This co-occurrence of prefrontal and temporal-limbic abnormalities
across declarative memory, working memory (see Manoach, 2003, for review), and verbal fluency studies of schizophrenia clearly points to a problem
in intracortical functional connectivity (Frith et al., 1995; Friston et al., 1992)
rather than an isolated dysfunction of either the frontal or temporal lobe systems. However, the exact direction and mechanism of this network dysfunction have yet to be established.

Recent Research and Future Directions

This chapter focused primarily on studies of resting and activated metabolism and blood flow using [133]Xenon clearance and PET [15]O blood flow methods, because these somewhat older technologies formed the foundation of the leading pathophysiology models of schizophrenia. Since the middle of the 1990s there has been an exponential growth of functional imaging research with the widespread adoption of BOLD fMRI. fMRI is more available, less expensive and invasive than traditional radiological methods, and has the advantage of improved temporal and somewhat improved spatial resolution. fMRI methods also permit event-related studies that facilitate parametric designs that can provide a finer-grained analysis of task difficulty and performance effects. These fMRI studies have helped to better characterize the specific components of disrupted frontotemporal functioning in schizophrenia. For example, numerous studies of working memory and attentional processing (see Carter et al., 1999, for review) have established that the anterior cingulate plays an important role, as well as the prefrontal and hippocampal regions previously discussed. Although this more recent fMRI research has helped to refine the frontotemporal hypothesis, it has not led to widespread adoption of any new models of pathophysiology in schizophrenia. However, there is a growing literature on early information processing in schizophrenia that deserves comment, as it could lead to changes in how functional imaging studies are performed and may lead to a change in how brain dysfunction in schizophrenia is conceptualized.

What the previously reviewed research studies have in common is that most studies utilized neurobehavioral probes that tap higher-level cognitive abilities requiring frontal integration of a broad network of cortical and subcortical regions. It is therefore not surprising that results have converged on a model of impaired intracortical and cortical–subcortical frontotemporal connectivity. However, there is a smaller body of electrophysiology literature that is beginning to examine early information processing to determine whether functional deficits can be identified in the brains of individuals with schizophrenia during basic perceptual and sensory processing prior to engagement of higher-level executive control mechanisms. Such studies promise to establish whether or not there may be a "bottom-up" problem in information processing that could help explain the "top-down" deficits that have occupied center stage in the functional neuroimaging research on schizophrenia.

For example, a visual evoked potential study by Butler and colleagues (2001) examined components of early sensory visual processing to determine if they could explain higher-level problems in visual perception. The authors found that the ratio of signal-to-noise for visual evoked potentials was lower in patients for basic sensory visual tasks, which biased processing toward magnocellular rather than parvocellular visual pathways. These problems in early visual processing were viewed as consistent with later problems in eye movement and visual identification during backward masking. In another EEG study, Winterer and colleagues (2000) examined the signal-to-noise characteristics of auditory evoked potentials and found that reduced signal-to-noise in patients' responses to auditory stimuli may be due to an increase in noise following stimulus presentation, rather than a signaling failure in auditory cortex activation. If there is a fundamental problem in early information processing that reduces the signal-to-noise characteristics of neural responses to visual and auditory stimuli, it is possible that the pathophysiology of schizophrenia is even less focal and more widespread than previous theories have led us to believe. Given this framework, it may be that the reason that the functional imaging literature has converged on a frontotemporal model is that most studies have utilized neurobehavioral probes requiring frontotemporal integration. It will therefore be important in future imaging studies to integrate more basic sensory paradigms to test the specificity of the frontotemporal model.

REFERENCES

Anderson, J., Fawdry, R., Gordon, E., et al. (1991). SPECT asymmetry of left temporal lobe in hallucinated schizophrenics. *Biological Psychiatry, 29,* 291.

Andreasen, N. C., O'Leary, D. S., Cizadlo, T., et al. (1996). Schizophrenia and cognitive dysmetria: A positron-emission tomography study of dysfunctional prefrontal–thalamic–cerebellar circuitry. *Proceedings of the National Academy of Sciences of the United States of America, 93,* 9985–9990.

Andreasen, N. C., Rezai, K., Alliger, R., et al. (1992). Hypofrontality in neuroleptic-naïve patients and in patients with chronic schizophrenia. *Archives of General Psychiatry, 49,* 943–958.

Berg, E. A. (1948). A simple, objective technique for measuring flexibility in thinking. *Journal of General Psychology, 39,* 15–22.

Berman, K. F., Illowsky, B. P., & Weinberger, D. R. (1988). Physiological dysfunction of dorsolateral prefrontal cortex in schizophrenia: IV. Further evidence for regional and behavioral specificity. *Archives of General Psychiatry, 45,* 616–622.

Berman, K. F., Torrey, E. F., Daniel, D. G., et al. (1992). Regional cerebral blood flow in monozygotic twins discordant and concordant for schizophrenia. *Archives of General Psychiatry, 49,* 927–934.

Berman, K. F., Zec, R. F., & Weinberger, D. R. (1986). Physiologic dysfunction of dorsolateral prefrontal cortex in schizophrenia: II. Role of neuroleptic treatment, attention, and mental effort. *Archives of General Psychiatry, 43,* 126–135.

Blanchard, J. J., & Neale, J. M. (1994). The neuropsychological signature of schizophrenia: Generalized or differential deficit? *American Journal of Psychiatry, 151,* 40–48.

Buchsbaum, M. S., Ingvar, D. H., Kessler, R., et al. (1982). Cerebral glucography with positron tomography: Use in normal subjects and in patients with schizophrenia. *Archives of General Psychiatry, 39,* 251–259.

Butler, P. D., Schechter, I., Zemon, V., et al. (2001). Dysfunction of early-stage visual processing in schizophrenia. *American Journal of Psychiatry, 158,* 1126–1133.

Carter, C. S., Botvinick, M. M., & Cohen, J. D. (1999). The contribution of the anterior cingulate cortex to executive processes in cognition. *Reviews in the Neurosciences, 10*, 49–57.

Catafau, A. M., Parellada, E., Lomena, F. J., et al. (1994). Prefrontal and temporal blood flow in schizophrenia: Resting and activation technetium-99m-HMPAO SPECT patterns in young neuroleptic-naïve patients with acute disease. *Journal of Nuclear Medicine, 35*, 935–941.

DeLisi, L. E., Buchsbaum, M. S., & Holcomb, H. H. (1989). Increased temporal lobe glucose use in chronic schizophrenic patients. *Biological Psychiatry, 25*, 835–851.

Ebmeier, K. P., Lawrie, S. M., Blackwood, D. H. R., et al. (1995). Hypofrontality revisited: A high resolution single photon emission computed tomography study in schizophrenia. *Journal of Neurology and Neurosurgery in Psychiatry, 58*, 452–456.

Frankle, W. G., & Laruelle, M. (2002). Neuroreceptor imaging in psychiatric disorders. *Annals of Nuclear Medicine, 16*, 437–446.

Franzen, G., & Ingvar, D. H. (1975). Absence of activation in frontal structures during psychological testing of chronic schizophrenics. *Journal of Neurology and Neurosurgery in Psychiatry, 38*, 1027–1032.

Friston, K. J., Liddle, P. F., Frith, C. D., et al. (1992). The left medial temporal region and schizophrenia. A PET study. *Brain, 115*, 367–382.

Frith, C. D., & Done, D. J. (1988). Towards a neuropsychology of schizophrenia. *British Journal of Psychiatry, 153*, 437–443.

Frith, C. D., Kapur, N., Friston, K. J., et al. (1995). Regional cerebral activity associated with the incidental processing of pseudo-words. *Human Brain Mapping, 3*, 153–160.

Fuster, J. M. (1999). Synopsis of function and dysfunction of the frontal lobe. *Acta Psychiatrica Scandinavia, 99*, 51–57.

Fuster, J. M. (1980). *The prefrontal cortex: Anatomy, physiology, and neuropsychology of the frontal lobe.* New York: Raven Press.

Goldberg, E. (1985). Akinesia, tardive dysmentia, and frontal lobe disorder in schizophrenia. *Schizophrenia Bulletin, 11*, 255–263.

Goldberg, T. E., Weinberger, D. R., Berman, K. F., et al. (1987). Further evidence for dementia of the prefrontal type in schizophrenia? A controlled study of teaching the Wisconsin Card Sorting Test. *Archives of General Psychiatry, 44*, 1008–1014.

Goldman-Rakic, P. S., Selemon, L. D., & Schwartz, M. L. (1984). Dual pathways connecting the dorsolateral prefrontal cortex with the hippocampal formation and parahippocampal cortex in the rhesus monkey. *Neuroscience, 12*, 719–743.

Grant, D. A., & Berg, E. A. (1948). A behavioral analysis of degree of reinforcement and ease of shifting to a new response in a Weigl-type card-sorting problem. *Journal of Experimental Psychology, 38*, 404–411.

Gur, R. C., Erwin, R. J., & Gur, R. E. (1992). Neurobehavioral probes for physiologic neuroimaging studies. *Archives of General Psychiatry, 49*, 409–414.

Gur, R. C., & Gur, R. E. (1995). Hypofrontality in schizophrenia: RIP. *Lancet, 345*, 1383–1384.

Gur, R. C., Jaggi, J. L., Ragland, J. D., et al. (1993). Effects of memory processing on regional brain activation: Cerebral blood flow in normal subjects. *International Journal of Neuroscience, 72*, 31–44.

Gur, R. E., Gur, R. C., Skolnick, B. E., et al. (1985). Brain function in psychiatric disorders: III. Regional cerebral blood flow in unmedicated schizophrenics. *Archives of General Psychiatry, 42,* 329–334.

Gur, R. E., Jaggi, J., Shtasel, D., et al. (1994). Cerebral blood flow in schizophrenia: Effects of memory processing on regional activation. *Biological Psychiatry, 35,* 3–15.

Gur, R. E., Mozley, P. D., Resnick, S. M., et al. (1995). Resting cerebral glucose metabolism in first-episode and previously treated patients with schizophrenia relates to clinical features. *Archives of General Psychiatry, 52,* 657–667.

Gur, R. E., Resnick, S. M., Alavi, A., et al. (1987a). Regional brain function in schizophrenia: I. A positron emission tomography study. *Archives of General Psychiatry, 44,* 119–125.

Gur, R. E., Resnick S. M., Gur, R. C., et al. (1987b). Regional brain function in schizophrenia: II. Repeated evaluation with positron emission tomography. *Archives of General Psychiatry, 44,*126–129.

Gur, R. E., Skolnick, B. E., Gur, R. C., et al. (1983). Brain function in psychiatric disorders: I. Regional cerebral blood flow in medicated schizophrenics. *Archives of General Psychiatry, 40,* 1250–1254.

Harrison, P. J., & Roberts, G. W. (Eds.). (2000). *The neuropathology of schizophrenia: Progress and interpretation.* New York: Oxford University Press.

Heckers, S. (2001). Neuroimaging studies of the hippocampus in schizophrenia. *Hippocampus, 11,* 520–528.

Heckers, S., Rauch, S. L., Goff, D., et al. (1998). Impaired recruitment of the hippocampus during conscious recollection in schizophrenia. *Nature Neuroscience, 1,* 318–323.

Ingvar, D. H., & Franzen, G. (1974). Distribution of cerebral activity in chronic schizophrenia. *Lancet, 2,* 1484–1486.

Keshavan, M. S. (1999). Development, disease and degeneration in schizophrenia: A unitary pathophysiological model. *Journal of Psychiatric Research, 33,* 513–521.

Lewis, S. W., Ford, R. A., Syed, G. M., et al. (1992). A controlled study of ^{99m}Tc-HMPAO single-photon emission imaging in chronic schizophrenia. *British Journal of Psychiatry, 160,* 179–186.

Liddle, P. F., Friston, K. J., Frith, C. D., et al. (1992). Patterns of cerebral blood flow in schizophrenia. *British Journal of Psychiatry, 158,* 340–345.

Light, G. A., & Braff, D. L. (1999). Human and animal studies of schizophrenia-related gating deficits. *Current Psychiatry Reports, 1,* 31–40.

Manoach, D. S. (2003). Prefrontal cortex dysfunction during working memory performance in schizophrenia: Reconciling discrepant findings. *Schizophrenia Research, 60,* 285–298.

Mathew, R. J., Wilson, W. H., Tant, S. R., et al. (1988). Abnormal resting regional cerebral blood flow patterns and their correlates in schizophrenia. *Archives of General Psychiatry, 45,* 542–549.

McCarley, R. W., Faux, S. F., Shenton, M. E., et al. (1991). Event-related potentials in schizophrenia: Their biological and clinical correlates and a new model of schizophrenic pathophysiology. *Schizophrenia Research, 4,* 209–231.

Mozley, L. H., Gur, R. C., Gur, R. E., et al. (1996). Relationships between verbal memory performance and the cerebral distribution of flurodeoxyglucose in patients with schizophrenia. *Biological Psychiatry, 40,* 443–451.

Nauta, W. J. H. (1971). The problem of the frontal lobe: A reinterpretation. *Journal of Psychiatry Research*, 8, 167–187.

Pearlson, G. D., & Marsh, L. (1999). Structural brain imaging in schizophrenia: A selective review. *Biological Psychiatry*, 46, 627–649.

Ragland, J. D., Censits, D. M., Gur, R. E., et al. (1996). Assessing declarative memory in schizophrenia using Wisconsin Card Sorting Test stimuli: The Paired Associate Recognition Test. *Psychiatry Research* 60, 135–145.

Ragland, J. D., Glahn, D. C., Gur, R. C., et al. (1997). PET regional cerebral blood flow change during working and declarative memory: Relationship with task performance. *Neuropsychology*, 11, 222–231.

Ragland, J. D., Gur, R. C., Deutsch, G. K., et al. (1995). Reliability and construct validity of the paired-associate recognition test: A test of declarative memory using Wisconsin Card Sorting stimuli. *Psychological Assessment*, 7, 25–32.

Ragland, J. D., Gur, R. C., Glahn, D. C., et al. (1998). Fronto-temporal cerebral blood flow change during executive and declarative memory tasks in schizophrenia: A positron emission tomography study. *Neuropsychology*, 12, 399–413.

Ragland, J. D., Gur, R. C., Valdez, J. N., et al. (2005). Levels-of-processing effect on frontotemporal function in schizophrenia during word encoding and recognition. *American Journal of Psychiatry*, 162, 1840–1848.

Saykin, A. J., Gur, R. C., Gur, R. E., et al. (1991). Neuropsychological function in schizophrenia: Selective impairment in memory and learning. *Archives of General Psychiatry*, 48, 618–624.

Shenton, M. E., Dickey, C. C., Frumin, M., et al. (2001). A review of MRI findings in schizophrenia. *Schizophrenia Research*, 49, 1–52.

Squire, L. R. (1992). Memory and the hippocampus: A synthesis from findings with rats, monkeys, and humans. *Psychiatry Review*, 99, 195–231.

Strub, R. L., & Black, F. W. (1985). Higher cognitive functions. In R. L. Strub & F. W. Black (Eds.), *The Mental Status Examination in neurology* (pp. 125–138). Philadelphia: Davis.

Trimble, M. R. (1990). Psychopathology of frontal lobe syndromes. *Seminars in Neurology*, 10, 287–294.

Vita, A., Giobbo, G. M., Dieci, M., et al. (1991). Frontal lobe dysfunction in schizophrenia: Evident from neuropsychological testing and brain imaging techniques. *Biological Psychiatry*, 29, 647S.

Volkow, N. D., Brodie, J. D., Wolf, A. P., et al. (1986). Brain organization in schizophrenia. *Journal of Cerebral Blood Flow and Metabolism*, 6, 441–446.

Volkow, N. D., Wolf, A. P., Van Gelder, P., et al. (1987). Phenomenological correlates of metabolic activity in 18 patients with chronic schizophrenia. *American Journal of Psychiatry*, 144, 151–158.

Weinberger, D. R. (1988). Schizophrenia and the frontal lobes. *Trends in Neuroscience*, 11, 367–370.

Weinberger, D. R. (1987). Implications of normal brain development for the pathogenesis of schizophrenia. *Archives of General Psychiatry*, 44, 660–669.

Weinberger, D. R., & Berman, K. F. (1996). Prefrontal function in schizophrenia: Confounds and controversies. *Philosophical Transactions: Biological Sciences*, 351, 1495–1503.

Weinberger, D. R., Berman, K. F., & Daniel, D. G. (1991). Prefrontal cortex dysfunction in schizophrenia. In H. S. Levin, H. M. Eisenberg, & A. L. Benton (Eds.),

Frontal lobe function and dysfunction (pp. 275–287). New York: Oxford University Press.

Weinberger, D. R., Berman, K. F., & Illowsky, B. P. (1988). Physiological dysfunction of dorsolateral prefrontal cortex in schizophrenia: III. A new cohort and evidence from a monoaminergic mechanism. *Archives of General Psychiatry, 45*, 609–615.

Weinberger, D. R., Berman, K. F., Suddath, R., et al. (1992). Evidence of dysfunction of a prefrontal–limbic network in schizophrenia: A magnetic resonance imaging and rCBF flow study of discordant monozygotic twins. *American Journal of Psychiatry, 7*, 890–897.

Weinberger, D. R., Berman, K. F., & Zec, R. F. (1986). Physiological dysfunction of dorsolateral prefrontal cortex in schizophrenia: I. Regional cerebral blood flow (rCBF) evidence. *Archives of General Psychiatry, 43*, 114–125.

Weiss, A. P., & Heckers, S. (2001). Neuroimaging of declarative memory in schizophrenia. *Scandinavian Journal of Psychology, 42*, 239–250.

Weiss, A. P., Schacter, D. L., Goff, D. C., et al. (2003). Impaired hippocampal recruitment during normal modulation of memory performance in schizophrenia. *Biological Psychiatry, 53*, 48–55.

Winterer, G., Ziller, M., Dorn, H., et al. (2000). Schizophrenia: Reduced signal-to-noise ratio and impaired phase-locking during information processing. *Clinical Neurophysiology, 111*, 837–849.

Wood, F. B., & Flowers, L. (1990). Hypofrontal vs. hypo-sylvian blood flow in schizophrenia. *Schizophrenia Bulletin, 16*, 413–424.

Yurgelun-Todd, D. A., Waternaux, C. M, Bruce, B. C., et al. (1996). Functional magnetic resonance imaging of schizophrenic patients and comparison subjects during word production. *American Journal of Psychiatry, 153*, 200–205.

CHAPTER 13

Testing Hypotheses
of Age-Related Performance Changes
Using Functional Magnetic Resonance Imaging

Bart Rypma

Since its inception, cognitive aging research has indicated that increasing age is associated with lower performance on a broad range of cognitive tasks (e.g., Foster & Taylor, 1920; Jones & Conrad, 1933). These changes are mediated by deterioration of the physiological mechanisms that give rise to information-processing capabilities. Indeed, the entire stream of information processing, from peripheral perceptual processes to central cognitive processes, appears to undergo profound age-related change. In this chapter, I present evidence to support the notion that the cognitive consequence of age-associated changes to peripheral and central nervous system structures is a reduction in the efficiency of information processing.

Structural Changes in the Periphery
and Their Relations to Cognitive Aging

Perceptually, auditory and visual deficits increase with age. Hearing loss is among the most prevalent and disabling symptoms that older adults encounter. Changes in the human cochlear structure lead to age-related hearing impairment. Focal inner hair cell loss in the basilar membrane leads to diminution of sensitivity to higher frequencies, and diffuse outer hair cell loss in the basilar membrane leads to reduced processing of low frequencies. In addition, age-related changes to auditory brainstem lead to more profound changes in frequency discrimination, temporal discrimination, localization, and speech perception (e.g., Willot, 1991; Hellstrom & Schmeidt, 1996; Schneider, 1997; Schneider & Pichora-Fuller, 2000).

The human visual system also exhibits age-related changes that lead to information-processing difficulties. Changes to the cornea, iris, lens, and vitreous and aqueous humors adversely affect the quality of the image projected to the retina (e.g., Michaels, 1993). These structural changes lead to increases in retinal blurring, light scatter that decreases retinal contrast (Sloane et al., 1988), and reductions in contrast sensitivity, which have been associated with age-related changes in object recognition performance (Owsley & Sloane, 1987).

Second- and third-order brain regions in the visual pathway appear to be less affected by aging. Structural studies of lateral geniculate nucleus (LGN) suggest age-equivalent neuron density and minimal changes in size, and functional studies suggest minimal age changes in LGN-cell response properties (Ahmad & Spear, 1993; Spear, 1993; Spear et al., 1994). The striate cortex similarly undergoes minimal age-related structural changes in neuron density or cellular response properties (Haug et al., 1984; Vincent et al., 1989). The apparent sparing of these higher-order visual structures implicates reduced functions in the visual periphery as a causal factor in age-related performance changes.

A number of investigators have explored the effects of peripheral function changes on age-related changes in cognitive performance. In one study, for instance, Salthouse and colleagues (1998) demonstrated that changes in visual acuity accounted for about one-half of the age-related variance in cognitive measures. Similarly, about one-third of age-related variance in Raven Advanced Progressive Matrices performance has been shown to be related to visual acuity deficits. Furthermore, results from several large-scale studies have supported the notion that age-related changes in sensory acuity are intimately related to changes in higher cognitive functions. In a study of 516 70- to 103-yr-olds, threshold measures of visual and auditory acuity accounted for 93% of the age-related variance in intellectual functioning, as measured by a comprehensive battery of tests (Lindenberger & Baltes, 1994). Subsequent work has tied changes in visual acuity to a fundamental index of cognitive efficiency, processing speed (Salthouse et al., 1996).

Central Structural Changes and Their Relations to Cognitive Aging

In addition to peripheral visual structures, central brain regions undergo progressive age-related tissue loss. This loss is marked by neocortical atrophy, widening sulci, and ventricular dilation. The progressive tissue volume decrease culminates in brain mass shrinkage of as much as 10% by 80 years of age (Minckler & Boyd, 1968; Wisniewski & Terry, 1976). Tissue loss is not evenly distributed across the cortex. Disproportionate tissue decline has been observed in the prefrontal cortex, as compared with other structures, in both humans and other primates (e.g., Corsellis, 1976; Haug & Eggers, 1991; Raz, 2000; Raz et al., 1997).

There has been considerable controversy concerning the relative contributions of grey and white brain matter to such deterioration. Grey matter is composed of neural cell bodies in the cortex and in subcortical structures. White matter is composed of tightly packed axons that connect neurons to each other in the cortex and that connect cortical neurons to the periphery. Studies in both humans and nonhuman primates suggest a primary role for white matter deterioration in age-related brain changes, possibly especially in the prefrontal cortex (Madden et al., 2004; Peters, 2002; Peters & Sethares, 2002, 2004). Further, age-related white matter loss without axonal loss suggests that the observed changes may be related specifically to decreases in nonneural cells, particularly myelinating oligodendroglia (Franklin et al., 2002; Sim et al., 2002; Tang et al., 1997). These changes could lead to disruptions of transcortical information flow and suggest a plausible neural mechanism for processing-efficiency models of age-related cognitive slowing.

Other research has suggested that age-related brain volume changes may result from grey matter degeneration. Early brain aging hypotheses maintained that cortical atrophy resulted from widespread neuron loss (e.g., Brody, 1955) in adulthood and senescence (Kemper, 2002; Turlejski & Djavadian, 2002). Recent studies in humans using voxel-based morphometric (VBM) analysis are in agreement with these early hypotheses in suggesting that age-related changes result more from *grey* matter tissue loss, than white matter loss, although evidence for white matter change is sometimes also observed in these studies. Tisserand and colleagues (2002) reported a significant age-associated decline in grey matter volume with VBM, but they did not evaluate white matter and analyzed only anterior regions. Good and colleagues (2001) examined grey matter, white matter, and cerebrospinal fluid (CSF) volumes in 465 adults ranging in age from 18 to 79 years. They found linear age-related declines in grey matter volume concentrated in several regions. These regions included the parietal, anterior cingulate, and middle frontal gyri corresponding to the dorsal prefrontal cortex (PFC). Other aging studies have revealed selective grey matter decline in the absence of white matter decline (Taki et al., 2004; Tisserand et al., 2004). Resnick et al. (2000) longitudinally examined grey and white matter changes in older adults (59–85 years old). Total grey and white matter volume loss was approximately 5.4 cm^3 and 2.4 cm^3, respectively. The greatest changes were observed in frontal and parietal lobes (see also Resnick et al., 2003).

Precise relationships between age-related anatomical changes and age-related cognitive decline are not yet well understood. On one hand, anatomical, histological, neurochemical, and neuroimaging data implicate principally white matter change with relative sparing of grey matter. On the other hand, VBM studies implicate either mainly grey matter or both grey and white matter changes. Thus, the weight of evidence supports the notion that age-related brain volume loss is predominantly due to white matter changes. Future research will be required to disentangle the differences between these studies and ascertain the effects of different measurement techniques on these discrepant results.

Although the evidence reviewed above indicates that many brain regions suffer deleterious aging effects, PFC may be especially susceptible to such effects. Histological studies have shown the greatest age-related decrements in cortical volume in PFC as compared with other brain regions (Haug & Eggers, 1991). PET studies in older subjects have found reduced metabolism within PFC (e.g., Kuhl et al, 1982). Neuropsychological tests show that older adults are more impaired on tasks that depend on PFC function than on those depending on other brain regions (West, 1996). In addition, MRI studies have found that age-related structural decline in PFC correlates with executive task impairment (Raz et al., 1997, 1998; Raz, 2000; West, 1996). Together, these results suggest that those cognitive processes that depend on PFC function are especially susceptible to deleterious aging effects.

One process known to depend on PFC function is working memory (WM). WM can be defined as the cognitive apparatus that allows individuals to temporarily maintain and manipulate information in mind. Because WM is considered fundamental to many higher cognitive processes (e.g., reasoning, text comprehension, problem solving), findings of age-related WM changes may plausibly explain the performance changes observed across a broad array of such higher cognitive tasks.

There are several theoretical conceptions of WM, but one prominent theory holds that it can be divided into separate components. "Slave system" buffers mediate the short-term retention of small amounts of information. An additional "supervisory attentional system," or "central executive," controls allocation of attention to the slave system buffers (Baddeley, 1986; Norman & Shallice, 1980; Baddley & Hitch, 1974). Neuropsychological studies in humans and unit-recording studies in monkeys have indicated an intimate connection between prefrontal cortex function and WM performance (e.g., Funahashi et al., 1989; Fuster & Alexander, 1971; Goldman-Rakic, 1987; Goldman-Rakic & Friedman, 1991; Kubota & Niki, 1971). Single-cell recordings of monkey brains have shown persistent activity in dorsolateral PFC cells during the delay period of a delayed-match-to-sample task. Moreover, monkeys with principal sulcus lesions show location-specific deficits in delayed-response performance (Goldman-Rakic & Friedman, 1991).

Age-Related Behavioral Changes in WM

Evidence from behavioral research with animals and humans indicates declines in WM with advancing age. For example, behavioral studies with older monkeys show performance deficits, as compared with their younger counterparts, on delayed-response WM tasks (e.g., Bachevalier et al., 1991; Bartus et al., 1979; Presty et al., 1987). The observation of these declines is considered critical to an understanding of the widespread cognitive changes that accompany human aging, because much evidence from a variety of research domains suggests that WM function is central to many human cognitive functions (Baddeley, 1986; Norman & Shallice, 1980).

Like older monkeys, older humans show behavioral deficits in WM. Age-related performance differences are often observed in delayed-response WM tasks. Moreover, greater performance declines are observed with increasing delay intervals (e.g., Craik, 1977; Nielsen-Bohlman & Knight, 1995; Poon & Fozard, 1980; Smith, 1975). The amount of information that must be held in mind (i.e., memory load) can also exacerbate age-related differences in WM performance. A number of studies examining the effects of varying memory loads on delayed-response task performance have shown greater age differences with higher than with lower memory loads (Anders et al., 1972; Anders & Fozard, 1973; Eriksen et al., 1973; Marsh, 1975). Anders et al. (1972), for instance, examined age-differential performance when subjects had to remember various numbers of digits across an unfilled delay interval. They observed increasing age differences in performance with increasing memory load, indicating faster memory retrieval rates in younger than in older participants.

The factors that mediate age-differential or age-equivalent WM performance are not yet clearly understood. For example, other studies using designs similar to those employed by Anders et al. (1972) did not observe age differences in memory retrieval rate (e.g., Boaz & Denney, 1993; Kirsner, 1972). Such variance may be related to task factors that vary between studies. Indeed, as compared with memory tasks that involve delays of at least several seconds, those with minimal delays often show minimal age-related performance differences. One such task is digit span, in which participants recall a digit string immediately following presentation. Performance on this task often appears unaffected by healthy aging (Botwinick & Storandt, 1974; Bromley, 1958; Craik, 1968; Drachman & Leavitt, 1972; Friedman, 1974; Gilbert, 1941; Gilbert & Levee, 1971; Kriauciunas, 1968; Taub, 1973).

The observation of greater age differences with increases in delay time or memory load suggests that different components of WM may be differentially susceptible to the deleterious effects of advancing age. It may be that WM slave systems, which allow maintenance of lower memory loads at shorter intervals, are relatively unaffected by aging. However, executive WM mechanisms, those believed to facilitate maintenance of higher memory loads over long delay intervals, may be differentially affected by advancing age.

Age-Related Changes in Neural Activity: Data and Theories

The advent of functional neuroimaging techniques has permitted the testing of hypotheses regarding age-related brain changes, developed through behavioral comparisons of younger and older adults, and older normal adults with older patients with neurological deficits (such as those with Alzheimer's or Parkinson's disease or focal brain injury; e.g., Gabrieli, 1991, 1996). These hypotheses may now be further tested and extended by observation of the intact human brain (Prull et al., 2000; Raz, 2000; Rypma & Gabrieli, 2000).

Patterns of neural activity do appear to change with age. Regions of increased activity in older adults, relative to younger adults, have been observed in a number of studies using positron emission tomography (PET) and functional magnetic resonance imaging (fMRI) (e.g., Cabeza et al. 1997; Grady et al., 1992; Madden et al., 1999; Park, 2002; Park et al., 2002; Reuter-Lorenz et al., 2000; Rypma et al., 2001). The observation of age-related activation increases have led to the proposal of several hypotheses of how neural activity increases are related to age-related behavioral changes.

"Dedifferentiation" hypotheses suggest that the increased activation observed in older adults reflects age-related neural deterioration. Dedifferentiation hypotheses concerning brain–behavior relationships arose from the proposal that ability structures differentiate during development, are maintained in adulthood, and "dedifferentiate" in advanced age (Reinert, 1970). Several studies have shown support for the dedifferentiation hypothesis in the form of age-related increases in intercorrelations among basic abilities measures (e.g., Babcock et al., 1997; Baltes et al., 1980), but strong behavioral support, in the form of reduced numbers of factors for old, as compared with young subjects, is lacking (Hertzog, 1985).

Some researchers have suggested that the age-related activation increases observed in neuroimaging studies reflect the physiological deterioration that underlies dedifferentiation (e.g., Park et al., 2004; Grady et al., 1992, 1994). In one study for instance, Grady and her colleagues (1992, 1994) showed an age-related reduction in the dorsoventral segregation of parietal and temporal activity during performance of spatial (i.e., dot-location matching) and object-based (i.e., face discrimination) tasks. Similarly, Park and her colleagues (2004) observed that in voxels selected for their unique activation to different categories (faces, houses, and chairs), older adults showed less distinctive activity between the categories than younger adults.

Dedifferentiation interpretations of age-related changes in neural activity are, interestingly, consistent, with increased intercorrelations among basic abilities measures. However, they remain less than entirely compelling for at least two reasons. First, they do not account for all neuroimaging results. That is, when one looks across studies, a relatively complex relationship between neural activity and age emerges (see below). Second, the extent to which age-related increases in neural activity are related to dedifferentiation of basic abilities remains to be explicitly tested because, to date, no studies of neural dedifferentiation have linked the age-related neural changes they have observed to age-related behavioral changes.

Other theories have focused on observations of activation increases across cerebral hemispheres or "hemispheric-asymmetry reduction in older adults" (HAROLD; Cabeza, 2002). This phenomenon has been interpreted as reflecting compensation mechanisms that account for neural deterioration. Thus, "compensation" hypotheses suggest that the increased activation observed in older adults reflects age-related acceleration of neural activity in the service of correcting for neural or cognitive deterioration. One form of this hypothesis may be referred to as a "brain compensation" hypothesis. In this view, the older brain "compensates" for affected regions with presumably less affected regions that, in a sense, "take over" the functions of the affected regions. Support for the hypothesis that relatively intact regions can assume the functions of regions that suffer from deterioration or trauma comes from studies showing functional plasticity following traumatic injury (Finger et al., 2003; Buckner et al., 1996). The observation that high-demand tasks involve brain regions that do not appear to be active in low-demand forms of these tasks also supports compensation hypotheses (e.g., Awh et al., 1996; Manoach et al., 1997; Rypma & D'Esposito, 1999, 2000; Rypma et al., 1999).

Problems with age-related compensation hypotheses arise from observations that activation increases and decreases do not appear to be systematically related. That is, age-related activation increases are not consistently accompanied by decreases in those regions activated in younger adults. More generally, activation decreases are not consistently accompanied by increases in other regions. Thus, although brain compensation is advanced as a general principle to explain age-related differences in neural activity, the data do not support a specific mechanism by which such a process may occur.

Another form of compensation hypothesis with clearer behavioral implications may be referred to as "cognitive compensation." In this view, older adults cognitively "compensate" for affected functions by using strategies that are different from those they used as young adults. This strategic shift presumably accommodates age-related changes to the "wetware" platform that yields the "young" strategies untenable.

Observations of increasing age-related performance differences with memory load increases and age-related activation differences with increases in memory load in the dorsal PFC could reflect differences in the susceptibility of slave system WM components and executive components to the deleterious effects of age. The notion that rehearsal mechanisms are engaged by low memory-demand tasks, and that additional memory mechanisms are engaged by high memory demands to compress or "chunk" to-be-maintained information, has been supported in a number of studies of short-term memory capacity (e.g., Baddeley & Hitch, 1974; Glanzer & Razel, 1974; Waugh & Norman, 1965). These behavioral results, coupled with findings of load-related increases in dorsal PFC (e.g., Rypma et al., 1999; Rypma & D'Esposito 1999, 2001) suggest (1) that activation increases in this region reflect cognitive strategy changes aimed at accommodation of supracapacity memory demand (i.e., recruitment of executive processes) and (2) that the age-related changes in this region reflect age-related differences in the cognitive strategies employed by younger and older adults under conditions of supracapacity memory demand.

Indeed, the observation of age-related increases in other PFC regions in the Rypma et al. (1999) study further suggests that this difference reflects age-related strategy differences (cf. Cabeza, 2002; Grady et al., 1995, 2003).

Problems with these hypotheses arise from observations that debriefing protocols and analyses of errors show minimal evidence for age-related strategy differences. In addition, age-related activation increases have not been consistently linked to performance improvements, a prediction that the "cognitive compensation" hypothesis would seem to predict. Reuter-Lorenz (2001) reviewed studies that show age-related increases in activity that have been accompanied by age-equivalent performance in some cases (Cabeza et al., 1997), and age-differential performances in others (Reuter-Lorenz et al., 2000, 2001). She and her colleagues (Jonides et al., 2000) have observed still a third relationship between performance and neural activity, age-related reductions in PET activation associated with reduced cognitive performance in elderly relative to young persons. Finally, in tasks that restrict the available strategies, age-related activation differences are still observed (for instance, by limiting the task to simple visual search; e.g., McIntosh et al., 1999; Eldreth et al., 2004).

Age-Related Brain–Behavior Changes: An Individual-Differences Approach

The literature reviewed above suggests that, although they are intuitively appealing, dedifferentiation and compensation hypotheses may not account well for the observed patterns of age-related changes in neural activity. Moreover, there is little evidence to suggest that they provide any insight regarding age-related performance changes. One feature of these hypotheses is that most of the evidence used to support them is based on mean or median observations of age-related performance changes in neural activity. Better understanding of age changes in complex brain–behavior relationships may be gained by more closely examining the relationship between neural activity and performance at the level of individual subjects. That is, understanding the neural factors that underlie age-related changes in performance may best be approached by the study of individual differences in brain–behavior relationships. Support for this notion comes from fMRI studies that use event-related methods. Event-related methodology has the advantage of permitting analyses that emphasize relationships between individual subjects' performance and their neural activity (Rypma & D'Esposito, 2001).

In an event-related study, Rypma and D'Esposito (2000) sought to determine possible sources of age-related differences in activation by using an event-related fMRI methodology in which age differences in activation could be isolated to the encoding, maintenance, and retrieval portions of a delayed-response item recognition task. Their results suggest that the age-related activation differences in dorsal PFC were isolated to memory retrieval. In their experiments, subjects were required to (1) encode either two or six letters, (2) maintain them over an unfilled delay interval, and (3) determine whether a single letter was or was not part of the memory set. The results of their studies indicated age-equivalent load-dependent effects in the encoding and delay periods of the task. In the retrieval period, however, large and significant differences in PFC activation were observed only in dorsal regions. These results indicated that PFC mechanisms related to encoding and maintenance of WM may be relatively robust to the deleterious effects of age. Those PFC mechanisms that mediate WM executive processes related to memory retrieval, however, may suffer in the aging process.

In addition to these region- and task-period-dependent age-related effects, Rypma and D'Esposito (1999) noticed that there was a considerable role for subject factors in explaining the variability of fMRI data. When they tested the relationship between subjects' performance and PFC activation in all task periods and PFC regions, they observed that individual subjects' reaction times accounted for most of the variability in fMRI data only in dorsal PFC regions and only during the response period. Specifically, for younger subjects, response period activation showed a significant positive correlation between individual subjects' reaction times (RT) and dorsal PFC cortical activity, which accounted for 71% of the variance. In contrast, for older subjects, response period activation showed a significant negative correlation between individual subjects' RT and dorsal PFC activation, which accounted for 72% of the variance.

These results suggest an alternative to the notion that age-related activation changes reflect some form of dedifferentiation or compensation. One possibility suggested by these data is that age-related activation increases are related to differences in the efficiency of transmission mechanisms required for the implementation of cognitive processes. Thus, decreased speed of information processing among younger adults may be related to relative increases in activation, but to decreases in activation among older adults. One model that could account for such a pattern of activation–performance relationships is based on findings of overall age-related reductions in baseline levels of activation in humans (e.g., De Santi et al., 1995; Eberling et al,. 1995; Moeller et al., 1996; Rypma & D'Esposito, 2000). For instance, Moeller and his colleagues (1996) examined age-related changes in "metabolic topography." In a sample of 130 adults ranging in age from 21 to 90 yr, they observed relative frontal hypometabolism in the brains of older, as compared with younger, adults. Such overall activation reductions could alter the relationship between neural activation and response probability. This relationship is known to be sigmoid in nature; middle ranges of neural activation result in optimal performance, and increases above or below this optimal range result in performance-level decrements (i.e., a shift in the bias parameter of the sigmoid function; Kimberg et al., 1997: Rypma & D'Esposito, 2000; Servan-Schreiber et al., 1990).

In summary, findings of age-differential PFC activation patterns, and age-differential functions relating PFC activation levels to performance, suggest two possible hypotheses to explain age-related increases in neural activity during WM performance. The first hypothesis is that the age-related differences in patterns of PFC activation reflect differences in the cognitive strategies employed by younger and older adults. The second hypothesis is that age-related differences in patterns of PFC activation reflect changes in the neural integrity of direct-processing links between nodes that must make contact for WM processing to occur. Such changes lead to age-related differences in the optimal neural activation level required for optimal task performance.

To date, no studies have attempted to directly test these competing hypotheses concerning age-related changes in neural activity. In one study, my colleagues and I (Rypma et al., 2005) sought to test these hypotheses with the same set of subjects performing a single task during fMRI scanning. We tested the hypothesis of age-related differences in strategy by comparing PFC activation levels of younger and older adults performing a WM task with a broad range (one to eight letters) of memory-demand levels. Findings of age-related differences in the functions relating PFC activation to memory demand would suggest a fundamental shift in the strategies used by younger and older adults to optimize WM task performance. We tested the hypothesis of age-related differences in neural efficiency by comparing PFC activation across performance levels of younger and older adults performing a delayed-response WM task. Findings of age-related differences in relationships between PFC activation and individual subjects' performance levels would suggest a fundamental shift in the volume of neural activity required by younger and older adults to optimize WM task performance.

Strategy Differences or Efficiency Differences? Studies of Age-Related Cerebral Activity Changes during WM Task Performance

For the aforementioned study, eight younger and six older adults were fMRI scanned while they performed a task in which, on each trial, letter strings, ranging in length from one to eight letters, were presented simultaneously in pseudorandom order for 4 s. This letter presentation was followed by a 12-s unfilled delay interval, during which subjects rehearsed the letters they saw at encoding. Then, a probe letter appeared for 2 s, during which the subject pressed a button with his or her right thumb if the probe item was part of the memory set or with the left thumb if the probe item was not part the memory set (Sternberg, 1966). This design allowed us to examine neural activity associated with stimulus encoding, associated with rehearsal processes in the delay period, and associated with memory retrieval during the response period.

To examine activity during specific task periods, we analyzed the data using event-related methods that permitted separate analyses of the neural activity that occurred during the encoding, delay, and retrieval portions of the task (Zarahn et al. 1997; Postle et al., 2000). We assessed cortical activation in each subject's dorsal (i.e., middle and superior frontal gyri) and ventral PFC (i.e., inferior frontal gyri). In the encoding, delay, and response periods in each of the eight memory load conditions (i.e., of one to eight letters) using the parameter estimates (nonthresholded) for the covariates that modeled each task period, in each memory load condition (D'Esposito, Zarahn, Aguirre, et al., 1999; Rypma & D'Esposito, 2000).

fMRI Signal: Tests of Age-Related Strategy Differences

Behavioral data analyses indicated that all subjects showed increasing RT and decreasing accuracy with increases in WM load, and older adults performed more slowly and less accurately than younger adults. In the fMRI data analyses, tests of strategy differences between the two age groups involved examination of differences in neural activity between memory load conditions across individual subjects, in each task period. To examine the relationship between PFC activation and memory load in each of the age groups, we determined, for each subject, the extent of activation change in each task period, by determining the regional activation in each memory load condition. Figure 13.1 shows the regional activation (based on median parameter estimates) of younger and older subjects plotted against memory load in each task period in dorsal and ventral PFC. In dorsal PFC, memory load-related changes in activity were apparent in all three task periods (formal tests of these changes were significant in the delay and retrieval periods). Visual inspection of the slope functions plotted in Figure 13.1 indicated minimal age-related differences (formal tests of the age differences were nonsignificant in all task periods). A similar pattern of results occurred in ventral PFC. Although significant memory load-related activity is apparent in all task periods, the slope functions plotted in Figure 13.1 indicated minimal age-related differences (formal tests of the age differences were nonsignificant in all task periods).

Tests of Age-Related Efficiency Differences

Tests of efficiency differences between the two subject groups involved examination of differences in activation–performance relationships between individual subjects across memory load conditions in each task period. To characterize the performance of individual subjects, we computed a performance composite score for each subject that was made up of the subject's z-standardized RT subtracted from his or her standardized accuracy scores. Thus, high-performance composite scores corresponded to high accuracy and low RT. Table 13.1 shows the subjects' performance scores by rank. To characterize each subject's activation level, we determined, for each subject, the extent of activation in each task period, independent of memory load, by determining the regional mean parameter estimate averaged over memory load. We could infer age-related differences in neural efficiency to the extent that we could

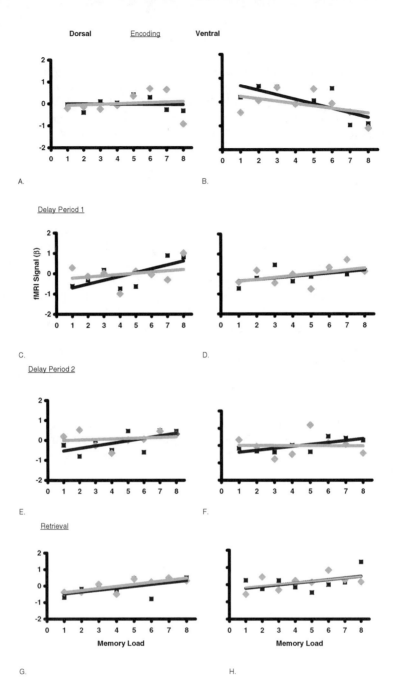

FIGURE 13.1. fMRI signal plotted against memory load for each task period in (A) dorsal PFC for Encoding, (B) ventral PFC Encoding, (C) dorsal PFC Delay Period 1, (D) ventral PFC for Delay Period 1, (E) dorsal PFC for Delay Period 2, (F) ventral PFC for Delay Period 2, (G) dorsal PFC for Response Period, (H) ventral PFC for Response Period. Younger subjects' results are illustrated as squares and older subjects' are illustrated as diamonds.

TABLE 13.1. Individual Subjects' Performance Scores

Subject	Performance score	Subject	Performance score
BB	1.58	ME	2.49
BH	1.00	JO	1.35
NO	0.27	DA	0.33
MP	0.11	PU	−0.61
JL	−0.40	SP	−1.45
TW	−0.52	WH	−2.94
IT	−0.59		
HL	−1.46		

Note. Higher performance scores correspond to better performance.

observe interactions between age group and performance score on activation. Thus, to test for age differences in performance–activation relationships, we performed analyses of variance in each task period, with age group, performance score, and activation as between-subjects factors.

Tables 13.2 and 13.3 show the standardized regression coefficients that characterize the relationship between performance-composite scores and regional activation in dorsal PFC and ventral PFC, and the results of the *F*-tests for age group by performance score interactions. Tables 13.2 and 13.3 indicate that, in general, the regression coefficients for younger adults were negative, indicating *decreases* in activation with increasing performance-composite scores, whereas regression coefficients for older adults were positive, indicating *increases* in activation with increasing performance-composite scores for older adults. In dorsal PFC, the observation of opposite linear trends between the younger and older adults was confirmed by significant age group by per-

TABLE 13.2. Dorsal PFC: Regression of Activation and Performance Composite

Task period	Slope	r^2	$F(1, 10)$	p
Encoding				
Younger	−.96	.91	10.88	.008*
Older	.71	.50		
Delay 1				
Younger	−.05	.003	.784	.40
Older	.43	.19		
Delay 2				
Younger	−.44	.19	.948	.35
Older	.56	.32		
Response				
Younger	−.75	.56	5.30	.04*
Older	.65	.42		

*$p < .05$

TABLE 13.3. Ventral PFC: Regression of Activation and Performance Composite

Task period	Slope	r^2	$F(1, 10)$	p
Encoding				
Younger	−.72	.52	6.81	.03*
Older	.37	.14		
Delay 1				
Younger	−.48	.23	.82	.39
Older	.04	.001		
Delay 2				
Younger	−.57	.32	7.60	.02*
Older	.82	.67		
Response				
Younger	−.45	.20	1.14	.31
Older	.11	.01		

*$p < .05$

formance score interactions in the Encoding and Response periods. In ventral PFC, similar effects occurred in the Encoding and Late-Delay Periods.

The results of this study (Rypma et al., 2005) replicated earlier findings from Rypma and D'Esposito (2000) showing age-differential activation–performance relationships that were limited to dorsal PFC in the Retrieval task period (see Figure 13.2). The results presented here, however, suggest that the age × performance interaction effects may be more widespread than our previous results indicated (e.g., Rypma & D'Esposito, 2000). To gain a

a.   b.

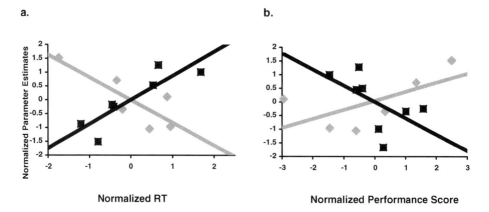

FIGURE 13.2. Scatterplots of normalized regional mean parameter estimates during the response period in dorsal PFC from (a) an earlier study, plotted against normalized RT for younger subjects (squares; slope = .87, r^2 = .76) and older subjects (diamonds; slope = −.82, r^2 = .68; Rypma & D'Esposito, 2000, 2001) and (b) from the present study plotted against normalized performance scores (for younger, slope = −.75, r^2 = .56; for older, slope = .65, r^2 = .42).

clearer understanding of the results, we performed further analyses in which we decomposed the performance-composite score into its accuracy and RT components. We then regressed the parameter estimates against accuracy and RT separately, in each task period and region of interest (ROI). In ventral PFC, the only significant result was the interaction of age group and accuracy on activation in the Delay period. In dorsal PFC, the only significant results were the interactions of age group and accuracy on activation in the Encoding period and the age group and RT on activation in the Response (see also Rypma et al., 2007). Thus, the performance–activation interaction at Encoding was due mainly to age differences in the relationship between performance *accuracy* and fMRI activation, whereas the performance–activation interaction we observed at Response was due to age differences in the relationship of individual subjects' performance *speed* and fMRI activation.

We observed large and significant age-related differences in the nature of the relationship between performance and activation in both dorsal and ventral PFC. These results suggest that the mechanisms underlying the observation of age-related differences in neural activity are related to age-related reductions in the efficiency of WM-critical PFC mechanisms. In dorsal PFC, there were significant interactions of age, performance, and fMRI activation in the Encoding and the Response periods. In ventral PFC such interactions also occurred in the Encoding period and during the second Delay period. Decomposition of the performance score indicated that the performance–activation interaction at Encoding was due mainly to age differences in the relationship between performance accuracy and fMRI activation. This decomposition analysis also indicated that the performance–activation interaction we observed in the Response period was mainly due to age differences in the relationship of individual subjects' performance speed and fMRI activation. These patterns of fMRI data suggest a central role for individual differences in processing efficiency in explanations of performance-activation relationships (see also Grady et al., 2003; Haier et al., 1992; Kosslyn et al., 1996; Mattay et al., 2000; Rypma & D'Esposito, 2000, 2001; Rypma et al., 2002; Zarahn et al., 2007).

Strategy Differences or Efficiency Differences?

Both younger and older adults showed increases in dorsal PFC activation with increasing memory load. These results are consistent with earlier studies showing increasing fMRI signal in dorsal PFC with increases in mnemonic demand. For example, in an fMRI study using a blocked design (i.e., signal collapsed across all task periods), Rypma et al. (1999) observed increasing activation in dorsal and ventral PFC with increasing memory loads. They proposed that ventral PFC is involved in maintenance of subcapacity WM loads, but when WM loads exceed memory capacity, dorsal PFC may be recruited to mediate strategic processes necessary for maintenance of high WM loads. The present results are consistent with this proposal and suggest that both younger and older adults utilize manipulation functions of dorsal PFC to implement strategic data compression or "chunking" operations (e.g., Miller, 1956; Cowan, 2001; Bor et al., 2003) for maintenance of large amounts of information (e.g., Rypma & Gabrieli, 2001; Rypma & D'Esposito, 1999). In the current study we also found increasing activation in dorsal PFC with increasing load, but in contrast to our earlier studies (which examined only two memory set sizes; Rypma & D'Esposito, 1999, 2000), these load-dependent activation increases occurred later in the task, during the retention and retrieval periods. A possible reason for this difference may be the increased and more varied memory load requirements of the present task as compared with those used in previous studies (Rypma & D'Esposito, 2001; Rypma et al., 2006). Indeed, strategic organization and strategy shifting may be among the processes mediated by dorsal PFC (Deiber et al., 1991; Jenkins et al., 1994; Prabhakaran et al., 1997, 2001).

Ventral PFC, which is proposed to mediate maintenance/rehearsal processes (Awh et al., 1996; Paulesu et al., 1993; Rypma et al., 1999; D'Esposito et al., 1999), showed decreases in activation with increasing memory demand during encoding, suggesting that it may play a larger role in memory encoding with subcapacity memory loads than with supracapacity memory loads. Ventral PFC may play an increasingly limited role in WM encoding functions with increasing memory loads, given its limited capacity. The qualitative difference between this activation pattern and those observed in dorsal PFC is consistent with proposals suggesting distinct roles for dorsal and ventral PFC in WM (e.g., D'Esposito et al., 1995, 1999a, 2000; Rypma et al., 1999; Rypma & D'Esposito, 1999, 2001). In other task periods, ventral PFC showed increases in activation with increasing memory load. This result is consistent with some earlier results (Rypma et al., 1999) but inconsistent with others (Rypma & D'Esposito, 1999). Further research will be required to determine when, and under what task conditions, ventral PFC is sensitive to memory load effects. In summary, in one set of subjects performing a single WM task, we observed that minimal age-related differences in the relationship between PFC activation and memory load provide little support for the notion that younger and older adults bring fundamentally different strategies to WM tasks.

Results of our regression analyses indicated that the age-equivalent load-dependent effects described above were imbedded within a pattern of age-differential activation performance patterns. These analyses suggested that, for younger adults, dorsal and ventral PFC activation was greater during the encoding, maintenance, and retrieval periods for those who performed more slowly and less accurately, relative to those who performed faster and more accurately. For older adults, we observed the opposite pattern. Specifically, dorsal and ventral PFC activation was reduced during the Encoding, Maintenance, and Retrieval periods for the slower and less accurate performers, relative to for those who were faster and more accurate.

These results replicate earlier results showing less PFC activation for faster and more accurate young adults during memory retrieval, but more PFC activation for faster and more accurate older adults (Rypma & D'Esposito,

1999, 2000, 2001; see Figure 13.2). They are at variance, however, with the results indicating that relationships between activation and performance were limited to dorsal regions of PFC and to retrieval periods of delayed-response WM tasks.

The disparity between this result and our earlier results is important because it suggests that where (i.e., in which brain regions) and when (i.e., in which WM task subcomponents) age-related differences in neural efficiency exert their effects depends on the relative importance of the WM sub-component and the brain region to the task. Thus, it may be that the current task taxed the encoding functions of dorsal PFC relatively more than the limited extreme-conditions designs we have previously employed. Similar variations in task complexity have been shown to influence neural activity in previous research (e.g., Johnson et al., 1997; Schacter et al., 1996). An important implication of the present findings, therefore, is that differences in task structure play a vital, albeit poorly understood, role in neuroimaging results. A critical task for future research will be to more precisely identify the nature of neural processes underlying these differences.

The results presented here come from a single study in which one relatively small set of subjects performed a single cognitive task. Nonetheless, we were able to test two competing hypotheses of age differences in fMRI signal activity during cognitive task performance. The results suggested that younger and older adults rely on similar strategies during their cognitive performance. The volume of neural activity required for optimal implementation of those strategies appeared to differ, however. The observation of similar age differences in activation–performance relationships in other studies (Rypma & D'Esposito, 1999, 2000, 2001; Rypma et al., 2002; Rypma et al., 2006; Mattay et al., 2000; Grady et al., 2003; Persson et al., 2004; Zarahn et al., 2007) suggests that the pervasive age-related slowing observed across many different kinds of behavioral tasks (e.g., Myerson et al., 1990; Salthouse, 1996) may result from a fundamental change in brain–behavior relationships with age.

A Model of Age-Related Changes in Brain–Behavior Relationships

Our proposal is that age-related behavioral changes result from age-related decreases in neural efficiency. Reductions in neural efficiency may begin with reductions in the quality of information relayed to central structures from peripheral structures. Subsequent deterioration of central structures, most notably PFC, could exacerbate slowing of central cognitive processes, including the speed with which information can be activated in WM. Slower WM activation may lead to degradation in the quality of information that is encoded, maintained, and available for memory retrieval.

Our proposed model of the age-related brain–behavior differences observed in this and other studies is an extension of models of performance based on the sigmoid (S-shaped) relationship between a neuron's input activation and its firing probability. Some researchers have proposed that this relationship influences performance (Kimberg & Farah, 1993; Kimberg et al., 1997; Servan-Schreiber et al., 1990). In these models, response selection is characterized as a signal detection mechanism in which the probability of a given response is determined by the relative strength of signal between representations in memory. Middle ranges of neural activation result in large differences in signal between representations and easy discrimination between potential responses. As neural activation levels move above or below this range, these signal differences become less discriminable and response selection becomes more difficult (Rypma & D'Esposito, 2000, 2001).

This model proposes that aging may result in baseline reductions in PFC activation levels (e.g., Moeller et al., 1996). One consequence of this reduced neural activity may be that higher activation levels are required to optimally encode, maintain, and retrieve information from WM. That is, the sigmoid function relating neural activation to optimal performance may require a higher level of activation for older adults to achieve optimal performance. Relative to older adults, younger adults function with higher baseline activation levels. Thus, they require relatively less activation to achieve optimal performance. This proposal is consistent with our observation that increased activation is associated with performance improvements for older adults, but to decrements for younger adults (see also Rypma & D'Esposito, 2000, 2001). The effects of these age-related changes in the sigmoid functions relating neural activity to performance may be implemented in transactions between nodes in a system such as that proposed by Cerella (1990). Such a system, cognitive task performance, depends on transmission across an array of interconnected nodes (e.g., McClelland & Rumelhart, 1986). Nodes may represent individual neurons or functionally connected cell assemblies (e.g., Hebb, 1949). These nodes may be connected by pathways that correspond to axonal processes. In this system, the fewer nodes that must be traversed, the more direct the processing paths and the quicker the information processing. Reductions in the integrity of direct processing connections (which may occur in aging) requires traversal of more indirect links for successful task performance. Greater internodal transmission may lead to greater neural activity but slower information processing. Thus, age-related changes in neural activity observed in these and other studies may result from age-related efficiency decreases in the interaction of neural cell assemblies during WM performance.

REFERENCES

Aguirre, G. K., Zarahn, E., & D'Esposito, M. (1998). The variability of the human BOLD hemodynamic responses. *NeuroImage, 8,* 360–369.

Ahmad, A., & Spear, P. D. (1993). Effects of aging on the size, density, and number of rhesus monkey lateral genicualte neurons. *Journal of Comparative Neurology, 334*, 631–643.

Anders, T. R., & Fozard, J. L. (1973). Effects of age upon retrieval from primary and secondary memory. *Developmental Psychology, 9*, 411–415.

Anders, T. R. Fozard, J. L., & Lillyquist, T. D. (1972). Effects of age upon retrieval from short-term memory. *Developmental Psychology, 6*, 214–217.

Awh, E., Jonides, J., Smith, E. E., et al. (1996). Dissociation of storage and rehearsal in working memory: Evidence from positron emission tomography. *Psychological Science, 7*, 25–31.

Babcock, R. L., Laguna, K. D., & Roesch, S. C. (1997). A comparison of the factor structure of processing speed for younger and older adults: Testing the assumption of measurement equivalence across age groups. *Psychology and Aging, 12*, 268–276.

Bachevalier, J. L., Landis, S., Walker, L. C., et al. (1991). Aged monkeys exhibit behavioral deficits indicative of widespread cerebral dysfunction. *Neurobiology of Aging, 12*, 99–111.

Baddeley, A. (1986). *Working memory*. New York: Oxford University Press.

Baddeley, A., & Hitch, G. J. (1974). Working memory. In G. Bower (Ed.), *Recent advances in learning and motivation* (Vol. 8, pp. 47–90). New York: Academic Press.

Baltes, P. B., Cornelius, S. W., Spiro, A., et al. (1980). Integration versus de-differentiation of fluid/crystallized intelligence in old age. *Developmental Psychology, 16*, 625–635.

Bartus, R. T., Dean, R. L., III, & Fleming, D. L. (1979). Aging in the rhesus monkey: Effects on visual discrimination learning and reversal learning. *Journal of Gerontology, 34*, 209–219.

Boaz, T. L., & Denney, D. R. (1993). Speed of scanning in primary memory in persons with dementia of the Alzheimer type. *Psychology and Aging, 2*, 294–300.

Bor, D., Duncan, J., Wiseman, R. J., et al. (2003). Encoding strategies dissociate prefrontal activity from working memory demand. *Neuron, 37*, 361–367.

Botwinick, J., & Storandt, M. (1974). *Memory, related functions, and age*. Springfield, IL: Thomas.

Brody, H. (1955). Organization of the cerebral cortex: III. A study of aging in the human cerebral cortex. *Journal of Comparative Neurology, 102*, 511–556.

Bromley, J. (1958). Some effects of age on short-term learning and memory. *Journal of Gerontology, 13*, 12–21.

Buckner, R. L., Corbetta, M., Schatz, J., et al. (1996). Preserved speech abilities and compensation following prefrontal damage. *Proceedings of the National Academy of Sciences of the United States of America, 93*, 1249–1253.

Cabeza, R. (2002). Hemispheric asymmetry reduction in older adults: The HAROLD model. *Psychology and Aging, 17*, 85–100.

Cabeza, R., Grady, C. L., Nyberg, L., et al. (1997). Age-related differences in neural activity during memory encoding and retrieval: A positron emission tomography study. *Journal of Neuroscience, 17*, 391–400.

Cerella, J. (1990). Aging and information processing rate. In J. E. Birren & K. W. Schaie (Eds.), *Handbook of the psychology of aging* (pp. 201–221). San Diego: Academic Press.

Corsellis, J. A. W. (1976). Some observations on the Purkinje cell population and on brain volume in human aging. In R. D. Terry & S. Gershon (Eds.), *Neurobiology of aging* (pp. 205–209). New York: Raven Press.

Cowan, N. (2001). The magical number 4 in short-term memory: A reconsideration of mental storage capacity. *Behavioral and Brain Sciences, 24,* 87–185.

Craik, F. I. M. (1977). Age differences in human memory. In J. E. Birren & K. W. Schaie (Eds.), *Handbook of the psychology of aging* (pp. 384–414). New York: Van Nostrand Reinhold.

Craik, F. I. M. (1968). Short-term memory and the aging process. In G. A. Talland (Ed.), *Human aging and behavior* (pp. 131–168). New York: Academic Press.

Deiber, M. P., Passingham, R. E., Colebatch, J. G., et al. (1991). Cortical areas and the selection of movement: A study with positron emission tomography *Experimental Brain Research, 84,* 393–402.

De Santi, S., de Leon, M. J., Convit, A., et al. (1995). Age-related changes in brain: II. Positron emission tomography of frontal and temporal lobe glucose metabolism in normal subjects. *Psychiatric Quarterly, 66,* 357–370.

D'Esposito, M., Aguirre, G. K., Zarahn, E., et al. (1998). Functional MRI studies of spatial and non-spatial working memory. *Cognitive Brain Research, 7,* 1–13.

D'Esposito, M., Detre, J. A., Alsop, D. C., et al. (1995). The neural basis of the central executive system of working memory. *Nature, 378,* 279–281.

D'Esposito, M., Postle, B. R., Ballard, D., et al. (1999a). Maintenance versus manipulation of information held in working memory: An event-related fMRI study. *Brain and Cognition, 41,* 66–86.

D'Esposito, M., Zarahn, E., Aguirre, G. K., et al. (1999b). The effect of normal aging on the coupling of neural activity to the BOLD hemodynamic response. *Neuro-Image, 10,* 6–14.

Drachman, D., & Leavitt, J. (1972). Memory impairment in the aged: Storage versus retrieval deficit. *Journal of Experimental Psychology, 93,* 302–308.

Eberling, J. L., Roberts, J. A., De Manincor, D. J., et al. (1995). Reduced temporal lobe glucose metabolism in aging. *Journal of Neuroimaging, 6,* 156–160.

Eldreth, D. A., Porcelli, A. J., Geneva, H. M., et al. (2004). *Neural correlates of age-related reduction in processing speed: An event-related fMRI study.* Paper presented at the Cognitive Aging Conference, Atlanta, Georgia.

Erikson, C. W., Hamlin, R. M., & Daye, C. (1973). Aging adults and rate of memory scan. *Bulletin of the Psychonomic Society, 1,* 259–260.

Finger S., Buckner R. L., & Buckingham H. (2003). Does the right hemisphere take over after damage to Broca's area? The Barlow case of 1877 and its history. *Brain and Language, 85,* 385–395.

Foster, J. C., & Taylor, G. A. (1920). The applicability of mental tests to persons over 50. *Journal of Applied Psychology, 4,* 39–58.

Franklin, R. J., Zhao, C., & Sim, F. J. (2002). Ageing and CNS remyelination. *Neuroreport, 13,* 923–928.

Friedman, H. (1974). Interrelation of two types of immediate memory in the aged. *Journal of Psychology, 87,* 177–181.

Funahashi, S., Bruce, C. J., & Goldman-Rakic, P. S. (1989). Mnemonic coding of visual space in the monkey's dorsolateral prefrontal cortex. *Journal of Neurophysiology, 61,* 331–349.

Fuster, J. M., & Alexander, G. E. (1971). Neuron activity related to short-term memory. *Science, 173,* 652–654.

Gabrieli, J. D. E. (1996). Memory systems analysis of mnemonic disorders in aging and age-related diseases. *Proceedings of the National Academy of Sciences of the United States of America, 93*, 13534–13540.

Gabrieli, J. D. E. (1991). Brain basis of changes in memory performance in aging and Alzheimer's disease. *Experimental Aging Research, 17*, 96–97.

Gilbert, J. G. (1941). Memory loss in senescence. *Journal of Abnormal and Social Psychology, 36*, 73–86.

Gilbert, J. G., & Levee, R. F. (1971). Patterns of declining memory. *Journal of Gerontology, 26*, 70–75.

Glanzer, M., & Razel, M. (1974). The size of the unit in short-term storage. *Journal of Verbal Learning and Verbal Behavior, 13*, 114–131.

Goldman-Rakic, P. S. (1987). Circuitry of primate prefrontal cortex and regulation of behavior by representational memory. In F. Plum (Ed.), *Handbook of physiology: The nervous system V* (pp. 373–417). New York: Oxford University Press.

Goldman-Rakic, P. S., & Friedman, H. (1991). Circuitry of the prefrontal cortex and the regulation of behavior by representational memory. In H. Levin, H. Eisenberg, & A. Benton (Eds.), *Frontal lobe function and dysfunction* (pp. 72–91). New York: Oxford University Press.

Good, C. D., Johnsrude, I. S., Ashburner, J., et al. (2001). A voxel-based morphometric study of ageing in 465 normal adult human brains. *NeuroImage, 14*, 21–36.

Grady, C. L., Haxby, J. V., Horwitz, B., et al. (1992). Dissociation of object and spatial vision in human extrastriate cortex: Age-related changes in activation of regional cerebral blood flow measured with ^{15}O water and positron emission tomography. *Journal of Cognitive Neuroscience, 4*, 23–34.

Grady, C. L., McIntosh, A. R., & Craik, F. I. M. (2003). Age-related differences in the functional connectivity of the hippocampus during memory encoding. *Hippocampus, 13*, 572–586.

Grady, C. L., McIntosh, A. R., Horwitz, B., et al. (1995). Age-related reductions in human recognition memory due to impaired encoding. *Science, 269*, 218–220.

Haier, R. J., Siegel, B., Tang, C., et al. (1992). Intelligence and changes in regional cerebral glucose metabolic-rate following learning. *Intelligence, 16*, 415–426.

Haug, H., & Eggers, R. (1991). Morphometry of the human cortex cerebri and corpus striatum during aging. *Neurobiology of Aging, 12*, 336–338.

Haug, H., Kuhl, S., Mecke, E., et al. (1984). The significance of morphometric procedures in the investigation of age changes in cytoarchitectonic structures of human brain. *Journal für Hirnforschung, 25*, 353–374.

Hebb, D. O. (1949). *The organization of behavior*. New York: Wiley.

Hellstrom, L. I., & Schmeidt, R. A. (1990). Compound action potential input/output functions in young and quiet-aged gerbils. *Hearing Research, 50*, 163–174.

Hertzog, C. (1985). An individual differences perspective: Implications for cognitive research in gerontology. *Research on Aging, 7*, 7–45.

Jenkins, I. H., Brooks, D. J., Nixon, P. D., et al. (1994). Motor sequence learning: A study with positron emission tomography. *Journal of Neuroscience, 14*, 3774–3790.

Johnson, M. K., Nolde, S. F., Mather, T. E. M., et al. (1997). Mental agendas can affect the similarity associated with true and false recognition memory. *Psychological Science, 8*, 250–257.

Jones, H. E., & Conrad, H. (1933). A study of a homogeneous group between the ages of ten and sixty. *Genetic Psychological Monographs, 13*, 223–298.

Jonides, J., Marshuetz, C., Smith, E. E., et al. (2000). Brain activation reveals changes with age in resolving interference in verbal working memory. *Journal of Cognitive Neuroscience, 12,* 188–196.

Kemper, T. L. (2002). Neuroanatomical and neuropathological changes during aging and in dementia. In M. L. Albert & E. J. E. Knoepfel (Eds.), *Clinical neurology of aging* (2nd ed., pp. 3–67). New York: Oxford University Press.

Kimberg, D. Y., D'Esposito, M., & Farah, M. T. (1997). Effects of bromocriptine on human subjects depend on working memory capacity. *Neuroreport, 8,* 3581–3585.

Kimberg, D. Y., & Farah, M. T. (1993). A unified account of cognitive impairments following frontal lobe damage: The role of working memory in complex organized behavior. *Journal of Experimental Psychology: General, 122,* 411–428.

Kirsner, K. (1972). Developmental changes in short-term recognition memory. *British Journal of Psychology, 63,* 109–117.

Kosslyn, S. M., Thompson, W. L., Kim, I. J., et al. (1996). Individual differences in cerebral blood flow in area 17 predict the time to evaluate visualized letters. *Journal of Cognitive Neuroscience, 8,* 78–82.

Kriauciunas, R. (1968). Short-term memory and age. *Journal of the American Geriatrics Society, 16,* 83–93.

Kubota, K., & Niki, H. (1971). Prefrontal cortical unit activity and delayed alternation performance in monkeys. *Journal of Neurophysiology, 34,* 337–347.

Kuhl, D. E., Metter, E. J., Riege, W. H., et al. (1982). Effect of human aging on patterns of local cerebral glucose utilization determined by 18-F-fluorodeoxyglucose method. *Journal of Cerebral Blood Flow and Metabolism, 2,* 163–171

Lindenberger, U., & Baltes, P. B. (1994). Sensory functioning and intelligence in old age: A strong connection. *Psychology and Aging, 9,* 339–355.

Madden, D. J., Turkington, T. G., Provenzale, J. M., et al. (1999). Adult age differences in functional neuroanatomy of verbal recognition memory. *Human Brain Mapping, 7,* 115–135.

Madden, D. J., Whiting, W. L., Huettel, S. A., et al. (2004). Diffusion tensor imaging of adult age differences in cerebral white matter: Relation to response time. *NeuroImage, 21,* 1174–1181.

Manoach, D. S., Schlaug, G., Siewert, B., et al. (1997). Prefrontal cortex fMRI signal changes are correlated with working memory load. *NeuroReport, 8,* 545–549.

Marsh, G. R. (1975). Age differences in evoked potential correlates of a memory scanning process. *Experimental Aging Research, 1,* 3–16.

Mattay, V. S., Callicott, J. H., Bertolino, A., et al. (2000). Effects of dextroamphetamine on cognitive performance and cortical activation. *NeuroImage, 12,* 268–275.

McIntosh, A. R., Sekuler, A. B., Penpeci, C., et al. (1999). Recruitment of unique neural systems to support visual memory in normal aging. *Current Biology, 9,* 1275–1278.

Michaels, D. D. (1993). Ocular disease in the elderly. In A. A. Rosenbloom & M. W. Morgan (Eds.), *Vision and aging* (pp. 111–159). Oxford, UK: Butterworth Heineman.

Miller, G. (1956). The magical number seven, plus or minus two: Some limits on our capacity for processing information. *Psychological Review, 63,* 81–97.

Minckler, T. M., & Boyd, E. (1968). Physical growth. In J. Minckler (Ed.), *Pathology of the nervous system* (pp. 98–122). New York: McGraw-Hill.

Moeller, J. R., Ishikawa, T., Dhawan, V., et al. (1996). The metabolic topography of normal aging. *Journal of Cerebral Blood Flow and Metabolism, 16,* 385–398.

Myerson, J., Hale, S., Wagstaff, D., et al. (1990). The information-loss model: A mathematical theory of age-related cognitive slowing. *Psychological Review, 97,* 475–487.

Nielsen-Bohlman, L., & Knight, R. T. (1995). Prefrontal alterations during memory processing in aging. *Cerebral Cortex, 5,* 541–549.

Norman, D., & Shallice, T. (1980). Attention to action: Willed automatic control of behavior. *University of California CHIP Report 99.*

Owsley, C., & Sloane, M. E. (1987). Contrast sensitivity, acuity and the perception of "real world" targets. *British Journal of Opthalmology, 71,* 791–796.

Park, D. C. (2002). Judging meaning improves function in the aging brain. *Trends in Cognitive Sciences, 6,* 227–229.

Park, D. C., Lautenschlager, G., Hedden, T., et al. (2002). Models of visuospatial and verbal working memory across the adult life span. *Psychology and Aging, 17,* 299–320.

Park, D. C., Polk, T. A., Park, R., et al. (2004). Aging reduces neural specialization in ventral visual cortex. *Proceedings of the National Academy of Sciences of the United States of America, 101,* 13091–13095.

Paulesu, E., Frith, C., & Frackowiak, R. (1993). The neural correlates of the verbal component of working memory. *Nature, 362,* 342–345.

Persson, J., Sylvester, C. Y., Nelson, J. K., et al. (2004). Selection requirements during verb generation: Differential recruitment in older and younger adults. *NeuroImage, 23,* 1382–1390.

Peters, A. (2002). The effects of normal aging on myelin and nerve fibers: A review. *Journal of Neurocytology, 8–9,* 581–593.

Peters, A., & Sethares, C. (2004). Oligodendrocytes, their progenitors, and other neuroglial cells in the aging primate cortex. *Cerebral Cortex, 14,* 995–1007.

Peters, A., & Sethares, C. (2002). Aging and the myelinated fibers in prefrontal cortex and corpus callosum of the monkey. *Journal of Comparative Neurology, 442,* 277–291.

Poon, L. W., & Fozard, J. L. (1980). Age and word frequency effects in continuous recognition memory. *Journal of Gerontology, 35,* 77–86.

Postle, B. R., Zarahn, E., & D'Esposito, M. (2000). Using event-related fMRI to assess delay-period activity during performance of saptial and nonspatial working memory tasks. *Brain Research Protocols, 5,* 57–66.

Prabhakaran, V., Rypma, B., & Gabrieli, J. D. E. (2001). Neural substrates of mathematical reasoning: An fMRI study of neocortical activation during performance of the Necessary Arithmetic Operations Test. *Neuropsychology, 15,* 115–127.

Prabhakaran, V., Smith, J. A. L., Desmond, J. E., et al. (1997). Neural substrates of fluid reasoning: An fMRI study of neocortical activation during performance of the Raven's Progressive Matrices Test. *Cognitive Psychology, 33,* 43–63.

Presty, S. K., Bachevalier, J., Walker, L. C., et al. (1987). Age differences in recognition memory of the rhesus monkey (*Macaca mulatta*). *Neurobiology of Aging, 8,* 435–440.

Prull, M., Bunge, S., & Gabrieli, J. D. E. (2000). In F. I. M. Craik & T. A. Salthouse (Eds.), *Handbook of aging and cognition* (pp. 91–153). Mahwah, NJ: Erlbaum.

Raz, N. (2000). Aging of the brain and its impact on cognitive performance: Integration of structural and functional findings. In F. I. M. Craik & T. A. Salthouse (Eds.), *The handbook of aging and cognition* (pp. 1–90). Mahwah, NJ: Erlbaum.

Raz, N., Gunning, F. M., Head, D. P., et al. (1997). Selective aging of human cerebral cortex observed *in vivo*: Differential vulnerability of the prefrontal gray matter. *Cerebral Cortex, 7,* 268–282.

Raz, N., Gunning-Dixon, F. M., Head, D., et al. (1998). Neuroanatomical correlates of cognitive aging: Evidence from structural magnetic resonance imaging. *Neuropsychology, 12,* 95–114.

Reinert, G. (1970). Comparative factor analytic studies of intelligence through the human life-span. In L. R. Goulet & P. B. Baltes (Eds.), *Life-span developmental psychology: Research and theory* (pp. 467–484). New York: Academic Press.

Resnick, S. M., Goldszal, A. F., Davatzikos, C., et al. (2000). One-year age changes in MRI brain volumes in older adults. *Cerebral Cortex, 10,* 464–472.

Resnick, S. M., Pham, D. L., Kraut, M. A., et al. (2003). Longitudinal magnetic resonance imaging studies of older adults: A shrinking brain. *Journal of Neuroscience, 23,* 3295–3301.

Reuter-Lorenz, P. A., Jonides, J., Smith, E., et al. (2000). Age differences in the frontal lateralization of verbal and spatial working memory revealed by PET. *Journal of Cognitive Neuroscience, 12,* 174–187.

Reuter-Lorenz, P. A., Marshuetz, C., Jonides, J., et al. (2001). Neurocognitive aging and storage of executive processes. *European Journal of Cognitive Psychology, 12,* 257–278.

Rypma, B. (2006). Factors controlling neural activity during delayed-response task performance: Testing a memory organization hypothesis of prefrontal function. *Neuroscience, 139,* 223–235.

Rypma, B., Berger, J. S., & D'Esposito, M. (2002). The influence of working-memory demand and subject performance on prefrontal cortical activity. *Journal of Cognitive Neuroscience, 14,* 721–731.

Rypma, B., Berger, J. S., Genova, H. M., et al. (2005). Dissociating age-related changes in cognitive strategy and neural efficiency using event-related fMRI. *Cortex, 41,* 582–594.

Rypma, B., & D'Esposito, M. (2001). Age-related changes in brain–behavior relationships: Evidence from event-related functional MRI studies. *European Journal of Cognitive Psychology, 13,* 235–256.

Rypma, B., & D'Esposito, M. (2000). Isolating the neural mechanisms of age-related changes in human working memory. *Nature Neuroscience, 3,* 509–515.

Rypma, B., & D'Esposito, M. (1999). The roles of prefrontal brain regions in components of working memory: Effects of memory load and individual differences. *Proceedings of the National Academy of Sciences of the United States of America, 96,* 6558–6563.

Rypma, B., Eldreth, D. A., & Rebbechi, D. (2006). Age-related differences in activation performance relations in delayed-response tasks: A multiple component analysis. *Cortex, 43,* 65–76.

Rypma, B., & Gabrieli, J. D. E. (2000). Functional neuroimaging of short-term memory: The neural mechanisms of mental storage. *Behavioral and Brain Sciences, 24,* 87–185.

Rypma, B., Prabhakaran, V., Desmond, J. E., et al. (2001). Age differences in prefrontal cortical activity in working memory. *Psychology and Aging, 16,* 371–384.

Rypma, B., Prabhakaran, V., Desmond, J. E., et al. (1999). Load-dependent roles of prefrontal cortical regions in the maintenance of working memory. *NeuroImage*, 9, 216–226.

Salthouse, T. A. (1996). The processing speed theory of adult age differences in cognition. *Psychological Review*, 103, 403–428.

Salthouse, T. A., Hambrick, D. Z., & McGuthry, K. E. (1998). Shared age-related influences on cognitive and non-cognitive variables. *Psychology and Aging*, 13, 486–500.

Salthouse, T. A., Hancock, H. E., Meinz, E. J., et al. (1996). Interrelations of age, visual acuity, and cognitive functioning. *Journal of Gerontology: Psychological Sciences*, 51B, P317–P330.

Schacter, D. L., Reiman, E., Curran, T., et al. (1996). Neuroanatomical correlates of veridical and illusory recognition memory: Evidence from positron emission tomography. *Neuron*, 17, 267–274.

Schneider, B. A. (1997). Psychoacoustics and aging: Implications for everyday listening. *Journal of Speech-Language Pathology and Audiology*, 21, 111–124.

Schneider, B. A., & Pichora-Fuller, M. K. (2000). Implications of perceptual deterioration for cognitive aging research. In F. I. M. Craik & T. A. Salthouse (Eds.), *Handbook of aging and cognition* (pp. 155–219). Mahwah, NJ: Erlbaum.

Servan-Schreiber, D., Printz, H., & Cohen, J. D. (1990). A network model of catecholamine effects: Gain, signal to noise ratio, and behavior. *Science*, 249, 892–895.

Sim, F. J., Zhao, C., Pendaris, J., et al. (2002). The age-related decrease in CNS remyelination efficiency is attributable to an impairment of both oligodendrocyte progenitor recruitment and differentiation. *Journal of Neuroscience*, 22, 2451–2459.

Sloane, M. E., Owsley, C., & Jackson, C. A. (1988). Aging and luminance-adaptation effects on spatial contrast sensitivity. *Journal of the Optical Society of America*, 5, 2181–2190.

Smith, A. D. (1975). Aging and interference with memory. *Journal of Gerontology*, 30, 319–325.

Spear, P. D. (1993). Neural bases of visual deficits during aging. *Vision Research*, 33, 2589–2609.

Spear, P. D., Moore, R. J., Kim, C. B., et al. (1994). Effects of aging on the primate visual system: Spatial and temporal processing by lateral geniculate neurons in young adult and old rhesus monkeys. *Journal of Neurophysiology*, 702, 402–420.

Sternberg, S. (1966). High-speed scanning in human memory. *Science*, 153, 652–654.

Taki, Y., Goto, R., Evans, A., et al. (2004). Voxel-based morphometry of human brain with age and cerebrovascular risk factors. *Neurobiology of Aging*, 25, 455–463.

Tang, Y., Nyengaard, J. R., Pakkenberg, B., et al. (1997). Age-induced white matter changes in the human brain: A stereological investigation. *Neurobiology of Aging*, 18, 609–615.

Taub, H. A. (1973). Memory span, practice and aging. *Journal of Gerontology*, 28, 335–338.

Tisserand, D. J., Pruessner, J. C., Sanz Arigita, E. J., et al. (2002). Regional frontal cortical volumes decrease differentially in aging: An fMRI study to compare volumetric approaches and voxel-based morphometry. *NeuroImage*, 17, 657–669.

Tisserand, D. J., van Boxtel, M. P., Pruessner, J. C., et al. (2004). A voxel-based morphometric study to determine individual differences in gray matter density associated with age and cognitive change over time. *Cerebral Cortex, 14,* 966–973.

Turlejski, K., & Djavadian, R. (2002). Life-long stability of neurons: A century of research on neurogenesis, neuronal death and neuron quantification in adult CNS. *Progress in Brain Research, 136,* 39–65.

Vincent, S. L., Peters, A., & Tigges, J. (1989). Effects of aging on the neurons within area 17 of rhesus monkey cerebral cortex. *Anatomical Record, 223,* 329–341.

Waugh, N. C., & Norman, D. A. (1965). Primary memory. *Psychological Review, 72,* 89–104.

West, R. L. (1996). An application of prefrontal cortex function theory to cognitive aging. *Psychological Bulletin, 2,* 272–292.

Willott, J. F. (1991). *Aging and the auditory system: Anatomy, physiology, and psychophysics.* San Diego: Singular Press.

Wisniewski, H. M., & Terry, R. D. (1976). Neuropathology of the aging brain. In R. D. Terry & S. Gershon (Eds.), *Neurobiology of aging* (pp. 65–78). New York: Raven Press.

Zarahn, E., Aguirre, G. K., & D'Esposito, M. (1997). Empirical analyses of BOLD fMRI statistics: I. Spatially unsmoothed data collected under null-hypothesis conditions. *NeuroImage, 5,* 179–195.

Zarahn, E., Rakitin, B., Abela, D., et al. (2007). Age-related changes in brain activation during a delayed item recognition task. *Neurobiology of Aging, 28,* 784–798.

CHAPTER 14

Functional Neuroimaging in Recovery from Stroke

Elizabeth R. Orr
Rachelle W. Rodriguez
Steven C. Cramer

Stroke and Stroke Recovery

Stroke remains a major source of human morbidity and mortality. Stroke is the third leading cause of death in the United States, with approximately 1 in 15 deaths attributable to stroke, and the second leading cause worldwide. Approximately 85% of patients in the United States survive an acute stroke, living an average of 7 yr thereafter. Most are left with significant disability (Gresham et al., 1995; Rathore et al., 2002), reducing activities and participation.

Stroke can affect all aspects of brain function. The nature and severity of poststroke deficits vary widely. Over the weeks to months following a stroke, most patients do show some spontaneous improvement in those behaviors affected by stroke (Duncan et al., 1992; Hier et al., 1983; Kertz & McCabe, 1977). However, this recovery is highly variable and generally incomplete. As a result, stroke is the leading cause of adult disability in the United States and many other countries.

Increasing investigation has explored the neurobiology of spontaneous poststroke recovery with the goal of using this information to improve patient outcomes. More recently studies have examined the brain events underlying experimentally derived poststroke gains. Most studies of stroke recovery have focused on recovery of motor or language function, two domains commonly affected by stroke (Gresham et al., 1995). A number of brain-mapping techniques has been used to investigate stroke recovery, each with its relative strengths. Functional magnetic resonance imaging (fMRI) has been the tool for many stroke recovery studies, given its relative safety and the accessibility of MRI machines, as well as this method's good temporal and excellent spatial resolution. Other investigative approaches have different strengths. Transcranial magnetic stimulation (TMS) is easier to use with patients and has excellent temporal resolution, but has reduced spatial resolution relative to fMRI. Positron emission tomography (PET) scanning has reduced temporal resolution and is generally less accessible but can measure many aspects of brain physiology.

This review is focused on fMRI, though results with other approaches have generally been concordant. The emphasis is on recovery of motor function, one of the major sources of impairment in patients with stroke. However, findings in motor recovery overlap substantially with investigations of recovery in other brain systems such as language (Baron et al., 2004).

The long-term goal of many studies, to better understand poststroke reorganization of brain function in order to improve patient outcomes, may be realized by better prediction of outcomes, patient triage to incipient restorative therapies, defining duration and intensity of restorative therapy, and measuring treatment effects. A number of restorative interventions are under study, including cell-based approaches (Bang et al., 2005; Kondziolka et al., 2005), selective serotonin reuptake inhibitors (Dam et al., 1996; Pariente et al., 2001), catecholaminergics (Grade et al., 1998; Scheidtman et al., 2001; Walker-Batson et al., 1995), brain stimulation (Khedr et al., 2005; Brown et al., 2006), robotic and other device-based interventions (Reinkensmeyer et al., 2004; Volpe et al., 2005), mental imagery-based protocols (Page et al., 2001), and constraint-induced and other intensive physical therapy regimens (Dromerick et al., 2000; Page et al., 2005; Wolf et al., 2002)—though currently none is approved for enhancing outcome after central nervous system (CNS) injury such as stroke. The maximum value of functional neuroimaging methods such as fMRI will be appreciated in the current context when applied in association with an established restorative intervention.

The Biology of Spontaneous Recovery after Stroke

A number of changes arise in the brain over the weeks following a stroke. These have been described at multiple levels. Cellular and molecular studies in animals undergoing an experimental unilateral infarct have characterized inflammation, angiogenesis, neurogenesis, synaptogenesis, changes in excitability, and cellular growth, many of which evolve bilaterally, during the days to weeks that follow a unilateral insult. A body of evidence suggests that many of these events contribute to spontaneous recovery of function after a stroke (Cramer & Chopp, 2000; Felling & Levison, 2003; Legos & Barone, 2003; Nudo, 1999; Schallert et al., 2000).

In animal studies, exogenous interventions have been found that amplify these molecular events and simultaneously improve behavioral outcome. Examples include amphetamine (Stroemer et al., 1998), growth factors (Kawamata et al., 1997; Ren et al., 2000), cellular therapies (Chen et al., 2003; Mahmood et al., 2004), brain stimulation (Adkins-Muir & Jones, 2003; Klein et al., 2003; Plantz et al., 2003), increased environmental complexity (Johansson & Belichenko, 2003; Johansson & Ohlsson, 1996), and increased physical activity level (Jones et al., 1999).

Thus, there are discrete molecular brain events that arise days to weeks after an infarct, these brain events likely underlie or substantially contribute to spontaneous recovery, and they can be therapeutically augmented in association with improved behavioral outcome in animals.

However, translating preclinical neurorestorative findings into improved therapeutics for human patients with stroke is hampered by a number of obstacles, some of which can be addressed with functional neuroimaging. The cellular-molecular measurements directly obtained in animal studies are not easily evaluated in human patients, where brain tissue is uncommonly available for examination. Human brain mapping with techniques such as fMRI can provide insights in this context. Human brain-mapping studies are also important because of the limitations of animal models in this context (Cramer, 2003). For example, rodent studies are of limited value because most of these creatures are quadrupeds with vastly different brain organization from humans, such as relative size of basal ganglia and white matter. Primate studies have been instructive; however, size and pathogenesis of brain injury has limited overlap with spontaneous human cerebrovascular disease. Animal models often lack the heterogeneity of injury found in the human condition, animals generally have a more uniform pre-infarct behavioral status, animals are generally at a much younger point in the lifespan, most if not all human stroke risk factors are absent in animal models, cognitive–affective features important to all aspects of recovery usually have limited correspondence with the human condition, and medical complications that, combined, affect a majority of human patients with stroke are generally absent in animal studies. Given some of these concerns related to animal models of stroke, it remains true that a complete animal model of human cerebrovascular disease is evasive, and functional neuroimaging methods remain among the most useful tools for measuring the neurobiological events of interest (Cramer, 2003).

Functional neuroimaging in human subjects provides insights not apparent with structural imaging or behavioral assessment. Behavioral changes do not consistently correspond tightly with the molecular–physiological events that constitute therapeutic targets. For example, there may be a variety of neural environments that produce a given behavioral phenotype, but only some of these brain states may be appropriate targets for therapeutic intervention. Moreover, behavioral assessments at times do not provide mechanistic insights or betray intersubject differences in underlying functional anatomy. Functional imaging, spanning molecular and behavioral levels, can be useful in regard to these issues because the data provide insights into brain changes at the systems level.

Functional imaging can provide improved insight beyond that obtained via anatomical measures. Human (Brott et al., 1989; Saver et al., 1999) and experimental animal (Lyden et al., 1997; Rogers et al., 1997) studies of brain infarction have consistently found that behavioral deficits correlate significantly with infarct volume, when measured during the acute or the chronic phase of stroke. However, these correlations are sometimes limited, especially in the chronic phase of stroke, as this approach to understanding brain injury assumes an equivalency of cortical function as described by theories of cerebral mass action (Lashley, 1950). Introduction of functional MRI measures into the analysis of injury can improve the correlation between injury and behavioral effects (Crafton et al., 2003), and thus this approach may have improved value for predicting stroke outcome versus using anatomical scans to measure total stroke volume (Plate 14.1). The use of a method such as structural or perfusion imaging characterizes an injury but provides limited insight as to how this injury will influence the final behavioral deficits resulting from the injury.

There are many other settings in which functional imaging can provide insights into a neurological condition when a behavioral exam or anatomical brain imaging provides limited information. For example, when a neurological exam is normal, expression of genetic risk for Alzheimer's disease (Bookheimer et al., 2000) can nevertheless be measured when a memory task is performed during fMRI. When neuropsychological testing is normal, fMRI identifies significant effects of HIV on brain function during a memory task performance (Ernst et al., 2002). When anatomical MRI is unrevealing, PET can be used to measure the relationship between cognitive deficits and decreased cortical metabolism after traumatic brain injury (Fontaine et al., 1999). When stroke renders a patient hemiplegic, and the exam is thus silent, functional MRI permits the measurement of activity across brain motor networks (Cramer et al., 2002) Even in patients without a neurological diagnosis, functional brain imaging studies suggest that the same behavioral phenotype can arise from varying patterns of brain activity; for example, some elderly patients may activate a greater fraction of their cognitive reserve to maintain normal function (Scarmeas et al., 2003).

It is possible that such human brain-mapping data may be used to derive neurophysiological data for improved clinical decision making at the level of the individual patient. This goal has precedence in medical practice. For example, when a patient presents with a ventricular tachyarrhythmia or a refractory epileptic disorder, current practice often incorporates electrophysiological data to guide specific decisions in treatment (Sheth, 2002; Wetzel et al., 2003). A recent study serves as an example of using data extracted from functional neuroimaging for decision making in the context of a clinical trial (Cramer et al., 2005). Motor maps via fMRI were used to localize the stroke hemisphere's hand motor area in patients with chronic stroke. This information was then used to guide targeted subthreshold cortical stimulation.

When considering clinical measures for clinical and brain mapping studies of stroke recovery, it is important to remember that neurorestorative therapeutics emphasizes specific brain systems. This is true at the behavioral level, where therapeutically reinforcing a specific behavior—for example, after exposure to a restorative drug—is critical to successfully improving the behavior of interest (Feeney et al., 1982). This is also true for functional imaging, in which many paradigms require a specific behavior to activate the brain. Thus, neurorestorative efforts emphasize specific brain systems at several levels. This is in contrast to the global clinical measures used in acute stroke trials.

Methodological Considerations and Sources of Bias

Many patterns of altered brain function have been described during the study of patients with stroke. These have been exhaustively compiled elsewhere (Baron et al., 2004; Calautti & Baron, 2003; Chen et al., 2002; Cramer & Bastingo, 2000; Rijntjes & Weiller, 2002).

Initial functional imaging studies were cross-sectional and observational in nature. Subsequent studies have examined subpopulations of patients with stroke, increased sample size, correlated features of brain activation with clinical measures, and performed serial studies during the period of behavioral gains poststroke. However, the overall understanding of changes in brain function after stroke, and the relationship between these changes and clinical measures, remains limited. The reason is, in part, the relative dearth of such investigations.

However, at least three groups of issues limit the current understanding of brain events underlying spontaneous return of function following a stroke. The first is the heterogeneity of stroke. There are a number of variables that likely modify brain function after stroke (Table 14.1). Some are related to the injury, such as pathogenesis, features of infarction, behavioral sequelae, and therapies. Some variables overlap with issues relevant to the study of brain function in health, such as age, hemispheric dominance, and medical comorbidity. Others are also important to the study of brain function in the setting of acute stroke, such as concomitant depression and prestroke disability. Each is a source of variance that can reduce power in functional imaging studies of stroke recovery.

Also a factor in this issue is that the behavioral experience during the process of brain mapping can be a source of variance in elderly or impaired subjects. Instructions sufficient for young control subjects may result in divergent behaviors or strategies among patients. In elderly and impaired subjects undergoing fMRI scanning, brain activity can be influenced by a number of common comorbidities such as cervical arthritis, bladder dysfunction, muscle spasms, reduced visual or auditory acuity, pain, anxiety, inattention, and cognitive dysfunction in domains apart from those being evaluated. These points also emphasize the need for particular care in screening for MRI-incompatible objects in the

TABLE 14.1. Clinical Variables That Potentially Influence Stroke Recovery and Its Measurement by Functional Imaging

• Stroke topography	• Medical comorbidities
• Time poststroke	• Prestroke disability
• Age	• Prestroke experience and education
• Hemispheric dominance	• Type of poststroke therapy
• Side of brain affected	• Amount poststroke therapy
• Depression	• Acute stroke interventions
• Injury to other brain network nodes	• Medications during stroke recovery
• Infarct volume	period
• Initial stroke deficits	• Medications at time of brain mapping
• Arterial patency	• Final clinical status
	• Stroke mechanism

Note. From Cramer (2004). Copyright 2004 by Lippincott Williams & Wilkins. Reprinted by permission.

body and clothing when scanning elderly or infirm subjects. Their endurance may be reduced, making a protocol that is appropriate for young subjects a challenge for those with neurological disease or advanced age. Polypharmacy may have a significant effect on subject status, as well as possibly neuronal–vascular coupling. A good bedside manner in the scanner room, a concept of reduced importance in most studies of healthy subjects, likely has a substantial effect on the results of fMRI studies of patients with stroke.

A second group of issues pertains to the divergence of investigative approaches. There is a lack of standardized methods for studying and reporting brain function across studies. For example, in the motor system, squeezing versus finger tapping activates different motor circuits (Cramer et al., 2001; Ehrsson et al., 2000). Differences in force (Cramer et al., 2002; Dettmers et al., 1995; Ward & Frackowiak, 2003), frequency (Blinkenberg et al., 1996; Rao et al., 1996; Schlaug et al., 1996; Van Meter et al., 1995), amplitude (Waldvogel et al., 1999), or complexity (Gerloff et al., 1998; Rao et al., 1993; Sadato et al., 1996) of finger movements can substantially impact activation in multiple brain sensorimotor areas. There is a similar degree of variability in clinical assessments used to measure stroke recovery (Duncan et al., 2000; Uchino et al., 2001). This situation in stroke recovery contrasts with that found in multiple sclerosis, in which the Multiple Sclerosis Functional Composite (Cutter et al., 1999) is routinely included across studies; and in spinal cord injury, in which the American Spinal Injury Association (ASIA) motor score, sensory scores, and Impairment Scale (Ditunno et al., 1994) are routinely reported. Adoption of a standardized approach to be included in studies of stroke recovery may reduce the impact of this latter issue.

A third group of issues pertains to brain and vascular changes common in patients with stroke. Vascular disease can modify neuronal–vascular coupling. Available data suggest this is most important with highly advanced stenosis or occlusion of cerebral arteries (Bilecen et al., 2002; Carusone et al., 2002; Cramer et al., 2002; Hamzei et al., 2003; Hund-Georgiadis et al., 2003; Rossini et al., 2004). Moreover, advanced large cerebral artery narrowing itself, in the absence of an MRI-resolvable infarct, can be associated with reorganization of brain function (Krakauer et al., 2004). Further studies are needed in this area. In addition, brain injury such as stroke can affect the intrinsic $T2^*$ property of brain tissue, the underlying measurement in blood-oxygen-level-dependent (BOLD) fMRI. Recent data from our lab (below) suggest that this may be important (Cramer et al., 2005). Multimodal assessment of brain function may be useful in addressing these concerns in contexts where they are most significant. Methods such as TMS, electroencephalography, and magnetoencephalography have reduced spatial resolution, relative to fMRI, but temporal resolution is improved and these vascular issues may not have the same impact on findings with these methods. Studies of the issue of neuronal–vascular coupling in the setting of vascular disease are ongoing (Krainik et al., 2005; Rossini et al., 2004).

Spontaneous Changes in Brain Function after Stroke

Despite current limitations, functional imaging studies examining spontaneous events related to stroke recovery converge in a number of findings.

Changes in Networks

The earliest study emphasized altered function within multiple nodes of relevant distributed networks (Brion et al., 1989). This finding has been replicated repeatedly. Clearly, altered function within one area changes function within interconnected areas within a distributed brain network after stroke, similar to multifocal, distant changes in brain function reported after a focal brain perturbation in the motor system of healthy subjects (Ilmoniemi et al., 1997; Lee et al., 2003; Siebner et al., 2000). A number of animal studies have been concordant with results in humans (see, for example, Biernaskie & Corbett, 2001; Dijkhuizen et al., 2003; Jones & Shallert, 1992; Kolb, 1995; Liu & Rouiller, 1999; Nudo et al., 1996; Xerri et al., 1998). Figure 14.1 presents a model that compiles these findings.

Changes in Laterality

One commonly reported effect of stroke on brain function in humans is a reduction in the laterality of activity (Cao et al., 1998; Chollet et al., 1991; Cramer et al., 1997; Hamdy et al., 1998; Seltz et al., 1998; Thulborn et al., 1999; Weiller et al., 1993). This issue has also received considerable attention in the study of normal aging (Cabeza, 2002) and has furthermore been described in a number of other neurological contexts, including epilepsy (Detre, 2004), traumatic brain injury (Christodoulou et al., 2001), and multiple sclerosis (Lee et al., 2000). Early reports emphasized a less lateralized pattern of activation after stroke than normal; that is, the effect of stroke on motor system function is to increase the extent to which both hemispheres are

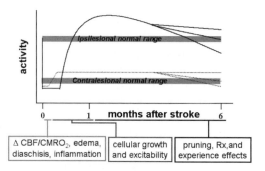

FIGURE 14.1. Changes in bilateral brain areas after unilateral stroke have been grouped into three time periods. From Cramer (2004). Copyright 2004 by Lippincott Williams & Wilkins. Reprinted by permission.

1. In the initial hours-days after a stroke, brain function and behavior can be globally deranged (Grotta & Bratina, 1995), and few restorative structural changes have started.

2. A period of growth then begins, lasting several weeks. Structural and functional changes in the contralesional hemisphere precede those of the ipsilesional hemisphere, and at such times activity in relevant contralesional areas can even exceed activity in the lesion hemisphere. This growth-related period may be a key target for certain restorative therapies.

3. Subsequently, there is pruning, reduction in functional overactivations, and establishment of a static pattern of brain activity and behavior. The final pattern may nevertheless remain accessible to plasticity-inducing, clinically meaningful, interventions (Carey et al., 2002; Liepert et al., 2000; Pariente et al., 2001). An excess of growth followed by pruning has precedence in human neurobiology, being a recapitulation of normal developmental events (Chugani et al., 1987). Supra- and subnormal activity levels in the ipsilesional and contralesional hemispheres correlate with features of behavioral outcome in specific patient populations, as described above.

recruited rather than just the hemisphere contralateral to movement. For example, a language task or a right-hand motor task that activates the left hemisphere in healthy controls will activate relevant regions within both the right and the left hemispheres in patients with a left-hemisphere stroke, and this added activation can be important to behavioral performance (Johansen-Berg et al., 2002).

A number of factors have been found to modify the extent to which stroke is associated with reduced laterality. Examples include time after stroke (laterality often increases toward normal as patients recover (Calautti et al., 2001; Feydy et al., 2002; Fujii & Nakada, 2003; Heiss et al., 1999; Marshall et al., 2000; Nhan et al., 2000), hemispheric dominance (motor task performance with the dominant hand is more lateralized than with the nondominant hand in both health and after stroke; Cramer et al., 1997; Kim et al., 1993; Zemke et al., 2003), and topography of injury (higher laterality may be more common with a subcortical, versus a cortical, infarct; Feydy et al., 2002; Luft et al., 2004). Other factors relevant to laterality in normal subjects are also likely important to the experience of stroke recovery, such as task complexity (higher laterality with less complex tasks; Just et al., 1996; Shibasaki et al., 1993; Wexler et al., 1997), subject age (higher laterality with lower age; Cabeza, 2002), task familiarity (higher laterality with novel behaviors; Lohmann et al., 2004), proximal versus distal (higher laterality with distal motor tasks; Colebatch et al., 1991; Cramer & Crafton, 2004; Cramer et al., 2001), and perhaps gender (Vikingstad et al., 2000). Note that the motor cortex activation site ipsilateral to movement that is recruited with reduced laterality is different from the site activated during movement of the contralateral hand and is on the anterior precentral gyrus, possibly representing the premotor cortex (Cramer et al., 1999).

Several studies suggest that the spontaneous increase in activity within the nonstroke hemisphere after stroke—that is, reduced laterality—reflects greater injury and/or deficits. This is particularly emphasized in the serial fMRI study by Fujii and Nakada (2003) and by TMS studies (Netz et al., 1997; Turton et al., 1996). TMS studies have further suggested possible mechanisms for this finding. In the primary motor cortex, stroke hemisphere inhibition upon the nonstroke hemisphere is reduced (Shimizu et al., 2002), and nonstroke hemisphere inhibition upon the stroke hemisphere is increased (Murase et al., 2004), though these inhibitory patterns may vary with the level of deficits (Butefisch et al., 2003).

Some studies suggest that changes in laterality of brain function may be important to whatever behavioral recovery is achieved after stroke (Cappa et al., 1997; Cardebat et al., 2003; Heiss et al., 1999; Johansen-Berg et al., 2002; Thulborn et al., 1999), even if the final behavior is less than normal. A number of cases have been published in which brain activation is mostly or completely restricted to the nonstroke hemisphere, contralateral to results in controls (Buckner et al., 1996; Cramer et al., 1997, 1999; Gold & Kertesz, 2000). When a patient has recovered from poststroke motor deficits, a second infarct affecting the side contralateral to the first infarct can reintroduce the initial weakness (Fisher, 1992; Song et al., 2005). Reduced laterality has behavioral significance, in at least some cases, and is not merely a marker of greater injury or passive disinhibition.

Changes in Activation Site

A spontaneous shift in the site of activation has also been reported after stroke, in all manner of directions, by fMRI, PET, and TMS. The most common changes described have been a ventral or a posterior shift in the contralateral (stroke hemisphere) activation site during unilateral motor task performance by the stroke-affected hand. Weiller et al., in a PET study of patients with subcortical stroke, described a ventral shift in the center of activation during motor task performance in recovered patients whose stroke affected the posterior aspect of the internal capsule, as opposed to more anterior sites, suggesting that topographic shifts in the cortical activation site may reflect survival of selected corticospinal tract fibers (Weller et al., 1993). An fMRI study of patients with a range of stroke topographies also reported the same finding among patients with complete motor recovery, as compared with patients with partial recovery (Zemke et al., 2003; Plate 14.2). This suggests that, at least for hand motor recovery, a ventral shift may be associated with better recovery of function. A posterior shift in the activation site has been described in motor studies of stroke recovery across multiple imaging modalities (Calautti et al., 2003; Cramer et al., 2000; Piniero et al., 2001; Rossini et al., 1998), and has also been described in the motor system of patients with multiple sclerosis (Lee et al., 2000) or spinal cord injury (Green et al., 1998; Turner et al., 2003). In most studies of patients with stroke, a posterior shift did not correlate with clinical status; however, a recent study suggests that degree of posterior shift is linearly related to degree of recovery, at least for proximal movements (Cramer & Crafton, 2004).

Changes in Activation Size

Studies have described changes in activation size in many brain areas in the setting of stroke recovery. Functional neuroimaging studies have emphasized that recovery of function is associated with increased activation over time in several areas within the stroke-affected hemisphere, accompanied by decreased activation over time in several areas, particularly within the nonstroke hemisphere (Heiss et al., 1999; Nelles et al., 1999; Nhan et al., 2004; Marshall et al., 2000; Tombari et al., 2004), consistent with TMS studies (Traversa et al., 1997, 2000). TMS studies converge in the conclusion that progressive expansion in the area of excitable primary motor cortex within the stroke hemisphere during the period of stroke recovery is a feature of patients with superior motor outcomes (Cicinelli et al., 1997; Traversa et al., 1997). It is important to note that although clinical status reaches a plateau in 3 mo or less for many functions such as motor function (Duncan et al., 1992; Nakayama et al., 1994), brain reorganization may continue to evolve for months beyond this (Tombari et al., 2004; Traversa et al., 2000).

The task used to probe activation can significantly influence the volume of activation. For example, contralateral activation volume during right-hand squeezing is significantly larger than the volume during right index finger tapping (Cramer et al., 2001). This illustrates one of the important principles of brain mapping of stroke recovery, that the results are highly influenced by the nature of the fMRI task used to address the questions.

Correlations between Behavior and Changes in Brain Activation

In some serial functional imaging studies, the correlate of better clinical outcome has been increased activation in key stroke-hemisphere areas (Fujli & Nakada, 2003; Heiss et al., 1999; Marshall et al., 2000; Nhan et al., 2004; Zemke et al., 2003), but in other studies, the correlate has been a reduction (Calautti et al., 2001; Ward et al., 2003). These differences across fMRI studies may arise from several sources. Several methodological issues may contribute, such as divergence in time after stroke at which investigations are performed, the task used to activate the brain, the patient populations enrolled, the nature of therapy given to patients after stroke, or in other variables. Indeed, when our lab applied the same fMRI probe, tapping the affected index finger at 2 Hz (driven by an auditory metronome) across a 25-degree range of motion with eyes closed, shoulder adducted, and elbow extended, at 1.5 tesla field strength), we found that, as compared with age-matched controls, activation volume is *decreased* after stroke (Zemke et al., 2003) and *increased* after spinal cord injury (Cramer et al., 2001). Together, these observations suggest that a particular brain-mapping method will have the best clinical validity when applied to a specific patient population and clinical context.

Across studies, results converge in certain likely relationships between behavior and brain function. First, for behaviors arising from a lateralized, *primary* cortex-driven brain area, increased activation in the primary cortex correlates with *better* outcome (Heiss et al., 1999; Traversa et al., 1997; Zemke et al., 2003) (Plate 14.2), indicating preservation of key substrate with optimal connections for supporting the behavior of interest. Second, in other brain areas such as the association cortex (e.g., *secondary* motor areas), greater activation correlates with *poorer* outcome, as in this case greater activation represents a compensatory event that is generally not able to support the full return of the behavior owing to the nature of the anatomical connections in these areas (Ward et al., 2003). Best outcomes are associated with the greatest return to the normal state of brain function (Ward et al., 2003).

Changes along Infarct Rim

Increased activity along the rim of a cortical infarct has been described in fMRI and PET studies (Cramer et al., 1997; Luft et al., 2004; Rosen et al., 2000). Butz et al. (2004), who found peri-infarct low-frequency activity in the majority of patients with cortical stroke, thought the functional significance of this finding was unclear. These observations may correspond to the increased levels of growth-related proteins found along the rim of an experimental infarct introduced into animals (Li et al., 1998; Stroemer et al., 1998). The clinical significance of the peri-infarct changes measured with functional neuroimaging requires further study. An important consideration in the interpretation of fMRI studies of this zone is that the intrinsic T2* property of brain tissue, changes in which underlie activation in BOLD fMRI, can be altered by stroke. Recent data from our lab suggest that the area surrounding an infarct might have increased T2* signal as compared with normal brain tissue, the impact of which on BOLD fMRI could be important.

Diaschisis

Diaschisis may also be an important process related to behavioral recovery after stroke. Brain areas connected to, but spatially distant from, the region of infarction show numerous changes poststroke (Baron et al., 1986; Nhan et al.,

2004; Seitz et al., 1999; Witte & Stoll, 1997). For example, we found several patients with a behavioral deficit early after stroke among whom areas that normally showed activation were near silent. These areas with reduced brain activation had no injury from stroke and showed normal resting cerebral blood flow. Behavioral recovery was associated with restitution of brain activity in these areas (Nhan et al., 2004). Indeed, in several cases an area of the brain had normal perfusion, was inactive early after stroke and highly active months later, and was sufficiently distant from the infarct so as to be in a separate vascular territory. Although numerous methods have been used to describe diaschisis, this process may be most directly measured using fluorodeoxyglucose-PET (FDG-PET; Cappa et al., 1997; Heiss et al., 1993). Further studies in humans are needed to understand this spontaneous distant suppression of function, its impact on behavioral status, and the extent to which it may be a therapeutic target.

Recovery Resulting from Therapeutic Intervention

fMRI and other brain-mapping methods have provided insights into the brain events underlying spontaneous return of function after stroke. These methods are also useful for understanding the brain events underlying behavioral gains arising from exogenous interventions. Furthermore, the promise of these methods extends beyond gaining neurobiological insight, as measures of brain function may provide useful information on prognosis, triage, and as a surrogate marker (Dobkin, 2003), as described above. In some therapeutic contexts, information derived from functional neuroimaging can guide certain treatment decisions (Cramer et al., 2005).

Several examples of brain-mapping treatment effects on stroke recovery have been published. Animal studies provide useful lessons in this regard (Biernaskie & Corbett, 2001; Johansson & Belichenko, 2002; Jones et al., 1999; Kleim et al., 2003; Nudo et al., 1996). Many human studies to date have focused on effects of increased physical activity (Carey et al., 2002; Johansen-Berg et al., 2002; Liepert et al., 1998; Luft et al., 2004; Wittenberg et al., 2003). Effects of pharmacological (Meinzer et al., 2004; Pariente et al., 2001) and other (Cramer et al., 2005; Meinzer et al., 2004) interventions have also been studied.

A number of adjuvant factors are important to reorganization of brain function after stroke, both in the spontaneous and treatment-induced settings, including repetitiveness of intervention, learning, sensorimotor integration, complexity, imagery, and attention. Restorative therapy will likely need to be graded to patient status with regard to such issues, such as by altering dose, context, demand level, and complexity of intervention. Such dosing adjustments might be based on features of behavior or, perhaps, of functional brain organization. These adjuvant aspects of restorative therapeutic interventions thus warrant consideration.

Active, Intense, Repetitive Content of Therapy

Active repetitive movement practice (Woldang & Hummelsheim, 2002) can enhance the strength and functional use of the affected limb in patients with chronic stroke. For instance, repetitive practice of hand and finger flexion and extension movements resulted in significant motor performance improvements during the therapy period (Butefisch et al., 1995). Intensity of therapy may be an important factor in the level of functional improvement (Kwakkel et al., 1999), and in this regard repetitive therapy may in part be based on events related to normal learning (Karni et al., 1996; Kleim et al., 2002; Nudo et al., 2001). Active participation has been found to be more effective in improving motor performance improvement as compared with passive training (Lotze et al., 2003). Constraint-induced movement therapy (CIMT) includes intense, active training. Changes in brain function have been described after CIMT, with the divergent functional neuroimaging results possibly reflecting differences in patients and study methods (Kopp et al., 1999; Liepert et al., 1998; Park et al., 2004; Schaechter et al., 2002; Wittenberg et al., 2003).

Sensorimotor Integration

Motor gains can be demonstrated when impaired voluntary movements are supplemented with some form of assistance, either through neuromuscular stimulation (Cauraugh et al., 2003; Cauraugh & Kim, 2002; Muellbacher et al., 2002) or by mechanical assistance (Lum et al., 2002; Volpe et al., 2000). Studies that utilize techniques to enhance somatosensory input have shown effectiveness at improving motor function in healthy (Muellbacher et al., 2002) and paretic limbs (Floel et al., 2004). Sensorimotor integration theory may provide insight into the basis for these motor gains: Motor output is inextricably linked to sensory input, and those unable to voluntarily complete movements cannot produce appropriate sensory patterns associated with motor effort (Bornschegl & Asanuma, 1987; Pavlides et al., 1993). This theory provides a rationale for active assistive therapy (Reinkensmeyer et al., 2004). The implementation of sensorimotor integration theory may be improved with measurement of function in key brain functional areas for integration (Huttunen et al., 1996; Thickbroom et al., 2001).

Environmental Complexity and Context

Environmental complexity or enrichment has been found to alter brain function and structure in normal (Diamond et al., 1977; Kempermann et al., 1997; van Praag et al., 2000) and neurologically impaired (Biernaskie & Corbett, 2001; Kolb et al., 1987, 1991) animals. Animals with experimental stroke have improved functional outcomes when exposed to enriched environments that allow social interaction and a broad range of activities (Johansson, 2003;

Will et al., 1977). Poststroke experience likely influences functional outcome similarly in humans. For example, specialized multidisciplinary stroke units show improved patient outcomes as compared with those of general wards (Langhorne et al., 1993; Ottenbacher & Jannell, 1993).

Computer, robotics, and motion tracking technology have recently been used to produce rich virtual reality environments (Holden et al., 2001; Jack et al., 2001; Ku et al., 2003). This technology can be utilized in a variety of settings and can influence environment in numerous ways, such as by augmenting sensory feedback (Sisto et al., 2002). Deriving maximum clinical gains from implementing environmental complexity in restorative therapies may be achieved by incorporating findings from brain-mapping studies in the neurobiology of complexity (Dhamala et al., 2003; Gerloff et al., 1998; Just et al., 1996; Stowe et al., 1998; Verstynen et al., 2005). In addition, virtual reality approaches lend themselves readily to incorporation into most brain mapping protocols.

The context in which restorative therapy is administered influences clinical gains. Task-specific training (Alon et al., 2003; Carey et al., 2002; Muellbacher et al., 2002; Nelson et al., 1996; Schaechter, 2004; Trombly & Wu, 1999), use of a functionally rich task ecology (Ma et al., 1999; Wu et al., 1998, 2000), and increased purpose of practiced exercise (Hsieh et al., 1996) can each improve clinical gains. Functional imaging can maximize the clinical gains derived from implementing such therapies by providing insight into the mechanism of effect on the injured brain.

Imagery

Imagery and observation reflect the planning and preparation stages of movement (Grezes & Decety, 2001; Jeannerod, 2001). Various forms of covert rehearsal, such as motor imagery or action observation, may be effective in producing increased recovery. This may be particularly true in patients among whom stroke-induced behavioral loss is complete, such as those with hemiplegia who are unable to perform the repetitive goal-directed movements important to recovery (Page et al., 2001; Pomeroy et al., 2005).

Brain-mapping studies in human subjects have found that motor imagery and action observation are each associated with widespread activation of a distributed motor control network (van Mier, 2000). A range of movement-related areas, such as the contralateral primary motor cortex, supplementary motor area, premotor cortex, and parietal cortex, are also active during motor imagery and during movements observation (Gerardin et al., 2000; Grezes & Decety, 2001; Jeannerod, 2001; Lacourse et al., 2004; Lotze et al., 1999; Porro et al., 1996). Mere observation of a movement can activate complex motor output circuits in healthy (Gangitano et al., 2004) or in hemiplegic (Cramer et al., 2002) human subjects.

Primate studies by Rizzolatti et al. have identified a cortical action–observation matching system with ties to physical movement, in which cells termed "mirror neurons" fire during both action observation and action execution (di Pelligrino et al., 1992; Rizzolatti et al., 1996). Brain-mapping studies suggest that a similar system exists in humans (Buccino et al., 2001; Decety et al., 1997; Fadiga et al., 1995; Hari et al., 1998) with preservation of substantial somatotopic specificity (Maeda et al., 2002). These observations add strength to the suggestion that action observation can give rise to a covert experience of that same action, including premovement planning and preparation stages.

Attention

Practice conditions that make performance more difficult have the potential to enhance the cognitive and motor processes involved with improving long-term performance (Lee et al., 1991). For instance, contextual interference, which incorporates random practice conditions, is known to stimulate attention and cognition. This pattern of practice conditions has been shown to enhance the retention and transfer of motor skill learning (Hall & Magill, 1995; Immink & Wright, 2001; Lee et al., 1991; Shea et al., 2001; Ste.-Marie et al., 2004; Wulf & Schmidt, 1988). Associative plasticity also depends on attention (Stefan et al., 2004). Indeed, simply looking at one's tapping finger, versus looking away, increases by 50% the volume of motor cortex activated (Baker et al., 1999). Studies examining the effect of attention on brain function in healthy subjects (Immink & Wright, 2001; Li & Wright, 2000; Stefan et al., 2004) may be of guiding value in understanding how to manipulate attention in order to maximize therapeutic gains in patients with stroke.

Summary

Functional imaging of stroke recovery is a unique source of information that provides insights into spontaneous recovery of function after stroke and may also be useful in the development of restorative treatments. A number of features of brain function change spontaneously after stroke. Current studies have defined many of the most common events. Key challenges for the future are to develop standardized approaches to help address certain questions, determine the psychometric qualities of these measures, and define the clinical utility of these methods.

REFERENCES

Adkins-Muir, D., & Jones, T. (2003). Cortical electrical stimulation combined with rehabilitative training: Enhanced functional recovery and dendritic plasticity following focal cortical ischemia in rats. *Neurological Research*, 25, 780–788.

Alon, G., Sunnerhagen, K. S., Geurts, A. C., et al. (2003). A home-based, self-administered stimulation program to improve selected hand functions of chronic stroke. *NeuroRehabilitation, 18,* 215–225.

Baker, J., Donoghue, J., & Sanes, J. (1999). Gaze direction modulates finger movement activation patterns in human cerebral cortex. *Journal of Neuroscience, 19,* 10044–10052.

Bang, O. Y., Lee, J. S., Lee, P. H., et al. (2005). Autologous mesenchymal stem cell transplantation in stroke patients. *Annals of Neurology, 57,* 874–882.

Baron, J., Cohen, L., Cramer, S., et al. (2004). Neuroimaging in stroke recovery: A position paper from the First International Workshop on Neuroimaging and Stroke Recovery. *Cerebrovascular Diseases, 18,* 260–267.

Baron, J., D'Antona, R., Pantano, P., et al. (1986). Effects of thalamic stroke on energy metabolism of the cerebral cortex: A positron tomography study in man. *Brain, 109,* 1243–1259.

Biernaskie, J., & Corbett, D. (2001). Enriched rehabilitative training promotes improved forelimb motor function and enhanced dendritic growth after focal ischemic injury. *Journal of Neuroscience, 21,* 5272–5280.

Bilecen, D., Radu, E., Schulte, A., et al. (2002). fMRI of the auditory cortex in patients with unilateral carotid artery steno-occlusive disease. *Journal of Magnetic Resonance Imaging, 15,* 621–627.

Blinkenberg, M., Bonde, C., Holm, S., et al. (1996). Rate dependence of regional cerebral activation during performance of a repetitive motor task: A PET study. *Journal of Cerebral Blood Flow and Metabolism, 16,* 794–803.

Bookheimer, S., Strojwas, M., Cohen, M., et al. (2000). Patterns of brain activation in people at risk for Alzheimer's disease. *New England Journal of Medicine, 343,* 450–456.

Bornschlegl, M., & Asanuma, H. (1987). Importance of the projection from the sensory to the motor cortex for recovery of motor function following partial thalamic lesion in the monkey. *Brain Research, 437,* 121–130.

Brion, J.-P., Demeurisse, G., & Capon, A. (1989). Evidence of cortical reorganization in hemiparetic patients. *Stroke, 20,* 1079–1084.

Brott, T., Marler, J., Olinger, C., et al. (1989). Measurements of acute cerebral infarction: Lesion size by computed tomography. *Stroke, 20,* 871–875.

Brown, J., Lutsep, H., Weinand, M., et al. (2006). Motor cortex stimulation for the enhancement of recovery from stroke: A prospective multicenter safety study. *Neurosurgery, 58,* 464–473.

Buccino, G., Binkofski, F., Fink, G., et al. (2001). Action observation activates premotor and parietal areas in a somatotopic manner: An fMRI study. *European Journal of Neuroscience, 13,* 400–404.

Buckner, R., Corbetta, M., Schatz, J., et al. (1996). Preserved speech abilities and compensation following prefrontal damage. *Proceedings of the National Academy of Sciences of the United States of America, 93,* 1249–1253.

Butefisch, C., Hummelsheim, H., Denzler, P., et al. (1995). Repetitive training of isolated movements improves the outcome of motor rehabilitation of the centrally paretic hand. *Journal of the Neurological Sciences, 130,* 59–68.

Butefisch, C., Netz, J., Wessling, M., et al. (2003). Remote changes in cortical excitability after stroke. *Brain, 126,* 470–481.

Butz, M., Gross, J., Timmermann, L., et al. (2004). Perilesional pathological oscillatory activity in the magnetoencephalogram of patients with cortical brain lesions. *Neuroscience Letters, 355,* 93–96.

Cabeza, R. (2002). Hemispheric asymmetry reduction in older adults: The HAROLD model. *Psychological Aging, 17*, 85–100.

Calautti, C., & Baron, J. (2003). Functional neuroimaging studies of motor recovery after stroke in adults: A review. *Stroke, 34*, 1553–1566.

Calautti, C., Leroy, F., Guincestre, J., et al. (2003). Displacement of primary sensorimotor cortex activation after subcortical stroke: A longitudinal PET study with clinical correlation. *NeuroImage, 19*, 1650–1654.

Calautti, C., Leroy, F., Guincestre, J., et al. (2001). Dynamics of motor network overactivation after striatocapsular stroke: A longitudinal PET study using a fixed-performance paradigm. *Stroke, 32*, 2534–2542.

Cao, Y., D'Olhaberriague, L., Vikingstad, E., et al. (1998). Pilot study of functional MRI to assess cerebral activation of motor function after poststroke hemiparesis. *Stroke, 29*, 112–122.

Cappa, S., Perani, D., Grassi, F., et al. (1997). A PET follow-up study of recovery after stroke in acute aphasics. *Brain and Language, 56*, 55–67.

Cardebat, D., Demonet, J., De Boissezon, X., et al. (2003). Behavioral and neurofunctional changes over time in healthy and aphasic subjects: A PET language activation study. *Stroke, 34*, 2900–2906.

Carey, J. R., Kimberley, T. J., Lewis, S. M., et al. (2002). Analysis of fMRI and finger tracking training in subjects with chronic stroke. *Brain, 125*, 773–788.

Carusone, L., Srinivasan, J., Gitelman, D., et al. (2002). Hemodynamic response changes in cerebrovascular disease: Implications for functional MR imaging. *American Journal of Neuroradiology, 23*, 1222–1228.

Cauraugh, J., Light, K., Kim, S., et al. (2003). Chronic motor dysfunction after stroke: Recovering wrist and finger extension by electromyography-triggered neuromuscular stimulation. *Stroke, 31*, 1360–1364.

Cauraugh, J. H., & Kim, S. (2002). Two coupled motor recovery protocols are better than one: Electromyogram-triggered neuromuscular stimulation and bilateral movements. *Stroke, 33*, 1589–1594.

Chen, J., Li, Y., Katakowski, M., et al. (2003). Intravenous bone marrow stromal cell therapy reduces apoptosis and promotes endogenous cell proliferation after stroke in female rat. *Journal of Neuroscience Research, 73*, 778–786.

Chen, R., Cohen, L., & Hallett, M. (2002). Nervous system reorganization following injury. *Neuroscience, 111*, 761–773.

Chollet, F., DiPiero, V., Wise, R., et al. (1991). The functional anatomy of motor recovery after stroke in humans: A study with positron emission tomography. *Annals of Neurology, 29*, 63–71.

Christodoulou, C., DeLuca, J., Ricker, J., et al. (2001). Functional magnetic resonance imaging of working memory impairment after traumatic brain injury. *Journal of Neurology, Neurosurgery and Psychiatry, 71*, 161–168.

Chugani, H., Phelps, M., & Mazziotta, J. (1987). Positron emission tomography study of human brain functional development. *Annals of Neurology, 22*, 487–497.

Cicinelli, P., Traversa, R., & Rossini, P. (1997). Post-stroke reorganization of brain motor output to the hand: A 2–4 month follow-up with focal magnetic transcranial stimulation. *Electroencephalography and Clinical Neurophysiology, 105*, 438–450.

Colebatch, J., Deiber, M.-P., Passingham, R., et al. (1991). Regional cerebral blood flow during voluntary arm and hand movements in human subjects. *Journal of Neurophysics, 65*, 1392–1401.

Crafton, K., Mark, A., & Cramer, S. (2003). Improved understanding of cortical injury by incorporating measures of functional anatomy. *Brain, 126,* 1650–1659.

Cramer, S. (2003). Clinical issues in animal models of stroke and rehabilitation. *Ilar Journal, 44,* 83–84.

Cramer, S. (2004). Functional imaging in stroke recovery. *Stroke, 35,* 2695–2698.

Cramer, S., & Bastings, E. (2000). Mapping clinically relevant plasticity after stroke. *Neuropharmacology, 39,* 842–851.

Cramer, S., Benson, R., Himes, D., et al. (2005). Use of functional MRI to guide decisions in a clinical stroke trial. *Stroke, 36,* e50–e52.

Cramer, S., & Chopp, M. (2000). Recovery recapitulates ontogeny. *Trends in Neuroscience, 23,* 265–271.

Cramer, S., & Crafton, K. (2004). Changes in lateralization and somatotopic organization after cortical stroke. *Stroke, 35,* 240.

Cramer, S., Finklestein, S., Schaechter, J., et al. (1999). Distinct regions of motor cortex control ipsilateral and contralateral finger movements. *Journal of Neurophysiology, 81,* 383–387.

Cramer, S., Fray, E., Tievsky, A., et al. (2001). Changes in motor cortex activation after recovery from spinal cord inflammation. *Multiple Sclerosis, 7,* 364–370.

Cramer, S., Mark, A., Barquist, K., et al. (2002). Motor cortex activation is preserved in patients with chronic hemiplegic stroke. *Annals of Neurology, 52,* 607–616.

Cramer, S., Mark, A., & Maravilla, K. (2002). Preserved cortical function with reduced cerebral blood flow after stroke. *Stroke, 33,* 418.

Cramer, S., Moore, C., Finklestein, S., et al. (2000). A pilot study of somatotopic mapping after cortical infarct. *Stroke, 31,* 668–671.

Cramer, S., Nelles, G., Benson, R., et al. (1997). A functional MRI study of subjects recovered from hemiparetic stroke. *Stroke, 28,* 2518–2527.

Cramer, S., Nelles, G., Schaechter, J., et al. (2001). A functional MRI study of three motor tasks in the evaluation of stroke recovery. *Neurorehabilitation and Neural Repair, 15,* 1–8.

Cramer, S., Weisskoff, R., Schaechter, J., et al. (2002). Motor cortex activation is related to force of squeezing. *Human Brain Mapping, 16,* 197–205.

Cramer, S. C., Shah, R., Juranek, J., et al. (2005). Activity in the peri-infarct rim in relation to recovery from stroke. *Stroke.*

Cutter, G., Baier, M., Rudick, R., et al. (1999). Development of a multiple sclerosis functional composite as a clinical trial outcome measure. *Brain, 122,* 871–882.

Dam, M., Tonin, P., De Boni, A., et al. (1996). Effects of fluoxetine and maprotiline on functional recovery in poststroke hemiplegic patients undergoing rehabilitation therapy. *Stroke, 27,* 1211–1214.

Decety, J., Grèzes, J., Costes, N., et al. (1997). Brain activity during observation of actions: Influence of action content and subject's strategy. *Brain, 120,* 1763–1777.

Detre, J. (2004). fMRI: Applications in epilepsy. *Epilepsia, 45*(Suppl. 4), 26–31.

Dettmers, C., Fink, G., Lemon, R., et al. (1995). Relation between cerebral activity and force in the motor areas of the human brain. *Journal of Neurophysiology, 74,* 802–815.

Dhamala, M., Pagnoni, G., Wiesenfeld, K., et al. (2003). Neural correlates of the complexity of rhythmic finger tapping. *NeuroImage, 20,* 918–926.

Diamond, M. C., Johnson, R. E., & Gold, M. W. (1977). Changes in neuron number and size and glia number in the young, adult, and aging rat medial occipital cortex. *Behavioral Biology, 20,* 409–418.

Dijkhuizen, R., Singhal, A., Mandeville, J., et al. (2003). Correlation between brain reorganization, ischemic damage, and neurologic status after transient focal cerebral ischemia in rats: A functional magnetic resonance imaging study. *Journal of Neuroscience, 23,* 510–517.

di Pellegrino, G., Fadiga, L., Fogassi, L., et al. (1992). Understanding motor events: A neurophysiological study. *Experimental Brain Research, 91,* 176–180.

Ditunno, J., Young, W., & Donovan, W. (1994). The international standards booklet for neurological and functional classification of spinal cord injury. American Spinal Injury Association. *Paraplegia, 32,* 70–80.

Dobkin, B. (2003). *The clinical science of neurologic rehabilitation.* New York: Oxford University Press.

Dromerick, A., Edwards, D., & Hahn, M. (2000). Does the application of constraint-induced movement therapy during acute rehabilitation reduce arm impairment after ischemic stroke? *Stroke, 31,* 2984–2988.

Duncan, P., Goldstein, L., Matchar, D., et al. (1992). Measurement of motor recovery after stroke. *Stroke, 23,* 1084–1089.

Duncan, P., Jorgensen, H., & Wade, D. (2000). Outcome measures in acute stroke trials: A systematic review and some recommendations to improve practice. *Stroke, 31,* 1429–1438.

Ehrsson, H., Fagergren, A., Jonsson, T., et al. (2000). Cortical activity in precision- versus power-grip tasks: An fMRI study. *Journal of Neurophysiology, 83,* 528–536.

Ernst, T., Chang, L., Jovicich, J., et al. (2002). Abnormal brain activation on functional MRI in cognitively asymptomatic HIV patients. *Neurology, 59,* 1343–1349.

Fadiga, L., Fogassi, L., Pavesi, G., et al. (1995). Motor facilitation during action observation: A magnetic stimulation study. *Journal of Neurophysiology, 73,* 2608–2611.

Feeney, D., Gonzalez, A., & Law, W. (1982). Amphetamine, halperidol, and experience interact to affect the rate of recovery after motor cortex injury. *Science, 217,* 855–857.

Felling, R. J., & Levison, S. W. (2003). Enhanced neurogenesis following stroke. *Journal of Neuroscience Research, 73,* 277–283.

Feydy, A., Carlier, R., Roby-Brami, A., et al. (2002). Longitudinal study of motor recovery after stroke: Recruitment and focusing of brain activation. *Stroke, 33,* 1610–1617.

Fisher, C. (1992). Concerning the mechanism of recovery in stroke hemiplegia. *Canadian Journal of Neurological Sciences, 19,* 57–63.

Floel, A., Nagorsen, U., Werhahn, K. J., et al. (2004). Influence of somatosensory input on motor function in patients with chronic stroke. *Annals of Neurology, 56,* 206–212.

Fontaine, A., Azouvi, P., Remy, P., et al. (1999). Functional anatomy of neuropsychological deficits after severe traumatic brain injury. *Neurology, 53,* 1963–1968.

Fujii, Y., & Nakada, T. (2003). Cortical reorganization in patients with subcortical hemiparesis: Neural mechanisms of functional recovery and prognostic implication. *Journal of Neurosurgery, 98,* 64–73.

Gangitano, M., Mottaghy, F., & Pascual-Leone, A. (2004). Modulation of premotor mirror neuron activity during observation of unpredictable grasping movements. *European Journal of Neuroscience, 20,* 2193–2202.

Gerardin, E., Sirigu, A., Lehericy, S., et al. (2000). Partially overlapping neural networks for real and imagined hand movements. *Cerebral Cortex, 10,* 1093–1104.

Gerloff, C., Corwell, B., Chen, R., et al. (1998). The role of the human motor cortex in the control of complex and simple finger movement sequences. *Brain, 121*(Pt. 9), 1695–1709.

Gold, B., & Kertesz, A. (2000). Right hemisphere semantic processing of visual words in an aphasic patient: An fMRI study. *Brain and Language, 73*, 456–465.

Grade, C., Redford, B., Chrostowski, J., et al. (1998). Methylphenidate in early poststroke recovery: A double-blind, placebo- controlled study. *Archives of Physical and Medical Rehabilitation, 79*, 1047–1050.

Green, J., Sora, E., Bialy, Y., et al. (1998). Cortical sensorimotor reorganization after spinal cord injury: An electroencephalographic study. *Neurology, 50*, 1115–1121.

Gresham, G., Duncan, P., Stason, W., et al. (1995). *Post-stroke rehabilitation.* Rockville, MD: U.S. Department of Health and Human Services.

Grèzes, J., & Decety, J. (2001). Functional anatomy of execution, mental simulation, observation, and verb generation of actions: A meta-analysis. *Human Brain Mapping, 12*, 1–19.

Grotta, J., & Bratina, P. (1995). Subjective experiences of 24 patients dramatically recovering from stroke. *Stroke, 26*, 1285–1288.

Hall, K. G., & Magill, R. A. (1995). Variability of practice and contextual interference in motor skill learning. *Journal of Motor Behavior, 27*, 299–309.

Hamdy, S., Aziz, Q., Rothwell, J., et al. (1998). Recovery of swallowing after dysphagic stroke relates to functional reorganization in the intact motor cortex. *Gastroenterology, 115*, 1104–1112.

Hamzei, F., Knab, R., Weiller, C., et al. (2003). The influence of extra- and intracranial artery disease on the bold signal in fMRI. *NeuroImage, 20*, 1393–1399.

Hari, R., Forss, N., Avikainen, S., et al. (1998). Activation of human primary motor cortex during action observation: A neuromagnetic study. *Proceedings of the National Academy of Sciences of the United States of America, 95*, 15061–15065.

Heiss, W., Emunds, H., & Herholz, K. (1993). Cerebral glucose metabolism as a predictor of rehabilitation after ischemic stroke. *Stroke, 24*, 1784–1788.

Heiss, W., Kessler, J., Thiel, A., et al. (1999). Differential capacity of left and right hemispheric areas for compensation of poststroke aphasia. *Annals of Neurology, 45*, 430–438.

Hier, D., Mondlock, J., & Caplan, L. (1983). Recovery of behavioral abnormalities after right hemisphere stroke. *Neurology, 33*, 345–350.

Holden, M. K., Dettwiler, A., Dyar, T., et al. (2001). Retraining movement in patients with acquired brain injury using a virtual environment. *Studies in Health Technology and Informatics, 81*, 192–198.

Hsieh, C. L., Nelson, D. L., Smith, D. A., et al. (1996). A comparison of performance in added-purpose occupations and rote exercise for dynamic standing balance in persons with hemiplegia. *American Journal of Occupational Therapy, 50*, 10–16.

Hund-Georgiadis, M., Mildner, T., Georgiadis, D., et al. (2003). Impaired hemodynamics and neural activation? A fMRI study of major cerebral artery stenosis. *Neurology, 61*, 1276–1279.

Huttunen, J., Wikstrom, H., Korvenoja, A., et al. (1996). Significance of the second somatosensory cortex in sensorimotor integration: Enhancement of sensory responses during finger movements. *NeuroReport, 7*, 1009–1012.

Ilmoniemi, R., Virtanen, J., Ruohonen, J., et al. (1997). Neuronal responses to magnetic stimulation reveal cortical reactivity and connectivity. *NeuroReport, 8,* 3537–3540.

Immink, M. A., & Wright, D. L. (2001). Motor programming during practice conditions high and low in contextual interference. *Journal of Experimental Psychology: Human Perception and Performance, 27,* 423–437.

Jack, D., Boian, R., Merians, A. S., et al. (2001). Virtual reality-enhanced stroke rehabilitation. *IEEE Transactions on Neural Systems and Rehabilitation Engineering, 9,* 308–318.

Jeannerod, M. (2001). Neural simulation of action: A unifying mechanism for motor cognition. *NeuroImage, 14,* S103–S109.

Johansen-Berg, H., Dawes, H., Guy, C., et al. (2002). Correlation between motor improvements and altered fMRI activity after rehabilitative therapy. *Brain, 125,* 2731–2742.

Johansen-Berg, H., Rushworth, M., Bogdanovic, M., et al. (2002). The role of ipsilateral premotor cortex in hand movement after stroke. *Proceedings of the National Academy of Sciences of the United States of America, 99,* 14518–14523.

Johansson, B., & Belichenko, P. (2002). Neuronal plasticity and dendritic spines: Effect of environmental enrichment on intact and postischemic rat brain. *Journal of Cerebral Blood Flow and Metabolism, 22,* 89–96.

Johansson, B., & Ohlsson, A. (1996). Environment, social interaction, and physical activity as determinants of functional outcome after cerebral infarction in the rat. *Experimental Neurology, 139,* 322–327.

Johansson, B. B. (2003). Environmental influence on recovery after brain lesions— experimental and clinical data. *Journal of Rehabilitation Medicine,* 11–16.

Jones, T., Chu, C., Grande, L., et al. (1999). Motor skills training enhances lesion-induced structural plasticity in the motor cortex of adult rats. *Journal of Neuroscience, 19,* 10153–10163.

Jones, T., Kleim, J., & Greenough, W. (1996). Synaptogenesis and dendritic growth in the cortex opposite unilateral sensorimotor cortex damage in adult rats: A quantitative electron microscopic examination. *Brain Research, 733,* 142–148.

Jones, T., & Schallert, T. (1992). Overgrowth and pruning of dendrites in adult rats recovering from neocortical damage. *Brain Research, 581,* 156–160.

Just, M., Carpenter, P., Keller, T., et al. (1996). Brain activation modulated by sentence comprehension. *Science, 274,* 114–116.

Karni, A., Meyer, G., Jezzard, P., et al. (1996). Functional MRI evidence for adult motor cortex plasticity during motor skill learning. *Nature, 377,* 155–158.

Kawamata, T., Dietrich, W., Schallert, T., et al. (1997). Intracisternal basic fibroblast growth factor (bfgf) enhances functional recovery and upregulates the expression of a molecular marker of neuronal sprouting following focal cerebral infarction. *Proceedings of the National Academy of Sciences in the United States of America, 94,* 8179–8184.

Kempermann, G., Kuhn, H. G., & Gage, F. H. (1997). More hippocampal neurons in adult mice living in an enriched environment. *Nature, 386,* 493–495.

Kertesz, A., & McCabe, P. (1977). Recovery patterns and prognosis in aphasia. *Brain, 100*(Pt. 1), 1–18.

Khedr, E. M., Ahmed, M. A., Fathy, N., et al. (2005). Therapeutic trial of repetitive transcranial magnetic stimulation after acute ischemic stroke. *Neurology, 65,* 466–468.

Kim, S.-G., Ashe, J., Hendrich, K., et al. (1993). Functional magnetic resonance imaging of motor cortex: Hemispheric asymmetry and handedness. *Science*, *261*, 615–617.

Kleim, J., Barbay, S., Cooper, N., et al. (2002). Motor learning-dependent synaptogenesis is localized to functionally reorganized motor cortex. *Neurobiology of Learning and Memory*, *77*, 63–77.

Kleim, J., Bruneau, R., VandenBerg, P., et al. (2003). Motor cortex stimulation enhances motor recovery and reduces peri-infarct dysfunction following ischemic insult. *Neurological Research*, *25*, 789–793.

Kolb, B. (1995). Plasticity and recovery in adulthood. *Brain plasticity and behavior* (pp. 95–112). Mahwah, NJ: Erlbaum.

Kolb, B., & Gibb, R. (1991). Environmental enrichment and cortical injury: Behavioral and anatomical consequences of frontal cortex lesions. *Cerebral Cortex*, *1*, 189–198.

Kolb, B., Holmes, C., & Whishaw, I. Q. (1987). Recovery from early cortical lesions in rats: III. Neonatal removal of posterior parietal cortex has greater behavioral and anatomical effects than similar removals in adulthood. *Behavioral Brain Research*, *26*, 119–137.

Kondziolka, D., Steinberg, G. K., Wechsler, L., et al. (1005). Neurotransplantation for patients with subcortical motor stroke: A phase 2 randomized trial. *Journal of Neurosurgery*, *103*, 38–45.

Kopp, B., Kunkel, A., Muhlnickel, W., et al. (1999). Plasticity in the motor system related to therapy-induced improvement of movement after stroke. *NeuroReport*, *10*, 807–810.

Krainik, A., Hund-Georgiadis, M., Zysset, S., et al. (2005). Regional impairment of cerebrovascular reactivity and bold signal in adults after stroke. *Stroke*, *36*, 1146–1152.

Krakauer, J. W., Radoeva, P. D., Zarahn, E., et al. (2004). Hypoperfusion without stroke alters motor activation in the opposite hemisphere. *Annals of Neurology*, *56*, 796–802.

Ku, J., Mraz, R., Baker, N., et al. (2003). A data glove with tactile feedback for fMRI of virtual reality experiments. *Cyberpsychology and Behavior*, *6*, 497–508.

Kwakkel, G., Wagenaar, R., Twisk, J., et al. (1999). Intensity of leg and arm training after primary middle-cerebral-artery stroke: A randomised trial. *Lancet*, *354*, 191–196.

Lacourse, M., Turner, J., Randolph-Orr, E., et al. (2004). Cerebral and cerebellar sensorimotor plasticity following motor imagery-based mental practice of a sequential movement. *Journal of Rehabilitation Research and Development*, *41*, 505–524.

Langhorne, P., Williams, B. O., Gilchrist, W., et al. (1993). Do stroke units save lives? *Lancet*, *342*, 395–398.

Lashley, K. (1950). In search of the engram. *Society of Experimental Biology*, *4*, 454–482.

Lee, L., Siebner, H., Rowe, J., et al. (2003). Acute remapping within the motor system induced by low-frequency repetitive transcranial magnetic stimulation. *Journal of Neuroscience*, *23*, 5308–5318.

Lee, M., Reddy, H., Johansen-Berg, H., et al. (2000). The motor cortex shows adaptive functional changes to brain injury from multiple sclerosis. *Annals of Neurology*, *47*, 606–613.

Lee, T. D., Swanson, L. R., & Hall, A. L. (1991). What is repeated in a repetition? Effects of practice conditions on motor skill acquisition. *Physical Therapy, 71*, 150–156.

Legos, J. J., & Barone, F. C. (2003). Update on pharmacological strategies for stroke: Prevention, acute intervention and regeneration. *Current Opinion in Investigational Drugs, 4*, 847–858.

Li, Y., Jiang, N., Powers, C., et al. (1998). Neuronal damage and plasticity identified by map-2, gap-43 and cyclin d1 immunoreactivity after focal cerebral ischemia in rat. *Stroke, 29*, 1972–1981.

Li, Y., & Wright, D. L. (2000). An assessment of the attention demands during random- and blocked-practice schedules. *Quarterly Journal of Experimental Psychology: A. Human Experimental Psychology, 53*, 591–606.

Liepert, J., Bauder, H., Wolfgang, H., et al. (2000). Treatment-induced cortical reorganization after stroke in humans. *Stroke, 31*, 1210–1216.

Liepert, J., Miltner, W., Bauder, H., et al. (1998). Motor cortex plasticity during constraint-induced movement therapy in stroke patients. *Neuroscience Letters, 250*, 5–8.

Liu, Y., & Rouiller, E. (1999). Mechanisms of recovery of dexterity following unilateral lesion of the sensorimotor cortex in adult monkeys. *Experimental Brain Research, 128*, 149–159.

Lohmann, H., Deppe, M., Jansen, A., et al. (2004). Task repetition can affect functional magnetic resonance imaging-based measures of language lateralization and lead to pseudoincreases in bilaterality. *Journal of Cerebral Blood Flow and Metabolism, 24*, 179–187.

Lotze, M., Braun, C., Birbaumer, N., et al. (2003). Motor learning elicited by voluntary drive. *Brain, 126*, 866–872.

Lotze, M., Montoya, P., Erb, M., et al. (1999). Activation of cortical and cerebellar motor areas during executed and imagined hand movements: An fMRI study. *Journal of Cognitive Neuroscience, 11*, 491–501.

Luft, A., McCombe-Waller, S., Whitall, J., et al. (2004). Repetitive bilateral arm training and motor cortex activation in chronic stroke: A randomized controlled trial. *Journal of the American Medical Association, 292*, 1853–1861.

Luft, A., Waller, S., Forrester, L., et al. (2004). Lesion location alters brain activation in chronically impaired stroke survivors. *NeuroImage, 21*, 924–935.

Lum, P. S., Burgar, C. G., Shor, P. C., et al. (2002). Robot-assisted movement training compared with conventional therapy techniques for the rehabilitation of upper-limb motor function after stroke. *Archives of Physical Medicine and Rehabilitation, 83*, 952–959.

Lyden, P., Lonzo, L., Nunez, S., et al. (1997). Effect of ischemic cerebral volume changes on behavior. *Behavioral Brain Research, 87*, 59–67.

Ma, H. I., Trombly, C. A., & Robinson-Podolski, C. (1999). The effect of context on skill acquisition and transfer. *American Journal of Occupational Therapy, 53*, 138–144.

Maeda, F., Kleiner-Fisman, G., & Pascual-Leone, A. (2002). Motor facilitation while observing hand actions: Specificity of the effect and role of observer's orientation. *Journal of Neurophysiology, 87*, 3129–1335.

Mahmood, A., Lu, D., & Chopp, M. (2004). Intravenous administration of marrow stromal cells (mscs) increases the expression of growth factors in rat brain after traumatic brain injury. *Journal of Neurotrauma, 21*, 33–39.

Marshall, R., Perera, G., Lazar, R., et al. (2000). Evolution of cortical activation during recovery from corticospinal tract infarction. *Stroke, 31,* 656–661.

Meinzer, M., Elbert, T., Wienbruch, C., et al. (2004). Intensive language training enhances brain plasticity in chronic aphasia. *BMC Biology, 2,* 20–28.

Muellbacher, W., Richards, C., Ziemann, U., et al. (2002). Improving hand function in chronic stroke. *Archives of Neurology, 59,* 1278–1282.

Murase, N., Duque, J., Mazzocchio, R., et al. (2004). Influence of interhemispheric interactions on motor function in chronic stroke. *Annals of Neurology, 55,* 400–409.

Nakayama, H., Jorgensen, H., Raaschou, H., et al. (1994). Recovery of upper extremity function in stroke patients: The Copenhagen Stroke Study. *Archives of Physical Medicine and Rehabilitation, 75,* 394–398.

Nelles, G., Spiekermann, G., Jueptner, M., et al. (1999). Evolution of functional reorganization in hemiplegic stroke: A serial positron emission tomographic activation study. *Annals of Neurology, 46,* 901–909.

Nelson, D. L., Konosky, K., Fleharty, K., et al. (1996). The effects of an occupationally embedded exercise on bilaterally assisted supination in persons with hemiplegia. *American Journal of Occupational Therapy, 50,* 639–646.

Netz, J., Lammers, T., & Homberg, V. (1997). Reorganization of motor output in the nonaffected hemisphere after stroke. *Brain, 120,* 1579–1586.

Nhan, H., Barquist, K., Bell, K., et al. (2004). Brain function early after stroke in relation to subsequent recovery. *Journal of Cerebral Blood Flow and Metabolism, 24,* 756–763.

Nudo, R. (1999). Recovery after damage to motor cortical areas. *Current Opinion in Neurobiology, 9,* 740–747.

Nudo, R., Plautz, E., & Frost, S. (2001). Role of adaptive plasticity in recovery of function after damage to motor cortex. *Muscle and Nerve, 24,* 1000–1019.

Nudo, R., Wise, B., SiFuentes, F., et al. (1996). Neural substrates for the effects of rehabilitative training on motor recovery after ischemic infarct. *Science, 272,* 1791–1794.

Ottenbacher, K. J., & Jannell, S. (1993). The results of clinical trials in stroke rehabilitation research. *Archives of Neurology, 50,* 37–44.

Page, S. J., Levine, P., & Leonard, A. C. (2005). Modified constraint-induced therapy in acute stroke: A randomized controlled pilot study. *Neurorehabilitation and Neural Repair, 19,* 27–32.

Page, S. J., Levine, P., Sisto, S. A., et al. (2001). Mental practice combined with physical practice for upper-limb motor deficit in subacute stroke. *Physical Therapy, 81,* 1455–1462.

Pariente, J., Loubinoux, I., Carel, C., et al. (2001). Fluoxetine modulates motor performance and cerebral activation of patients recovering from stroke. *Annals of Neurology, 50,* 718–729.

Park, S. W., Butler, A. J., Cavalheiro, V., et al. (2004). Changes in serial optical topography and TMS during task performance after constraint-induced movement therapy in stroke: A case study. *Neurorehabilitation and Neural Repair, 18,* 95–105.

Pavlides, C., Miyashita, E., & Asanuma, H. (1993). Projection from the sensory to the motor cortex is important in learning motor skills in the monkey. *Journal of Neurophysiology, 70,* 733–741.

Pineiro, R., Pendlebury, S., Johansen-Berg, H., et al. (2001). Functional MRI detects posterior shifts in primary sensorimotor cortex activation after stroke: Evidence of local adaptive reorganization? *Stroke, 32,* 1134–1139.

Plautz, E., Barbay, S., Frost, S., et al. (2003). Post-infarct cortical plasticity and behavioral recovery using concurrent cortical stimulation and rehabilitative training: A feasibility study in primates. *Neurological Research, 25,* 801–810.

Pomeroy, V., Clark, C., Miller, J., et al. (2005). The potential for utilizing the "mirror neurone system" to enhance recovery of the severely affected upper limb early after stroke: A review and hypothesis. *Neurorehabilitation and Neural Repair, 19,* 4–13.

Porro, C., Francescato, M., Cettolo, V., et al. (1996). Primary motor and sensory cortex activation during motor performance and motor imagery: A functional magnetic resonance imaging study. *Journal of the Neuroscience, 16,* 7688–7698.

Rao, S., Bandettini, P., Binder, J., et al. (1996). Relationship between finger movement rate and functional magnetic resonance signal change in human primary motor cortex. *Journal of Cerebral Blood Flow and Metabolism, 16,* 1250–1254.

Rao, S., Binder, J., Bandettini, P., et al. (1993). Functional magnetic resonance imaging of complex human movements. *Neurology, 43,* 2311–2318.

Rathore, S., Hinn, A., Cooper, L., et al. (2002). Characterization of incident stroke signs and symptoms: Findings from the atherosclerosis risk in communities study. *Stroke, 33,* 2718–2721.

Reinkensmeyer, D. J., Emken, J. L., & Cramer, S. C. (2004). Robotics, motor learning, and neurologic recovery. *Annual Review of Biomedical Engineering, 6,* 497–525.

Ren, J., Kaplan, P., Charette, M., et al. (2000). Time window of intracisternal osteogenic protein-1 in enhancing functional recovery after stroke. *Neuropharmacology, 39,* 860–865.

Rijntjes, M., & Weiller, C. (2002). Recovery of motor and language abilities after stroke: The contribution of functional imaging. *Progress in Neurobiology, 66,* 109–122.

Rogers, D., Campbell, C., Stretton, J., et al. (1997). Correlation between motor impairment and infarct volume after permanent and transient middle cerebral artery occlusion in the rat. *Stroke, 28,* 2060–2065.

Rossini, P., Altamura, C., Ferretti, A., et al. (2004). Does cerebrovascular disease affect the coupling between neuronal activity and local haemodynamics? *Brain, 127,* 99–110.

Rizzolatti, G., Fadiga, L., Gallese, V., et al. (1996). Premotor cortex and the recognition of motor actions. *Brain Research: Cognitive Brain Research, 3,* 131–141.

Rosen, H., Petersen, S., Linenweber, M., et al. (2000). Neural correlates of recovery from aphasia after damage to left inferior frontal cortex. *Neurology, 55,* 1883–1894.

Rossini, P. M., Caltagirone, C., Castriota-Scanderbeg, A., et al. (1998). Hand motor cortical area reorganization in stroke: A study with fMRI, MEG and TCS maps. *Neuroreport, 9,* 2141–2146.

Sadato, N., Campbell, G., Ibanez, V., et al. (1996). Complexity affects regional cerebral blood flow change during sequential finger movements. *Journal of Neuroscience, 16,* 2691–2700.

Saver, J., Johnston, K., Homer, D., et al. (1999). Infarct volume as a surrogate or auxiliary outcome measure in ischemic stroke clinical trials: The RANTTAS investigators. *Stroke, 30,* 293–298.

Scarmeas, N., Zarahn, E., Anderson, K., et al. (2003). Cognitive reserve modulates functional brain responses during memory tasks: A PET study in healthy young and elderly subjects. *NeuroImage, 19,* 1215–1227.

Schaechter, J. D. (2004). Motor rehabilitation and brain plasticity after hemiparetic stroke. *Progress in Neurobiology, 73,* 61–72.

Schaechter, J. D., Kraft, E., Hilliard, T., et al. (2002). Motor recovery and cortical reorganization after constraint-induced movement therapy in stroke patients: A preliminary study. *Neurorehabilitation and Neural Repair, 16,* 326–338.

Schallert, T., Leasure, J. L., & Kolb, B. (2000). Experience-associated structural events, subependymal cellular proliferative activity, and functional recovery after injury to the central nervous system. *Journal of Cerebral Blood Flow and Metabolism, 20,* 1513–1528.

Scheidtmann, K., Fries, W., Muller, F., et al. (2001). Effect of levodopa in combination with physiotherapy on functional motor recovery after stroke: A prospective, randomised, double-blind study. *Lancet, 358,* 787–790.

Schlaug, G., Sanes, J., Thangaraj, V., et al. (1996). Cerebral activation covaries with movement rate. *NeuroReport, 7,* 879–883.

Seitz, R., Azari, N., Knorr, U., et al. (1999). The role of diaschisis in stroke recovery. *Stroke, 30,* 1844–1850.

Seitz, R., Hoflich, P., Binkofski, F., et al. (1998). Role of the premotor cortex in recovery from middle cerebral artery infarction. *Archives of Neurology, 55,* 1081–1088.

Shea, C. H., Lai, Q., Wright, D. L., et al. (2001). Consistent and variable practice conditions: Effects on relative and absolute timing. *Journal of Motor Behavior, 33,* 139–152.

Sheth, R. (2002). Epilepsy surgery. Presurgical evaluation. *Neurological Clinics, 20,* 1195–1215.

Shibasaki, H., Sadato, N., Lyshkow, H., et al. (1993). Both primary motor cortex and supplementary motor area play an important role in complex finger movement. *Brain, 116,* 1387–1398.

Shimizu, T., Hosaki, A., Hino, T., et al. (2002). Motor cortical disinhibition in the unaffected hemisphere after unilateral cortical stroke. *Brain, 125,* 1896–1907.

Siebner, H., Peller, M., Willoch, F., et al. (2000). Lasting cortical activation after repetitive TMS of the motor cortex: A glucose metabolic study. *Neurology, 54,* 956–963.

Sisto, S. A., Forrest, G. F., & Glendinning, D. (2002). Virtual reality applications for motor rehabilitation after stroke. *Topics in Stroke Rehabilitation, 8,* 11–23.

Song, Y., Lee, J., Park, J., et al. (2005). Ipsilateral hemiparesis caused by a corona radiata infarct after a previous stroke on the opposite side. *Archives of Neurology, 62,* 809–811.

Stefan, K., Wycislo, M., & Classen, J. (2004). Modulation of associative human motor cortical plasticity by attention. *Journal of Neurophysiology, 92,* 66–72.

Ste.-Marie, D. M., Clark, S. E., Findlay, L. C., et al. (2004). High levels of contextual interference enhance handwriting skill acquisition. *Journal of Motor Behavior, 36,* 115–126.

Stowe, L., Broere, C., Paans, A., et al. (1998). Localizing components of a complex task: Sentence processing and working memory. *NeuroReport, 9,* 2995–2999.

Stroemer, R., Kent, T., & Hulsebosch, C. (1998). Enhanced neocortical neural sprouting, synaptogenesis, and behavioral recovery with d-amphetamine therapy after neocortical infarction in rats. *Stroke, 29,* 2381–2395.

Thickbroom, G., Byrnes, M., Archer, S., et al. (2001). Differences in sensory and motor cortical organization following brain injury early in life. *Annals of Neurology*, 49, 320–327.

Thulborn, K., Carpenter, P., & Just, M. (1999). Plasticity of language-related brain function during recovery from stroke. *Stroke*, 30, 749–754.

Tombari, D., Loubinoux, I., Pariente, J., et al. (2004). A longitudinal fMRI study: In recovering and then in clinically stable sub-cortical stroke patients. *NeuroImage*, 23, 827–839.

Traversa, R., Cicinelli, P., Bassi, A., et al. (1997). Mapping of motor cortical reorganization after stroke: A brain stimulation study with focal magnetic pulses. *Stroke*, 28, 110–117.

Traversa, R., Cicinelli, P., Oliveri, M., et al. (2000). Neurophysiological follow-up of motor cortical output in stroke patients. *Clinical Neurophysiology*, 111, 1695–1703.

Trombly, C. A., & Wu, C. Y. (1999). Effect of rehabilitation tasks on organization of movement after stroke. *American Journal of Occupational Therapy*, 53, 333–344.

Turner, J., Lee, J., Schandler, S., et al. (2003). An fMRI investigation of hand representation in paraplegic humans. *Neurorehabilitation and Neural Repair*, 17, 37–47.

Turton, A., Wroe, S., Trepte, N., et al. (1996). Contralateral and ipsilateral EMG responses to transcranial magnetic stimulation during recovery of arm and hand function after stroke. *Electroencephalography and Clinical Neurophysiology*, 101, 316–328.

Uchino, K., Billheimer, D., & Cramer, S. (2001). Entry criteria and baseline characteristics predict outcome in acute stroke trials. *Stroke*, 32, 909–916.

VanMeter, J., Maisog, J., Zeffiro, T., et al. (1995). Parametric analysis of functional neuroimages: Application to a variable-rate motor task. *NeuroImage*, 2, 273–283.

van Mier, H. (2000). Human learning. In A. W. Toga & J. C. Mazziotta (Eds.), *Brain mapping: The systems* (pp. 605–617). Orlando: Academic Press.

van Praag, H., Kempermann, G., & Gage, F. H. (2000). Neural consequences of environmental enrichment. *Nature Reviews Neuroscience*, 1, 191–198.

Verstynen, T., Diedrichsen, J., Albert, N., et al. (2005). Ipsilateral motor cortex activity during unimanual hand movements relates to task complexity. *Journal of Neurophysiology*, 93, 1209–1222.

Vikingstad, E. M., George, K. P., Johnson, A. F., et al. (2000). Cortical language lateralization in right handed normal subjects using functional magnetic resonance imaging. *Journal of the Neurological Sciences*, 175, 17–27.

Volpe, B. T., Ferraro, M., Lynch, D., et al. (2005). Robotics and other devices in the treatment of patients recovering from stroke. *Current Neurology and Neuroscience Reports*, 5, 465–470.

Volpe, B. T., Krebs, H. I., Hogan, N., et al. (2000). A novel approach to stroke rehabilitation: Robot-aided sensorimotor stimulation. *Neurology*, 54, 1938–1944.

Waldvogel, D., van Gelderen, P., Ishii, K., et al. (1999). The effect of movement amplitude on activation in functional magnetic resonance imaging studies. *Journal of Cerebral Blood Flow and Metabolism*, 19, 1209–1212.

Walker-Batson, D., Smith, P., Curtis, S., et al. (1995). Amphetamine paired with physical therapy accelerates motor recovery after stroke: Further evidence. *Stroke*, 26, 2254–2259.

Ward, N., Brown, M., Thompson, A., et al. (2003). Neural correlates of motor recovery after stroke: A longitudinal fMRI study. *Brain, 126,* 2476–2496.

Ward, N., Brown, M., Thompson, A., et al. (2000). Neural correlates of outcome after stroke: A cross-sectional fMRI study. *Brain, 126,* 1430–1448.

Ward, N., & Frackowiak, R. (2003). Age-related changes in the neural correlates of motor performance. *Brain, 126,* 873–888.

Weiller, C., Ramsay, S., Wise, R., et al. (1993). Individual patterns of functional reorganization in the human cerebral cortex after capsular infarction. *Annals of Neurology, 33,* 181–189.

Wetzel, U., Hindricks, G., Dorszewski, A., et al. (2003). Electroanatomic mapping of the endocardium. Implication for catheter ablation of ventricular tachycardia. *Herz, 28,* 583–590.

Wexler, B., Fulbright, R., Lacadie, C., et al. (1997). An fMRI study of the human cortical motor system response to increasing functional demands. *Magnetic Resonance Imaging, 15,* 385–396.

Will, B. E., Rosenzweig, M. R., Bennett, E. L., et al. (1977). Relatively brief environmental enrichment aids recovery of learning capacity and alters brain measures after postweaning brain lesions in rats. *Journal of Comparative and Physiological Psychology, 91,* 33–50.

Witte, O., & Stoll, G. (1997). Delayed and remote effects of focal cortical infarctions: Secondary damage and reactive plasticity. *Advances in Neurology, 73,* 207–227.

Wittenberg, G., Chen, R., Ishii, K., et al. (2003). Constraint-induced therapy in stroke: Magnetic-stimulation motor maps and cerebral activation. *Neurorehabilitation and Neural Repair, 17,* 48–57.

Woldag, H., & Hummelsheim, H. (2002). Evidence-based physiotherapeutic concepts for improving arm and hand function in stroke patients: A review. *Journal of Neurology, 249,* 518–528.

Wolf, S., Blanton, S., Baer, H., et al. (2002). Repetitive task practice: A critical review of constraint-induced movement therapy in stroke. *Neurology, 8,* 325–338.

Wu, C., Trombly, C. A., Lin, K., et al. (2000). A kinematic study of contextual effects on reaching performance in persons with and without stroke: Influences of object availability. *Archives of Physical Medicine and Rehabilitation, 81,* 95–101.

Wu, C., Trombly, C. A., Lin, K., et al. (1998). Effects of object affordances on reaching performance in persons with and without cerebrovascular accident. *American Journal of Occupational Therapy, 52,* 447–456.

Wulf, G., & Schmidt, R. A. (1988). Variability in practice: Facilitation in retention and transfer through schema formation or context effects? *Journal of Motor Behavior, 20,* 133–149.

Xerri, C., Merzenich, M., Peterson, B., et al. (1998). Plasticity of primary somatosensory cortex paralleling sensorimotor skill recovery from stroke in adult monkeys. *Journal of Neurophysiology, 79,* 2119–2148.

Zemke, A., Heagerty, P., Lee, C., et al. (2003). Motor cortex organization after stroke is related to side of stroke and level of recovery. *Stroke, 34,* E23–E28.

CHAPTER 15

Implications of Functional Neuroimaging in Neurorehabilitation

Joseph H. Ricker

The concept of "neurorehabilitation" is potentially quite broad in scope, but for the purposes of this chapter it is used as an umbrella term that encompasses structured intervention (as contrasted with the natural history of recovery) for persons experiencing acquired neurologic dysfunction, with the ultimate goals of increasing their participation in functional activities of daily living and decreasing their disability. Thus, the very nature of many functional imaging technologies and paradigms (e.g., use of tasks and paradigms designed to cause a change in brain activity) provides a great deal of "face validity" for their use in populations in neurorehabilitation. The potential utility of specific functional neuroimaging techniques, such as functional magnetic resonance imaging (fMRI), in assessment, intervention, and rehabilitation has been formally acknowledged (Bobholz et al., 2004), but before this potential may be realized in clinical neurorehabilitation, however, a great deal of research that takes into account neurorehabilitation-specific issues must be conducted (Ricker & Arenth, 2006; Strangman et al., 2005).

Although much of the content of this chapter would be applicable to virtually any clinical population, the topics it presents were selected because of their particular relevance to those individuals who are receiving repeated or ongoing interventions that ostensibly lead to improvement in functional status and whose dysfunctions could be addressed (or at least studied) through the use of current functional neuroimaging technologies. To date, the primary populations receiving neurorehabilitation that have been examined using functional neuroimaging are those with stroke and traumatic brain injury.

However, there is an increasing literature demonstrating the effects of spinal cord injury on motor and somatosensory representation in the brain (see Ricker, 2005 for review), and individuals with such injury may also be so examined.

Interpretation of Change

The primary dependent variable of neurorehabilitation is a positive change (assumed to be an improvement) in the functional status of an individual with acquired brain dysfunction. There are, of course, multiple means of observing such change—for example, through the observation of functional status changes over the natural history of recovery or more systematic examinations of outcome after specified interventions. Nonetheless, reliable and valid characterization of true change in the individual must be a goal of rehabilitation research and practice. Many terms are utilized in neurorehabilitation that attempt to characterize changes at multiple levels, including behavioral and cerebral, and many of these terms invoke (either implicitly or explicitly) the concept of neural plasticity or brain reorganization.

As eloquently discussed by Stein (2000), constructs such as "plasticity" and "reorganization" are actually quite nebulous, do not necessarily refer to any specific processes, and are usually strongly inferred, based primarily on behavior. Thus, researchers and clinicians must be cautious when using these words, making sure that they are not actually applying them to between-group *differences*, which may simply reflect response to injury or natural recovery, rather than actual *changes* in the brain relative to its baseline that reflect the development of novel neurally mediated processes. Animal studies of neural plasticity have an inherent advantage, as one can actually obtain a preinjury baseline of radiotracer-uptake or cerebral hemodynamics. Such an experimental design is, of course, not possible in human studies; thus, other correlative approaches are necessary in order to examine change in cerebral activity.

There are a number of potential sources of measurement error (e.g., the instrumentation, the participants, or even the method of statistical analysis). The same participant repeating a task under identical experimental conditions may still yield very different data sets from one time to the next (Lange, 2000). To date, however, there are relatively few published studies of test–retest reliability and reproducibility of functional imaging results. Even when the task is one of simple fine motor movement, both systematic and random changes are likely when movements are repeated over time (Loubinoux et al., 2001). The neural correlates of cognitive change as a function of learning or specific interventions becomes even more difficult to characterize.

Changes that occur as the result of a rehabilitation intervention, or for that matter, spontaneous natural recovery over time, may be reflected through various types of neural changes, many of which could impact the data derived from functional neuroimaging studies (Stein, 2000). Sensory and motor learning can cause changes in gene expression (Hou et al., 2004) or through remodeling of receptors (Rosenzweig & Barnes, 2003). Cellular changes also occur, through increased dendritic arborization, synaptogenesis, or synaptic pruning, and such changes may differ in the injured brain (Keyvani & Schallert, 2002). The biophysical effects of these neurobiological changes on the signals obtained through functional neuroimaging technologies, however, remain unknown. Given the present lack of data that demonstrate a biophysical correlation between neural changes and imaging signal, it is very challenging at present to attribute changes during imaging solely to recovery, reorganization, or plasticity. Thus, changes in activation from preintervention to postintervention may reflect changes in factors other than those involved in a permanent change in the underlying neural architecture of the task (Poldrack, 2000).

Changes in the biophysical signal-to-noise ratio (SNR) in functional neuroimaging procedures are known to occur over time. Artifactually derived decreases in activation may result from reduced SNR, both across a single session and between sessions when using radioisotope-based procedures such as positron emission tomography (PET; Shadmehr & Holcomb, 1997), and in fMRI (Poldrack, 2000). Furthermore, even when one has a paradigm that yields reliable results over time among healthy participants, one may still obtain differential or unreliable signal changes over time within a clinical population. For example, Manoach and colleagues (2001) utilized a working memory paradigm in a study of patients with schizophrenia and healthy individuals. Changes over time were reliable in the healthy control group, but cognitive activations were not reliable over time among the persons with schizophrenia.

It is also important to recognize that performance-related changes extend beyond simple linear changes in the level or location of cerebral activation. For example, the prefrontal cortex may be activated in relation to task difficulty (Bookheimer, 2000). Thus, if task difficulty changes significantly following an intervention or task repetition over time (as would occur from simple carryover, practice, or test familiarity effects), then such brain regions could certainly exhibit activity changes during functional neuroimaging that may potentially be misattributed to brain reorganization or effects of retraining.

Interpretation of Lateralized Imaging Findings

Individuals with stroke represent the largest single population in neurorehabilitation (Brandstater, 2004). Most individuals with stroke present with lateralized lesions, and there is little doubt that such lateralized brain changes may affect the laterality of cerebral activations in functional imaging studies. In addition, even individuals in neurorehabilitation with diffuse injury or disease processes likely present with lateralized activations. Thus, it is important to consider the meaning of lateralized findings. Historically, laterality of function has been represented in brain-mapping studies through the use of a "laterality index" (e.g., Wilkus & Dodrill, 1975). The laterality index has been extended to other brain-imaging approaches, such as fMRI (Desmond et al, 1995; Thulborn et al., 1999). A laterality index is derived by taking the difference in the number of active pixels found between the hemispheres (i.e., left minus right), dividing it by the summed number of active pixels in both hemispheres (i.e., left plus right), and multiplying the results by 100. This yields a "score" that can range from −100 to +100. Although laterality indexes are routinely used in neuroimaging and brain mapping, it is not known whether the inferred (and *relative*) lateralization of a function is a fundamental feature of the cognitive process being examined, or whether it is more a direct function of the task design or statistical method. For example, it has been suggested that different fMRI language tasks result in different language laterality indexes, even in the same participants, and that the resulting brain activity depends heavily on statistical threshholding (Benson et al., 1999; Binder, 2000; Lehericy et al., 2000). Specifying regions of interest (ROI) a priori and then examining laterality differences between homologous ROIs may provide more accurate laterality indexes. It has been recommended that valid conclusions about lateralization of activations for techniques such as fMRI or ^{15}O PET first require that the activations of interest be present in each individual participant (Rutten et al., 2002).

Patient/Participant Characteristics

It should be apparent to all imaging researchers that not every individual is an appropriate candidate for functional imaging studies. Many individuals experience claustrophobia or, in the case of magnetic resonance (MR)-based technologies, sensitivity to the noise of the scanner (Hammeke, 2000). In addition, in populations of people in neurorehabilitation there are common presentations or aspects of an individual's clinical condition (e.g., agitation, visual neglect, motor restlessness, emotional lability, or fatigue) that may preclude the level of compliance necessary to obtain reliable imaging results (Ricker, 2005).

The presence of stroke or brain injury does not mitigate or override issues of premorbid educational achievement, language, learning style (including the presence of a formal learning disability), or preexisting psychopathology. Many premorbid or comorbid factors have significant effects on functional neuroimaging findings. For example, there are between-group differences in activated functional imaging studies of persons with and without learning disabilities (Papanicolaou et al., 2003) or with and without mood disorders (Haldane & Frangou, 2004). These critically relevant issues of pre-injury considerations and even differential diagnosis are extensive and beyond the scope of this chapter; thus, the reader is referred to other reviews of the topic (e.g., Hanks et al., 2004). In addition, consideration of participant characteristics is relevant not only for clinical populations of interest, but also for control groups. Control participants must be matched as closely as possible to the demographic and other aspects of the clinical group being examined.

By definition, members of neurorehabilitation populations have experienced some form of negative change affecting their central nervous systems. Although much of this involvement may be at a molecular or microscopic level (e.g., in the case of diffuse axonal injury), many individuals with more severe cerebral involvement may present with large focal lesions, particularly in regions of the brain that are of interest to cognitive neuroscientists (e.g., prefrontal cortex). In addition, many individuals with severe traumatic brain injury (TBI) undergo removal of brain tissue as part of decompressive procedures or other neurosurgical interventions. Furthermore, neuropathological features of some populations (e.g., focal or extensive regions of infarction, contusion, or surgical tissue removal) may result in methodological challenges in the image reconstruction process (Hillary et al., 2002). Such factors are critical to consider when designing studies of neurorehabilitation populations such as persons with stroke or severe TBI.

Patient safety is of primary and ultimate concern for any assessment technique, whether the goal is research or rehabilitation. Although contemporary radioligand-based imaging technologies expose participants to very minimal levels of ionizing radiation, frequent exposure to such radiation is not desirable nor is it readily supported by many institutional review boards without solid justification. Safety concerns for functional MR-based imaging technologies are the same as for structural MR procedures (e.g., removal of paramagnetic materials from the participant, avoiding the introduction of any such materials into the scanner room; Huettel et al., 2004). In members of neurorehabilitation populations, however, there may also be an increased likelihood of their having implanted medical devices, such as implanted pumps that control administration of antispasticity medications, or residual shrapnel from penetrating injuries.

At present, the most obvious and sound methodological approach is to take morphologic integrity, premorbid status, and potential medical device confounds into account during participant recruitment and selection. Such requirements may, however, put constraints on sample size or time to complete an investigation, thus slowing the rate of progress in the integration of neurorehabilitation and functional neuroimaging.

Examples of Applications of Functional Imaging in Neurorehabilitation Research

The vast majority of studies that integrate functional neuroimaging with neurorehabilitation have examined motor recovery and rehabilitation, primarily in the population of individuals with stroke (Strangman et al., 2005). Radioligand-based studies of stroke recovery have suggested that bilateral activation is more predictive of a positive outcome than ipsi- or contralesional activity alone. This finding contrasts with those of fMRI investigations, however, which generally have yielded data that puts greater emphasis on the compensatory role of preexisting uncrossed motor neural pathways. For example, among individuals who have sustained stroke, when moving the recovered hand, fMRI studies have shown that there is increased activation in *ipsilateral* motor regions, relative to individuals who have not sustained stroke (Cramer et al., 1997). Other fMRI studies have demonstrated relatively equal representation of contralateral and ipsilateral cerebral activations, but such studies typically include participants with great variability in recovery of motor function (Cao et al., 1998). Studies using multiple convergent brain-mapping modalities (e.g., fMRI combined with magnetoencephalography [MEG] and transcranial magnetic stimulation [TMS]) have suggested a role for the involvement of uncrossed motor pathways in functional recovery (Rossini et al., 1998). Brain-mapping studies using TMS, MEG, or fMRI have also provided interesting insights into motor recovery after stroke, particularly following rehabilitation intervention (Elbert et al., 1994; Levy et al., 2001; Nudo et al., 1996; Taub et al., 1999).

The aforementioned motor recovery studies, along with fMRI studies of poststroke language recovery (e.g., Kurland et al., 2004; Crosson et al., 2005; Vandenbulcke et al., 2005) emphasize that an increase in cerebral activation represents positive improvement in behavioral output—in other words, evidence for recovery of function. Yet studies of cognitive processes after illness or injury (see the next section for examples) consistently demonstrate that increases in brain activation indexed via functional neuroimaging are related to decreased levels of behavioral output and are thus suggestive of poorer outcome. Thus, one may encounter dissociable correlates of activation within the same clinical population (or even in the same individual) such that motor and language functions yield positive correlations with activation whereas more purely cognitive functions yield negative correlations.

The integration of functional imaging with cognitive rehabilitation after traumatic brain injury remains an open area for research. Activation paradigms have been used, however, to characterize the nature of episodic and working memory impairment following brain trauma (see Christodoulou et al., 2001; Levine et al., 2002; McAllister et al. 1999, 2001; Perlstein et al., 2004; Ricker et al., 2001; Scheibel et al., 2003). Taken together, these studies suggest increased recruitment of cerebral resources, particularly when task difficulty is increased or a response inhibition component is required. Such findings clearly provide a preliminary basis for additional research, but none have utilized interventional or repeated measures designs, thus making valid conclusions about change over time or brain reorganization impossible. In addition, the nature of this differential expenditure of cerebral resources after TBI may not be exclusively linked to cognitive impairment, as altered cerebral activations have been demonstrated in an fMRI study of simple motor performance (i.e., finger tapping) among persons with severe TBI even several years after injury (Prigatano et al., 2004).

At the time of this writing, there are no published prospective, systematically controlled studies that integrate functional neuroimaging with a cognitive rehabilitation intervention in an adequately large number of participants in any neurorehabilitation population. Nevertheless, there is great potential for such studies. At least one recently published case study (Laatsch et al., 2004) has demonstrated correlations between changes in fMRI activations and improvement in cognitive status following rehabilitation of an individual that sustained a severe TBI. It is anticipated that large-sample (and most likely multicenter) studies of individuals with TBI undergoing rehabilitation will yield data eventually supporting the integration of functional imaging and cognitive assessment after brain trauma.

Future Directions

Although functional neuroimaging is primarily a research tool at this time, there is clear justification for examining ways of translating this line of research into eventual clinical use. In an era of evidence-based practice, it is critical that empirical research be generated in support of interventions— whether these interventions be pharmacological, physical or cognitive—and that results be demonstrated through a variety of modalities (e.g., change in medical status, change in functional status, or change in the cerebral substrates of a function).

Functional neuroimaging has seen increased use in the study of cognitive and motor functions, but until more benchmarking research is conducted and lingering issues of reliability and validity in signal change are addressed, functional neuroimaging will remain investigational in diagnosis and intervention in many populations of individuals participating in neurorehabilitation (Davis et al., 2006). Although the need for rehabilitation of motor and cognitive processes following neurologic dysfunction is readily apparent, the vast majority of the principles underlying clinical approaches to rehabilitation have not been scientifically verified. Functional neuroimaging may assist in providing evidence of efficacy (National Institutes of Health, 1998; Strangman et al., 2005).

Functional neuroimaging is an innovative way to examine the precise mechanisms compromised in the efficiency of information processing and thus may be potentially useful in the process of measuring the effectiveness of cognitive rehabilitation. As outlined previously (e.g., Ricker, 2005; Strangman et al., 2005), contemporary functional neuroimaging techniques have the potential for the following applications in medical rehabilitation: (1) Functional imaging may be used to evaluate the efficacy of interventions (whether physical, behavioral, or pharmacological) by providing objective demonstration of long-term or permanent changes at the cerebral level; (2) functional imaging could eventually be used as an assessment tool in and of itself; once neurofunctional correlates or "markers" of specific cognitive impairments have been established, it would be possible to compare an individual's performance to that of populations who are known to be impaired; and (3) functional imaging may eventually be used clinically as a prognostic tool. For example, if, following an intervention that has a known therapeutic window, patients do not show change even at the cerebral level, future strategies and planning can be focused at the level of compensating for permanent deficits. This could form a basis for targeted and tailored approaches to rehabilitation.

The development of novel markers (for radioligand studies) and improvements in MR-based technologies will only strengthen imaging research in TBI. Novel agents that label specific neurotransmitter systems or precursors are beginning to see application in TBI (Donnemiller et al., 2000). Such biomarkers will not only allow for better characterization of TBI pathophysiology, but may also be used as a measure of response to pharmacological and other treatments.

The present array of imaging technologies provides researchers and, to a lesser degree, clinicians with an arsenal of ways to measure changes in the brain. Yet it is likely that emerging and yet-to-be-developed portable technologies will hold even greater promise for neurorehabilitation by bringing the imaging lab into the rehabilitation clinic. For example, near-infrared spectroscopy (NIRS), a technology originally developed for assessing the consistency of liquids sealed in containers (e.g., paints and solvents), has in recent years been applied to the study of human brain function. NIRS utilizes near-infrared light sources and detectors in order to measure many of the same physiological parameters as ^{15}O PET and fMRI (e.g., changes in oxy- and deoxy-hemoglobin ratios), but it has several advantages over these more established techniques. NIRS is noninvasive, uses no ionizing radiation, and does not require the use of high-field magnetization or the need for a stationary external scanner. At present, it has the unique advantage over other functional imaging technologies of being highly portable and far less affected by subject movement. NIRS has been used to describe human cerebral hemodynamic changes related to movement (Watanabe et al., 1996), language (Sato et al., 1999), executive control (Fallgatter & Strik, 1998), and working memory (Hoshi et al., 2000). The use of NIRS as a functional imaging tool in neurorehabilitation has been quite limited, however (Arenth et al., 2007), but several research groups are exploring its potential applications.

Conclusions

This chapter has reviewed some, but by no means all, of the issues to consider in the integration of functional neuroimaging with neurorehabilitation. Although it could be argued that some of the content is quite critical of the existing literature, this should not be surprising, given the very preliminary status of this line of research, much less its clinical application. Such a view must not be misinterpreted as fatalistic, however, as this has been the state of every research endeavor at some point in its development. Rather, it is hoped—and expected—that many of the points raised here will serve as heuristics for creative thinking and productivity in addressing the needs of individuals with acquired brain injuries and other forms of neurological compromise.

REFERENCES

Arenth, P. A., Ricker, J. H., & Schultheis, M. T. (2007). Functional near-infrared spectroscopy in neurorehabilitation. *Clinical Neuropsychologist, 21*(1), 38–57.

Benson, R. R., Fitzgerald, D. B., LeSueur, L. L., et al. (1999). Language dominance determined by whole brain functional MRI in patients with brain lesions. *Neurology, 52*(4), 798–809.

Binder, J. R. (2000). Functional MRI of the language system. In C. T. Moonen & P. A. Bandettini (Eds.), *Functional MRI* (pp. 407–419). Berlin: Springer-Verlag.

Bobholz, J., Bilder, R., Bookheimer, S., et al. (2004). Official position of the Division of Clinical Neuropsychology (APA Division 40) on the role of neuropsychologists in clinical use of fMRI. *Clinical Neuropsychologist, 18*, 349–351.

Bookheimer, S. Y. (2000). Methodological issues in pediatric imaging. *Mental Retardation and Developmental Disabilities Research Reviews, 6*, 161–165.

Brandstater, M. E. (2004). Stroke rehabilitation. In J. A. DeLisa & B. Gans (Eds.), *Rehabilitation medicine* (4th ed., pp. 1655–1676). Philadelphia: Lippincott Williams & Wilkins.

Cao, Y., D'Olhaberriague, L., Vikingstad, E. M., et al. (1998). Pilot study of functional MRI to assess cerebral activation of motor function after poststroke hemiparesis. *Stroke, 29*, 112–122.

Christodoulou, C., DeLuca, J., Ricker, J. H., et al. (2001). Functional magnetic resonance imaging of working memory impairment following traumatic brain injury. *Journal of Neurology, Neurosurgery and Psychiatry, 71*, 161–168.

Cramer, S. C., Nelles, G., Benson, R. R., et al. (1997). A functional MRI study of subjects recovered from hemiparetic stroke. *Stroke, 28*, 2518–2527.

Crosson, B., Moore, A. B., Gopinath, K., et al. (2005). Role of the right and left hemispheres in recovery of function during treatment of intention in aphasia. *Journal of Cognitive Neuroscience, 17*(3), 392–406.

Davis, P. C., Drayer, B. P., Anderson, R. E., et al. (1999). *American College of Radiology appropriateness criteria: Head trauma* (pp. 507–524). Reston, VA: American College of Radiology.

Davis, P. C., Seidenwurm, D. J., Brunberg, J. A., et al. (2006). *American College of Radiology Appropriateness Criteria* (pp. 1–12). Reston, VA: American College of Radiology.

Desmond, J. E., Sum, J. M., Wagner, A. D., et al. (1995). Functional MRI measurement of language lateralization in Wada-tested patients. *Brain, 118*(6), 1411–1419.

Donnemiller, E., Brenneis, C., Wissel, J., et al. (2000). Impaired dopaminergic neurotransmission in patients with traumatic brain injury: A SPET study using

123I-β-CIT and 123I-IBZM. *European Journal of Nuclear Medicine, 27*, 1410–1414.

Elbert, T., Flor, H., & Birbaumer N. (1994). Extensive reorganization of the somatosensory cortex in adult humans after nervous system injury. *NeuroReport, 5*, 2593–2597.

Fallgatter, A. J., & Strik, W. K. (1998). Frontal brain activation during the Wisconsin Card Sorting Test assessed with two-channel near-infrared spectroscopy. *European Archives of Psychiatry and Clinical Neurosciences, 248*, 245–249.

Haldane, M., & Frangou, S. (2004). New insights help define the pathophysiology of bipolar affective disorder: Neuroimaging and neuropathology findings. *Progress in Neuropsychopharmacology and Biological Psychiatry, 28*(6), 943–960.

Hammeke, T. (2000). Functional MRI in neurology. In C. T. Moonen & P. A. Bandettini (Eds.), *Functional MRI* (pp. 475–486). Berlin: Springer-Verlag.

Hanks, R. A., Ricker, J. H., & Millis, S. R. (2004). Empirical evidence in the neuropsychological assessment of moderate and severe traumatic brain injury. In J. H. Ricker (Ed.), *Differential diagnosis in adult neuropsychological assessment* (pp. 218–242). New York: Springer.

Hillary, F. G., Steffener, J., Biswal, B. B., et al. (2002). Functional magnetic resonance imaging technology and traumatic brain injury rehabilitation: Guidelines for methodological and conceptual pitfalls. *Journal of Head Trauma Rehabilitation, 17*(5), 411–430.

Hoshi, Y., Oda, I., Wada, Y., et al. (2000). Visuospatial imagery is a fruitful strategy for the digit span backward task: A study with near infrared optical tomography. *Cognitive Brain Research, 9*, 339–342.

Hou, Q., Gao, X., Zhang, X., et al. (2004). SNAP-25 in hippocampal CA1 region is involved in memory consolidation. *European Journal of Neuroscience, 20*(6), 1593–603.

Huettel, S. A., Song, A. W., & McCarthy, G. (2004). *Functional magnetic resonance imaging.* Sunderland, MA: Sinauer Associates.

Keyvani, K., & Schallert, T. (2002). Plasticity-associated molecular and structural events in the injured brain. *Journal of Neuropathology and Experimental Neurology, 61*(10), 831–840.

Kurland, J., Naeser, M. A., Baker, E. H., et al. (2004). Test–retest reliability of fMRI during nonverbal semantic decisions in moderate–severe nonfluent aphasia patients. *Behavioral Neurology, 15*(3–4), 87–97.

Laatsch, L., Little, D., & Thulborn, K. (2004). Changes in fMRI following cognitive rehabilitation in severe traumatic brain injury: A case study. *Rehabilitation Psychology, 49*(3), 262–267.

Lange, N. (2000). Statistical procedures for functional MRI. In C. T. Moonen & P. A. Bandettini (Eds.), *Functional MRI* (pp. 301–335). Berlin: Springer-Verlag.

Lehericy, S., Cohen, L., Bazin, B., et al. (2000). Functional MR evaluation of temporal and frontal language dominance compared with the Wada test. *Neurology, 54*(8), 1625–1633.

Levine, B., Cabeza, R., McIntosh, A. R., et al. (2002). Functional reorganisation of memory after traumatic brain injury: A study with H_2-^{15}O positron emission tomography. *Journal of Neurology, Neurosurgery and Psychiatry, 73*(2), 173–181.

Levy, C. E., Nichols, D. S., Schmalbrock, P. M., et al. (2001). Functional MRI evidence of cortical reorganization in upper-limb stroke hemiplegia treated with constraint-induced movement therapy. *American Journal of Physical Medicine and Rehabilitation, 80*(1), 4–12.

Loubinoux, I., Carel, C., Alary, F., et al. (2001). Within-session and between-session reproducibility of cerebral sensorimotor activation: A test–retest effect evidenced with functional magnetic resonance imaging. *Journal of Cerebral Blood Flow and Metabolism, 12*(5), 592–607.

Manoach, D. S., Halpern, E. F., Kramer, T. S., et al. (2001). Test–retest reliability of a functional MRI working memory paradigm in normal and schizophrenic subjects. *American Journal of Psychiatry, 158*(6), 955–958.

McAllister, T. W., Saykin, A. J., Flashman, L. A., et al. (1999). Brain activation during working memory 1 month after mild traumatic brain injury: A functional MRI study. *Neurology, 53,* 1300–1308.

McAllister, T. W., Sparling, M. B., Flashman, L. A., et al. (2001). Differential working memory load effects after mild traumatic brain injury. *NeuroImage, 14,* 1004–1012.

National Institutes of Health. (1998). *Rehabilitation of persons with traumatic brain injury: NIH consensus statement, 16*(1), 1–41.

Nudo, R. J., Wise, B. M., SiFuentes, F., et al. (1996). Neural substrates for the effects of rehabilitative training on motor recovery following ischemic infarct. *Science, 272,* 1791–1794.

Papanicolaou, A. C., Simos, P. G., Breier, J. I., et al. (2003). Brain mechanisms for reading in children with and without dyslexia. *Developmental Neuropsychology, 24*(2–3), 593–612.

Perlstein, W. M., Cole, M. A., Demery, J. A., et al. (2004). Parametric manipulation of working memory load in traumatic brain injury: Behavioral and neural correlates. *Journal of the International Neuropsychological Society, 10,* 724–741.

Poldrack, R. A. (2000). Imaging brain plasticity: Conceptual and methodological issues: A theoretical review. *NeuroImage, 12,* 1–13.

Prigatano, G. P., Johnson, S. C., & Gale, S. D. (2004). Neuroimaging correlates of the Halstead Finger Tapping Test several years post-traumatic brain injury. *Brain Injury, 18*(7), 661–669.

Ricker, J. H. (2005). Functional neuroimaging in medical rehabilitation populations. In J. A. DeLisa & B. Gans (Eds.), *Physical medicine and rehabilitation: Principles and practice* (4th ed., pp. 229–242). Philadelphia: Lippincott Williams & Wilkins.

Ricker, J. H., & Arenth, P. M. (2006). Traumatic brain injury. In M. D'Esposito (Ed.), *Functional MRI: Applications in clinical neurology and psychiatry* (pp. 197–206). London: Taylor & Francis.

Ricker, J. H., Müller, R. A., Zafonte, R. D., et al. (2001). Verbal recall and recognition following traumatic brain injury: A [^{15}O]-water positron emission tomography study. *Journal of Clinical and Experimental Neuropsychology, 23*(2), 196–206.

Rosenzweig, E. S., & Barnes, C. A. (2003). Impact of aging on hippocampal function: Plasticity, network dynamics, and cognition. *Progress in Neurobiology, 69*(3), 143–179.

Rossini, P. M., Caltagirone, C., Castriota-Scanderbeg, A., et al. (1998). Hand motor cortical area reorganization in stroke: A study with fMRI, MEG and TCS maps. *NeuroReport, 9,* 2141–2146.

Rutten, G. J. M., Ramsey, N. F., van Rijen, P. C., et al. (2002). Reproducibility of fMRI-determined language lateralization in individual subjects. *Brain and Language*, *80*, 421–437.

Sato, H., Takeuchi, T., & Sakai, K. L. (1999). Temporal cortex activation during speech recognition: An optical topography study. *Cognition*, *73*, 55–66.

Scheibel, R. S., Pearson, D. A., Faria, L. P., et al. (2003). An fMRI study of executive functioning after severe diffuse TBI. *Brain Injury*, *17*(11), 919–930.

Shadmehr, R., & Holcomb, H. H. (1997). Neural correlates of motor memory consolidation. *Science*, *277*, 821–825.

Stein, D. (2000). Brain injury and theories of recovery. In A.-L. Christensen & B. P. Uzzell (Eds.), *International handbook of neuropsychological rehabilitation* (pp. 9–32). New York: Kluwer Academic.

Strangman, G., O'Neil-Pirozzi, T. M., Burke, D., et al. (2005). Functional neuroimaging and cognitive rehabilitation for people with traumatic brain injury. *American Journal of Physical Medicine and Rehabilitation*, *84*, 62–75.

Taub, E., Uswatte, G., & Pidikiti, R. (1999). Constraint-induced movement therapy: A new family of techniques with broad application to physical rehabilitation. *Journal of Rehabilitation Research and Development*, *36*(3), 237–251.

Thulborn, K. R., Carpenter, P. A., & Just, M. A. (1999). Plasticity of language related brain function during recovery from stroke. *Stroke*, *30*, 749–754.

Vandenbulcke, M., Peeters, R., Van Hecke, P., et al. (2005). Anterior temporal laterality in primary progressive aphasia shifts to the right. *Annals of Neurology*, *58*(3), 362–370.

Watanabe, E., Yamashita, Y., Maki, A., et al. (1996). Noninvasive functional mapping with multi-channel near infra-red spectroscopy topography in humans. *Neuroscience Letters*, *205*, 41–44.

Wilkus, R. J., & Dodrill, C. B. (1975). Neuropsychological correlates of the electroencephalogram in epileptics: I. Topographic distribution and average rate of epileptiform activity. *Epilepsia*, *17*(1), 89–100.

Index